Intoxicating Manchuria

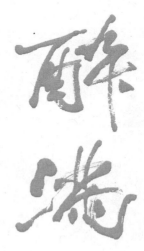

Contemporary Chinese Studies

This series provides new scholarship and perspectives on modern and contemporary China, including China's contested borderlands and minority peoples; ongoing social, cultural, and political changes; and the varied histories that animate China today.

A list of titles in this series appears at the end of this book.

Intoxicating Manchuria

Alcohol, Opium, and Culture in China's Northeast

Norman Smith

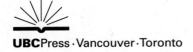

UBCPress · Vancouver · Toronto

20 19 18 17 16 15 14 13 12   5 4 3 2 1

Printed in Canada on FSC-certified ancient-forest-free paper
(100 percent post-consumer recycled) that is processed chlorine- and acid-free.

Library and Archives Canada Cataloguing in Publication

Smith, Norman (Norman Dennis)
    Intoxicating Manchuria : alcohol, opium, and culture in China's northeast /
Norman Smith.

(Contemporary Chinese studies, 1206-9523)
Includes bibliographical references and index.
Also issued in electronic format.
ISBN 978-0-7748-2428-6 (bound); ISBN 978-0-7748-2429-3 (pbk.)

    1. Drinking of alcoholic beverages – China – Manchuria – History – 20th century.
2. Opium abuse – China – Manchuria – History – 20th century. 3. Manchuria (China)
– Social condition – 20th century. 4. Manchuria (China) – Civilization – 20th century.
I. Title II. Series: Contemporary Chinese studies

HV5620.M35S65 2012   362.2920951809041   C2012-903631-5

Canadä

UBC Press gratefully acknowledges the financial support for our publishing program of the Government of Canada (through the Canada Book Fund) and the British Columbia Arts Council.

This book has been published with the help of a grant from the Canadian Federation for the Humanities and Social Sciences, through the Awards to Scholarly Publications Program, using funds provided by the Social Sciences and Humanities Research Council of Canada.

Illustration credit: *Front:* Image from Manchurian dance hostess postcard; *Back:* Chinese characters for "Intoxicating Manchuria," created by Li Zhengzhong for use on cover, inside book.

UBC Press
The University of British Columbia
2029 West Mall
Vancouver, BC V6T 1Z2
www.ubcpress.ca

Contents

List of Figures

Dedicated to
the memory of Zhang Xingjuan,
the author Zhu Ti

Acknowledgments

Intoxicating Manchuria would not have been possible without the guidance and inspiration provided by my mentors at the University of British Columbia, especially Diana Lary, Glen Peterson, and Catherine Swatek. The firm grounding that they gave me brought me to the University of Guelph, where the best of colleagues in history and women's studies fostered the supportive environment that enabled this volume to be completed.

This book has benefited from readings by, and conversations with, Junko Nakajima Agnew, Olga Bakich, Darryl Bryant, Richard Cheng, Annika Culver, James Flath, Miriam Kingsberg, Diana Lary, Kelly Lautt, Yan Li, Li Zhengzhong, Pan Wu, Robert Perrins, Glen Peterson, Ren Yuhua, Bill Sewell, Ron Suleski, Sun Jiarui, Takamitsu Yoshie, Wang Ning, Yang Suanzhi, Victor Zatsepine, Zhang Hong'en, Zhang Quan, Zhang Xingjuan, and Zhu Zhenhua. I am grateful for assistance from Holly Karibo and Sheena Marti. And I thank the anonymous readers at UBC Press, the Alcohol and Drugs Society, and the Social Sciences and Humanities Research Council of Canada.

International conferences have been invaluable. I especially thank the organizers and participants of the following conferences: Alcohol and Drugs Society (London, Ontario, 2004; Glasgow, 2009); Association for Asian Studies (Honolulu, 2011); Canadian Asian Studies Association (Waterloo, 2008); "Global Challenge, Regional Response" (Harbin, 2009); "Japan/China Cultural Relations from the Late Nineteenth Century to the Second World War" (Victoria, 2008); "The Social Impact of the Sino-Japanese War" (Vancouver, 2006); "Suffering Bodies during the Sino-Japanese War: 1931-1945" (Harvard, 2012); and "The Third International Workshop on Chinese-Japanese Relations during the Sino-Japanese War, 1937-45" (Hakone, 2006).

Material for portions of this work has appeared in "Writing Opium in Manchukuo," in James Flath and Norman Smith, eds., *Beyond Suffering: Recounting War in Modern China,* 13-35 (Vancouver: UBC Press, 2011); "Spirits in China," in M. Darrol Bryant, Yan Li, and Judith Maclean Miller, eds., *Along the Silk Road: Essays on History, Literature and Culture in China,* 128-38 (Kitchener: Pandora Press, 2011); trans. Takamitsu Yoshie, "Manshūkoku no Chūgokugobungaku ni okeru ahen, chūdoku, jendā" (Opiates, Addiction, and Gender in the Chinese Language Literature of Manchukuo) in Ezra Vogel and Hirano Kenichiro, eds., *Nicchū sensōki Chūgoku no shakai to bunka (Chinese Society and Culture during the Sino-Japanese War)*, 329-64 (Tokyo: Keio University Press, 2010) (in Japanese); trans. Ren Yuhua, "Wei Manzhouguo shiqi de yapian yu wenxue" (Opium and Literature in the Era of Bogus Manchukuo), in Li Jianping and Zhang Zhongliang, eds., *Kangzhan wenhua yanjiu: Di'er juan (Studies of the Occupied Areas during the Anti-Japanese War: Volume 2)*, 213-35 (Guilin: Guangxi shifan daxue chubanshe, 2008) (in Chinese); with Ren Yuhua, "Dongbei lunxian shiqi yapian suo chongdang de shehui juese" (The Social Roles Played by Opium in the Northeast Occupation Era), *Shehui kexue zhanxian (Social Science Front Monthly)* (July 2008): 113-15 (in Chinese); with Ren Yuhua, "Dongbei lunxi-anqu suzhu de 'nüren de beiju': 'Yapian' suo chongdang de zhongyao juese" (Venting "Women's Tragedy" in the Northeast Occupied Territory: The Significant Parts Played by "Opium"), *Wenyi zhengming (Literature and Art Contend)* (May 2008): 78-81 (in Chinese); and "Opiate Addiction and the Entanglements of Imperialism and Patriarchy in Manchukuo, 1932-45," *Social History of Alcohol and Drugs* 20, 1 (Fall 2005): 66-104. All material has been revised for the purposes of the current book.

I am delighted to acknowledge the following sources of funding: the Social Sciences and Humanities Research Council of Canada and the University of Guelph.

At UBC Press, I am grateful to Emily Andrew for her constant enthusiasm and support; Megan Brand, for an outstanding job of guiding me through the editing process with great care and good humour; David Drummond, for his artful and evocative design; Robert Lewis, for his careful eye for detail; Frank Chow, for his keen attention; and Valerie Nair, for her timely contribution.

My research in China could not have been accomplished without Ren Yuhua; Li Zhengzhong, Zhang Xingjuan, and Li Qian; Li Ruomu and Chang Guizhi; Liu Huijuan; and Pan Wu. I can never thank them enough for all of their help and friendship. During the writing of this book, I was terribly sad-dened by the passing of one of my mentors, Pan Wu – a pioneer in the study of Manchukuo literature who wrote under the pen name of Shangguan Ying. Changchun is not the same without him.

I thank all of the above as well as my family and other friends who unfail-ingly supported me on the journey that bore this book, especially Margaret Arseneau; Barbara, Danial, Dan, and Cassandra Bertrand; Richard Cheng; Jeremy and Spencer King; Don Smith; and Lorraine Smith. Their patience and support are inspiring.

Intoxicating Manchuria

Introduction

This sacrifice is truly terrifying
You've turned your blood into mud
The price is far too high.
If it were your lover
You'd have to let it go.
It goes without saying that your enemy
Is also my enemy.

"JIE YAN GE" (GET OFF OPIUM SONG)

In 1942 Li Xianglan (b. 1920), the most famous entertainer from the Japanese colonial state of Manchukuo (1932-45), sang the "Jie yan ge" to decry the "truly terrifying" price of using opium, which she described as a seducer that destroyed those who fell under its sway.[1] Li sang of a fateful relationship with the drug, her words echoing the sentiments of a restive population, health professionals, and officials who sought to wean users off intoxicants such as opium and alcohol despite the state's dependence on the revenues they raised and the resistance of supporters who profited from their sale. In the first half of the twentieth century, the Northeast of China was certainly famous for its "opium problem" *(yapian wenti),* which attracted considerable international attention. Alcohol, however, was also a constant but seemingly less controversial influence on health and culture in the region. Whereas opium has been central to understandings of the region's modern history and Japanese imperialism, alcohol has not been a particular focus of scholarly attention despite the region's development of what is now in China popularly called a "unique alcohol culture" *(dute de jiu wenhua).*[2] Both alcohol and opium have been used for centuries in the pursuit of health and leisure, while also being linked with personal and social decline. Despite the stress on opium, the impact of alcohol on the region has been even more pronounced, and it continues to this day, as attested to by the recent firing of China's most decorated Winter Olympics athlete, the Northeasterner Wang Meng, whose drunken fighting is argued to have "violated the team's disciplines and jeopardized the sport's image," resulting in her expulsion from her team and banning from international competitions.[3] This study examines the ways that recreational intoxicant consumption was understood and characterized in the first half of the twentieth century, especially by the 1940s prohibitionist platform in Manchukuo, which dominated official policy and Chinese popular culture during the Japanese Empire's Holy War *(sheng zhan)* (1941-45) against Anglo-American imperialism.[4]

Li Xianglan's "Jie yan ge" occupies an important space at the intersection of mid-twentieth-century Chinese national weakness, foreign imperialism, and the battle against the recreational consumption of intoxicants: it is the theme song of the 1942 Japanese-sponsored, Chinese-language movie *Wanshi liufang (Eternity)*, which dramatizes the Anglo-Chinese Opium War of 1839-42. *Wanshi liufang* was produced in Japanese-occupied Shanghai a century after the end of the Opium War and during the Japanese Empire's Holy War against England and the United States. Although the film was intended to incite anti-opium, anti-Western sentiment among Chinese audiences, it also issues a negative reflection on its producers. Although the Japanese publicly vowed to liberate China from the double yoke of Western degradation and drug addiction, they inflicted brutal colonial regimes that belied the ideological underpinnings of Holy War and imposed what Mark Driscoll has termed "anticolonial colonialism."[5] Japanese efforts to placate critics through the promotion of domestic Chinese popular culture, such as *Wanshi liufang,* ironically accentuated for audiences the "far too high" costs of the subjugation that Li so famously sang about.

Li Xianglan is an enduring symbol of the Chinese culture produced within Japanese-occupied Manchuria.[6] Li was born to Japanese parents in Fushun, Manchuria, and was raised in the region and in Beijing.[7] Reflecting her parents' admiration of Chinese culture, Li attended Chinese schools, adopted a Chinese name, and pursued a Chinese-language career. In her late teens and early twenties, Li starred in films produced for Chinese audiences by the Japanese-sponsored Manchuria Motion Picture Producing and Distributing Company (Chinese: Zhushi huishe Manzhou yinghua xiehui; Japanese: Manshū eiga kyōkai). Audiences were led to believe that Li was a pro-Japanese Chinese national.[8] Li also established a formidable career as a singer, popularizing several of the most beloved Chinese songs of the twentieth century.[9] Her rendition of the "Jie yan ge" was lauded not only in Japanese-occupied territories but also in Republican- and Communist-held areas, including the revolutionary stronghold of Yan'an; its anti-opiate message had a strong appeal in war-torn China. So, too, did Chinese-language literature that condemned alcohol addiction. Local writers in Manchukuo, such as Mei Niang and Xiao Jun, gained considerable fame for works that criticized intoxicant consumption at a time of such national peril. But in the post-occupation period, all those who produced popular culture – no matter how critical – under Japanese dominion were tainted by a presumed "traitorous" collaboration with the imperialist power. Following Japan's defeat in 1945, for example, the Republican regime condemned Li to death. Li escaped execution by producing a genealogy that proved her Japanese identity, and she then fled to the United States and Japan.[10] Others who stayed, including Mei Niang and Xiao Jun, were persecuted by the Maoist regime for decades. Those who worked in the controversial fields of drugs control or rehabilitation also faced persecution and, in some cases, death. Their legacies, like the state of Manchukuo itself, were wiped from the face of China but have left long shadows in the national psyche.

The prominent roles of intoxicants in Manchukuo raise important questions regarding Japanese imperialism, narratives of addiction, and Chinese popular culture. *Intoxicating Manchuria* analyzes alcohol and opium narratives in the region's most popular Chinese-language media during the first half of the twentieth century with three questions foremost:

1 How were intoxicants, and addiction, popularly understood and characterized?
2 In what ways were intoxicant industries impacted by Japanese occupation and war?
3 Were serious efforts made to reduce intoxicant consumption?

The answers to these questions shed new light on received interpretations of the region's history and Japanese imperialism. This study does not deny that Japanese committed atrocities in China's Northeast, including a voluminous drug trade.[11] It does, however, argue that to gain a more comprehensive appreciation of the region's recent history, historians need to more fully restore to public memory its complicated *(fuza)* nature, which necessitates a closer examination of the historic roles of intoxicants.

Intoxicating Manchuria demonstrates that throughout the first half of the twentieth century, opium may have been a major trade commodity in the Northeast, but it was also widely denounced. In the early 1940s, alcohol was also repudiated but not until after it had been heralded for decades as a marker of modernity. Expanding hostilities across the mainland, and the launch of Holy War, transformed narratives regarding the consumption of alcohol, and it was increasingly condemned as a gateway drug for opium, heroin, and morphine. From then, huge intoxicant industries existed alongside harsh criticism of recreational intoxicant consumption. This study argues that efforts to control and condemn intoxicants in the region were even more extensive, diverse, and nuanced than has previously been appreciated – and they demonstrate just one example of the significant socio-cultural roles that intoxicants have played in the history of the Northeast and in China more generally.

In China and Taiwan there is a growing literature on alcohol history, including most notably Guo Panxi, *Zhongguo yin jiu xisu (Chinese Drinking Alcohol Customs)*; Li Zhengping, *Zhongguo jiu wenhua (Chinese Wine Culture)*; Xuan Bingshan, *Minjian yinshi xisu (Popular Food and Drink Customs)*; and Gong Li, *Yin jiu shihua (History of Alcohol Drinking)*.[12] These works reflect growing interest in the role of China's "alcohol culture" *(jiu wenhua)* and the desire to legitimize claims to the expertise of domestic consumers and producers and appeal to foreign markets. To date, there has been no English-language counterpart to this boom in Chinese publishing on alcohol. Rather, discussion of alcohol in China has been limited to works on food or has occurred as part of international studies; especially relevant titles include K.C. Chang, *Food in Chinese Culture;* John E. Helzer and Glorisa J. Canino, eds., *Alcoholism in North America, Europe, and Asia;* and David T. Courtwright, *Forces of Habit.*[13] The only exception has been David Armstrong's *Alcohol and Altered States in Ancestor Veneration Rituals of Zhou Dynasty China and Iron Age Palestine.*[14] This volume seeks to begin to address the historical lacunae with a focus on alcohol in the Chinese region most famed for alcohol consumption. The volume centres on the Manchukuo context of the 1930s and 1940s and especially complements Zhang Huinuan's *Beifang shaoshu minzu de jiu wenhua (Northern National Minority Alcohol Culture)*, which focuses on national minorities in China's north in the imperial and contemporary periods.[15]

There is an even larger volume of scholarship on opium in Chinese and Japanese history. Jonathan Spence's seminal essay on opium consumption has demonstrated that it "radically affected all levels of Chinese society" and not just in terms of physical harm.[16] Relevant, more recent works that continue to question opium's roles in society include Kathryn Meyer, *Webs of Smoke;* Timothy Brook and Bob Tadashi Wakabayashi, eds., *Opium Regimes;* Frank Dikötter, Lars Laamann, and Zhou Xun, *Narcotic Culture;* Yamada Goichi, *Manshukoku No Ahensenbai (Opium Monopoly in Manchuria);* and Zheng Yangwen, *The Social Life of Opium.*[17] These works underline the importance of contextualizing opium and its varied socio-economic roles. The work of Zhou Yongming, *Anti-Drug Crusades in Twentieth Century China,* and Alan

Baumler, *The Chinese and Opium under the Republic*, is especially relevant to this project.[18] Both detail anti-opium campaigns in China but dismiss out of hand the efforts made in Japan's mainland regimes, and both reflect the continued ambiguity of post–Qing Dynasty Chinese nationalistists' rendering of the Northeast as an integral part of the Chinese nation. *Intoxicating Manchuria* argues that a clearer understanding of the local prohibitionist movement is essential to understanding the region's history and relations with China and Japan.

There have been extensive studies of Japanese imperialism, especially in terms of opium. The most relevant are John M. Jennings, *The Opium Empire;* Louise Young, *Japan's Total Empire;* Lü Yonghua, *Wei Man shiqi de dongbei yandu (Opium Poison in the Northeast during the Bogus Manchukuo Era);* Yamamuro Shin'ichi (trans. Joshua Fogel), *Manchuria under Japanese Dominion;* and most recently, Mark Driscoll, *Absolute Erotic, Absolute Grotesque.*[19] *Intoxicating Manchuria* adds to this scholarship through a focus on Manchukuo's anti-opium movement as well as on the aggressive promotion of alcohol and on the later efforts to restrict alcohol consumption in Manchukuo. Major, recent projects on Manchuria in the 1920s and 1930s include Ronald Suleski, *Civil Government in Warlord China;* James Carter, *Creating a Chinese Harbin;* Prasenjit Duara, *Sovereignty and Authenticity;* Liu Jinghui, *Minzu, xingbie yu jieceng (Nation, Gender, and Social Stratum);* Mariko Asano Tamanoi, ed., *Crossed Histories;* the Sino-Japanese collected volume *Wei Manzhouguo de zhenxiang (The Real Truth of the Puppet Manchukuo);* and Blaine Chiasson, *Administering the Colonizer.*[20] These works stress the need for increasingly complex readings of the multi-ethnic region's history to enhance understandings of local history and have made this volume possible.

Intoxicating Manchuria comprises eight chapters. Chapter 1, "Alcohol and Opium in China," describes the historical treatment of alcohol and opium in China to the mid-twentieth century. It outlines the longstanding roles that they have had in cultural practices and state policies, from mythmaking to tax regimes. In Chapter 2, "Manchurian Context," attention is directed to China's Northeast and major business and state developments in the region's intoxicant industries, from the end of the imperial period through the 1940s, to argue their significance to local life and governance. The chapter focuses on the business of intoxicant production, providing the general context for the discussion of intoxicants in subsequent chapters.

Chapter 3, "Evaluating Alcohol," interrogates dominant alcohol narratives as revealed in the region's leading newspapers and journals in the 1930s and 1940s, such as *Datong bao (Great Unity Herald), Jiankang Manzhou (Healthy*

Manchuria), Qilin (Unicorn), Shengjing shibao (Shengjing Times), and *Xin Manzhou (New Manchuria).* Throughout the 1930s the narratives were generally positive, stressing alcohol's roles in health regimes, cultural production, and entertaining. These narratives bolstered the regime's modernity claims while reflecting lengthy traditions of alcohol use in the Manchu, Mongol, and growing Han Chinese, Japanese, and Russian communities. In the 1940s, however, health concerns and socio-economic instability resulting from occupation, war, and poverty inspired increasingly aggressive denunciation of alcohol as the type of poisonous foe that Li Xianglan so famously decried.

Chapter 4, "Selling Alcohol, Selling Modernity," traces advertising practices from the promotion of alcohol consumption as a marker of modernity to calls for strict control or prohibition. The products examined include Chi yu pai putaojiu (Red Jade Brand Grape Wine), Gui pai haomeng putaojiu/Suppon Holmon (Soft-Shell Turtle Brand Grass Grape Wine), Yangming jiu (Life Support Wine), and Asahi beer. For those who consumed too much, the health supplement Ruosu (Basic Element) was promoted as the most modern antidote to intoxication. The advertisements feature illustrations and text that aimed to teach consumers about the products and how to consume them in the most modern ways, shedding light on changing business and consumer practices and on changing state policies.

Chapter 5, "Writing Intoxicant Consumption," analyzes Chinese-language fictional work of the 1930s and 1940s that describes the consumption of alcohol and opium. The chapter maps the writers' efforts to raise mass consciousness of the dangers of intoxicants as they established their literary careers. Work of high-profile local writers, including Bai Lang, Li Qiao, Li Zhengzhong, Mei Niang, Wang Qiuying, Xiao Jun, and Zhu Ti, is examined.

Chapter 6, "The Hostess Scare," interrogates the intense debate that erupted in the 1930s over women working in opium retail outlets and in service industries more generally. Discussion centred on the "accepted talents" of women and how they should be deployed in the workforce. Starkly divisive contemporary *Shengjing shibao* reportage provides insight into perceptions of hostesses and the industry as a whole. It also helped to shape fictional accounts of service-industry workers, such as Mei Niang's 1940 "Zhui" (The Chase) and Wei Cheng's 1942 "Kuilan de du shi" (The Festering, Poisoned Tongue). Locating hostess work within debates over early-twentieth-century "new women" reveals the conflicted nature of women's roles in the service and intoxicant industries, an issue that still resonates today.

Chapter 7, "Reasoning Addiction, Taking the Cures," describes contemporary efforts to define "addiction" and to delineate methods by which it might be overcome – by individuals in their homes or in institutional settings. Media promotion of anti-addiction products and descriptions of hospitals, clinics, and Healthy Life Institutes (Kangsheng yuan) and their staffs highlight the seriousness with which many viewed achieving the end of addiction. Received interpretations of the period reject or minimize the attempt to treat and eradicate addiction, yet the most popular media of the day were consistently, aggressively engaged with the issue.

Chapter 8, "The Opium Monopoly's 'Interesting Discussion,'" examines the 1942 Manchukuo Opium Monopoly (Yapian zhuanmai gongshu) publication *Qu tan conglin, di'yi ji (Interesting Discussion Thicket: Volume Number 1)*, a 126-page book that was distributed free of charge. The richly illustrated volume contains fourteen chapters that reveal the monopoly's stance on alcohol and opium and on how addiction should best be treated. This volume, once widely available, is now extremely rare and has not previously been the subject of scholarly inquiry. This examination of *Qu tan conglin* brings together the main strands of inquiry in *Intoxicating Manchuria* to demonstrate the historical significance of Manchuria's intoxicant industries and their undeniable impact on local culture.

1 Alcohol and Opium in China

Alcohol and opium have long played important roles in cultural practices and state policies in China, melding local influences with those from further afield. From their first appearances, both have attracted praise and censure, although alcohol has historically been more fully integrated into Chinese society than opium, which has been far more excoriated in modern narratives regarding individual and societal health. The extent of alcohol consumption in Chinese societies has been dismissed or overlooked for a wide variety of reasons, especially because of widely held beliefs that Asian peoples are allergic to it.[1] But predominant methods of alcohol consumption, most often in small cups or bowls accompanying meals and ritual occasions, encouraged long-term acceptance of alcohol. For most of its history, too, opium was accepted and used as a medicine, not as a recreational product.[2] But nineteenth- and twentieth-century imperialist aggression and shifting patterns of consumption and medical discourses changed the ways that both alcohol and opium were viewed, resulting in a more singular focus on them as dangerous, addictive intoxicants. As Bai He argued in 1939, alcohol and opium were to be considered the same: "they harbour a kind of poisonous nature" *(yi han you yi zhong duzhi).*[3] This chapter provides a broad outline of the historical treatment of alcohol and opium in China to the mid-twentieth century. As alcohol use is often dated to the dawn of Chinese civilization, it is discussed first, followed by opium.

Alcohol

The adage "alcohol is for ceremonies, alcohol is for curing illness, alcohol is for making merry" *(jiu yi cheng li, jiu yi zhi bing, jiu yi cheng huan)* suggests the broad roles alcohol has played in Chinese history.[4] In *Yin jiu shihua (History of Alcohol Drinking),* Gong Li argues that "wine poses the core of all Chinese custom."[5] Guo Panxi has termed alcohol culture "a very colourful kaleidoscope" *(secai banxian wanhuatong).*[6] Xu Xiaomin has labelled alcohol the "Water of History."[7] China has been called the "birthplace of alcohol" *(jiu de guxiang)*[8] and the "kingdom of alcohol" *(jiu de wangguo)*.[9] In 1926 the writer Zhou Zuoren (1885-1967) declared, "I am a native of alcohol country" *(Wo ji shi jiu xiang de yi ge tuzhu)*.[10] These assertions underline the depth and breadth of the history of alcohol, or *jiu*, the standard Mandarin pronunciation of the character used to refer to all forms of alcohol, from distilled spirits, such as yellow wine *(huangjiu)*, to grape wine *(putao jiu)* and beer *(pijiu)*.[11] The character has been found on oracle bones that date to the earliest forms of Chinese writing. Zhou Dynasty (1046-256 BCE) writing of the word *yi* (to cure), for example, was composed of two parts, with the lower half being the character *jiu*, illustrating the long existence of alcohol and an important reason for its consumption in Chinese culture.[12] The ordinariness of consuming alcohol with food is reflected by the existence of the compound word "food and drink" *(yinshi)*, which attests to a long-assumed complementarity that has helped to structure interpretations of alcohol's social roles in China.[13] Of the fifty-five national minorities in China, it is said that only the Islamic Hui do not drink alcohol,[14] although not even all Hui observe religious prohibitions against alcohol consumption.

Not surprisingly, the circumstances surrounding the discovery or invention of alcohol in China are hotly contested. In *Minjian yinshi xisu (Popular Food and Drink Customs)*, Xuan Bingshan details a history of over 5,000 years while citing a saying that argues for a much longer duration: "alcohol and the earth are contemporaries" *(jiu yu tiandi tongshi)*.[15] Gong Li defends a history of over 6,000 years, noting that it is now generally held that alcohol was discovered rather than invented.[16] Chang Chiung-fang pushes the date of human use to over 7,000 years.[17] Archaeological excavations have yielded alcohol-related implements 8,000 years old.[18] Zhu Baoyong has demonstrated how *li*, an early form of beer referenced on oracle bones but now long forgotten, was being produced in China at approximately the same time that it was in neolithic Babylon, circa 9500 BCE.[19] In 1937 archaeologist Wu Qichang mused that crops had been planted "at first not for the purpose of food but for the brewing of alcoholic drinks; eating domesticated crops eventuated from the drinking of alcohol."[20] Wu thus envisioned a history dating to over 10,000 years, with a transformative impact on human socio-economic development. Debate over these dates demonstrates the expanding parameters of historical research and the expanding awareness of China's "alcohol culture" *(jiu wenhua)* as well as the desire to legitimize claims to the expertise of domestic consumers and producers and claims to foreign markets.

The earliest alcohol history is shrouded in myth. Alcohol's "invention" has long been associated with the names Yi Di and Du Kang, two figures supposed to have lived in the Xia Dynasty (2070-1600 BCE). Yi Di is argued to have produced alcohol for her father, Yu the Great, the founder of the dynasty.[21] Yi's position in popular narratives, as "the mother of alcohol," was secured by arguments that she made yellow wine, *laozao* (a beverage of fermented glutinous rice), and yeast.[22] Chu Guoqing has argued, partly because of Yi Di, that women and alcohol once had a more intimate relationship than men and alcohol, one that was subsequently destroyed by dominant patriarchal norms.[23] In recent times at least, Du Kang has been accorded more credibility than Yi Di as the inventor of alcohol. Du is believed to have been the son of the fifth Xia king, and traces of his life in historical records have long been posited as proof of his existence and that of alcohol. Legend has it that one day while he was tending sheep, he placed some rice in the hollow of a mulberry tree, and when he returned later to eat it, the rice had fermented into wine.[24] His association with alcohol has been so extensive that his name is now synonymous with *jiu* and is even linked with alcohol in proverbs; for example, in the words of the redoubtable historical figure Cao Cao (155-220), "to relieve worries, only Du Kang will do" *(heyi jie you, wei you Du Kang).*[25] Both Yi and Du attest to the long relevance of alcohol in Chinese culture, although it is doubtful that either actually invented alcohol.

Alcohol's earliest historical stages may ultimately prove impossible to plot, but the subsequent development of various forms of alcohol has been outlined with some precision. By the Zhou Dynasty, four kinds of alcoholic beverages were known and considered "an indispensable part of every feast, many meals, and important ritual occasions of both Shang and [Zhou] periods."[26] Alcohol was so valued by the Zhou court that 60 percent of the 4,000 workers in the king's residential quarters handled food and alcohol; this number included 110 alcohol officers, 340 alcohol servers, and 170 specialists in the "six drinks."[27] The Duke of Zhou, brother of the dynasty's founder, is credited with writing the first treatise on alcohol's relevance to politics, arguing that indiscriminate drinking outside of rituals and auspicious occasions was dangerous and not to be condoned.[28] Alcohol was an important part of elite Zhou life, but intoxication was a privilege normally extended only to the elderly, not the young; it was also held that during sacrificial rituals, only ancestral spirits were expected to get intoxicated.[29] Alcohol was important to effective rituals and important in support of seniors and the service of guests within prescribed patterns that later Confucianists continued to advocate.[30]

Alcohol has been featured in formal rituals, less-structured activities, and daily life. Alcohol was used in the most symbolic state rituals performed by emperors and other elites.[31] Alcohol is featured in activities for most major festivals, including the Lantern Festival, Spring Festival, Tomb Sweeping

Day, Dragon Boat, Moon Festival, and Double Ninth, and in ceremonies of veneration for one's ancestors and elders.[32] The depth to which alcohol penetrated Chinese culture is attested to by the proverb "without wine, there is no etiquette" *(fei jiu wu yi cheng li)*.[33] Alcohol is considered by many to be an essential element of a banquet. Leisurely consumption led drinkers to variously compose poetry, play music, or engage in finger-guessing games.[34] In terms of health, alcohol was credited with combating rheumatism and exhaustion; increasing blood production and circulation; improving mental well-being, appetite, digestion, and complexion; and expelling unhealthy elements in the body.[35] As early as the Han Dynasty (206 BCE-220 CE), Wang Mang (c. 45 BCE-23 CE) wrote that alcohol was "the oldest of a hundred medicines" *(bai yao zhi zhang)*.[36] One's physical strength might also be augmented by consuming alcohol, as demonstrated by the legendary examples of the Xin Dynasty's (9-23 CE) founder, Liu Bang (r. 202-195 BCE), who killed a giant white snake while intoxicated, or by Wu Song, a character in *Shui hu zhuan (The Water Margin)*, who killed a tiger with his bare hands after drinking eighteen bowls of alcohol.[37] Alcohol also served political purposes. Guo Panxi has written of how government officials often drank while formulating policy, citing the saying "three glasses can solve every problem" *(san bei neng he wan shi)*.[38] In the Western Han Dynasty (206 BCE-9 CE), domestically produced alcohol was sent as tribute to the Xiongnu, and controversy still surrounds arguments that the Tang Dynasty princess Wencheng (d. 680) took rice-wine brewing technologies with her to Tibet when she married the Tibetan king Songtsän Gampo (d. 649).[39]

By the Western Han Dynasty, millet, wheat, and other cereal-based forms of alcohol had overtaken *li* in popularity, and by the Northern Wei Dynasty (386-534), alcohol use is believed to have spread to the masses, who frequently produced their own.[40] In the Tang Dynasty (618-907), popular cereal-based beverages were joined by grape- and rice-based counterparts as extension of the Grand Canal enabled the spread of alcohol-producing technologies.[41] A strong form of alcohol that developed was "frozen-out wine," which was produced through increasing alcohol levels by freezing fermented beverages; Joseph Needham identified this as "the predecessor of all 'strong liquor'" and traced the technique to the sixth or seventh century CE.[42] Distillation has been dated to the Song Dynasty (960-1279) or to the Jin Dynasty (1115-1234).[43] Some have credited Taoist alchemists who were trying to create pills of immortality, whereas others, including the Ming Dynasty (1368-1644) doctor Li Shizhen, date distilling later, to the Yuan Dynasty (1271-1368), whence, Chang Chiung-fang has argued, it travelled westward to Europe, where it inspired the invention of vodka.[44]

Grape wine has a lengthy history in China, dating to the Han Dynasty and the Silk Road travels of Zhang Qian (b. 200 BCE). In 138 BCE the emperor Han Wudi (r. 141-87 BCE) sent Zhang west on a diplomatic mission, where he was introduced to grape wine. Although grape wine was known from then, it did not enjoy widespread popularity until several centuries later in the Tang Dynasty, when wines were not only locally grown but also imported from areas such as Chāch (modern Tashkent).[45] Tang consumers esteemed grape wine produced in the Silk Road city of Liangzhou (present-day Wuwei, Gansu); it was reported that the celebrated beauty Yang Guifei (719-56) drank it from a jewelled cup.[46] Contemporary literature is replete with references to wine, noting how it appealed to all classes of people and was available in shops, hostels, and monasteries. Wine drinkers indulged in Persian myrobalan wines as well as in local ones flavoured with pepper or fagara or made from chrysanthemums, ginger, or pomegranates.[47] The Tang Taizong emperor (r. 626-49) was even rumoured to have produced seven varieties of grape wine in his palace.[48] The cosmopolitan Tang era witnessed exponential growth in the variety and availability of wine and left lasting impressions across Chinese cultures.

. Literati and other cultural producers have been famed for drinking. Arthur Cooper has shown that, during the Tang, "among specially talented people, drunkenness was universally recognized as a state of perfect, untrammelled receptivity to divine inspiration."[49] Jiang Hai has calculated that about 14 percent of the more than 7,700 extant Tang poems relate to alcohol.[50] Even earlier, in the Jin Dynasty (265-420), the Seven Sages of the Bamboo Grove drank wine while socializing, writing poetry, and playing musical instruments. The most famous of them, in terms of alcohol consumption, was the "drunken ghost" *(zui gui)* Liu Ling (221-300), whose love of drinking is immortalized in the poem "In Praise of the Virtue of Wine."[51] Liu once famously shocked visitors who found him naked – he explained that he considered the universe his home and his house his clothes; he turned the tables on his guests by asking what they were doing inside his clothing![52] Liu was also alleged to have had a servant who constantly carried a bottle of alcohol and a shovel – always ready to serve his master a glass or to bury him if he died. Tao Yuanming (365-427), one of China's most famous poets, was poverty-stricken yet famed for entertaining guests, no matter how lofty or humble, with alcohol, often made by his own hand.[53] Tsai Yu has recently argued that Tao was "the first to write extensively on the subject of the states and delights of drinking wine ... [and] used drinking as a path to 'return to nature.'"[54] Jiang Hai has calculated that in over 140 still existing Tao Yuanming poems, alcohol features in 56, or approximately 40 percent.[55] Tao even titled a series of poems "Yin jiu" (Drink Alcohol). The association between alcohol and cultural production extended to other types of artists as well. One of the most famous Yuan Dynasty painters, Huang Gongwang, for example, declared that "without being drunk, I can't paint" *(jiu bu zui, bu neng hua).*[56]

During the Tang Dynasty, alcohol and cultural production forged links that have stood to the present, especially through the "god of wine," Li Bai (701-62). Li boasted that he would gladly trade prized possessions for wine:

> My flower-dappled horse, my furs worth a thousand
> Hand them to the boy in exchange for good wine
> And we'll drown away the woes of ten thousand generations![57]

Li's love of wine and his extraordinarily rich contributions to China's literary canon helped to establish the belief that wine could not only "drown away" one's sorrow but could also give impetus and expression to artistic ability. Li's works relate to drinking so often, in fact, that the writer Guo Moruo (1892-1978) calculated that 17 percent of Li's poems concern alcohol.[58] Li's contemporary Du Fu (712-70) named him one of the "Eight Immortals of the Wine Cup."[59] In a poem, Du described Li as able to "produce 100 poems after drinking a whole *dou* of wine" *(dou jiu shi bai pian).*[60] Du also recounted how, under the influence of alcohol, Li declined an imperial summons, excusing himself as the "wine immortal" *(jiu xian).*[61] Li's death was even linked with alcohol, as he is alleged to have drowned while drunkenly reaching out from a boat to grab the moon. This view of Li's death provided a high-profile foil to positive alcohol narratives.

Despite the benefits of alcohol consumption outlined above, "excessive" or "reckless" use was scorned. The most negative association with alcohol must be attributed to the last Shang Dynasty king, Dixin (r. 1075-46 BCE), and his wife, Daji (d. 1046 BCE). Dixin is credited with having created a "Wine Pool and Meat Forest" *(jiu chi rou lin)* on which canoes floated around an island on which trees with branches made of meat skewers were planted.[62] As the king and his (often naked) guests lay about the allegedly five-square-kilometre pool or drifted aimlessly on it, they simply filled their cups in the pool and reached upward to pick the roasted meat. On occasion, he was rumoured to have 3,000 people crouch by the pool to drink like cows on command.[63] This behaviour has earned Dixin a place in the halls of the most decadent of China's rulers, and he is blamed for the destruction of the Shang Dynasty (1600-1046 BCE); his name is synonymous with alcohol abuse, extravagance, and waste. But Shang alcohol consumption had an even more sinister side to it – the bronze vessels in which alcohol was popularly contained poisoned it, as the tin in the alloy dissolved in the drink.[64] Beyond such dangers, alcohol also came to be popularly associated with the "nine-fold harm," which included impairment of intellect and morals, predisposition to physical illness, shortening of life span, decline of sexual performance and fertility, passing on of inherited defects, and increased risks of criminality and suicide.[65] Long-standing warnings about alcohol consumption were underlined by famous examples ranging from Dixin to the very end of the imperial period in the Qing Dynasty (1644-1912). During the Yuan Dynasty, for example, several emperors were alleged to have died of alcoholism.[66] During the Kangxi reign (1661-1722), Han Tan (1637-1704), president of the Board of Rites, reputedly drank himself to death, and a Qing official, Yu Huai, described drinking parties in Nanjing that went on until guests vomited and passed out on the ground.[67] Critics charged that such behaviour harmed individuals, destroyed families, and risked the very foundations of the state.

Both positive and negative understandings of alcohol consumption led to official efforts to control or prohibit it, although no regime was ever entirely successful in completely eradicating alcohol consumption.[68] The first ruler to whom prohibition has been attributed is Yu, founder of the Xia Dynasty. According to popular belief, as recounted above, his daughter Yi Di brewed an alcoholic drink, which she then presented to her father. His great enjoyment of it led him to warn, from what many have dated to the very beginnings of alcohol production, against alcohol and the dangerous overindulgence it could inspire.[69] Yu's warning and Dixin's infamous "Wine Pool and Meat Forest" ensured that by the time of the Zhou Dynasty it was widely believed that "overindulgence in food and drink is a sin of such proportions that dynasties could fall on its account."[70] Zhou rulers issued edicts prohibiting the general public from drinking wine, only allowing the "ritual" use of wine, a stipulation that left considerable leeway in application of the law. They established an organization to supervise the production and use of alcoholic beverages by the imperial family and for sacrifices to gods or ancestors. During the Qin (221-206 BCE) and Han Dynasties, alcohol was alternately restricted and banned. Perhaps the most famous law of all was promulgated during the Han, when Premier Xiao He (d. 193 BCE) prohibited three or more people from gathering to drink "for no reason."[71] In 139 BCE, the third year of Han Wudi's reign, the emperor mandated a state takeover of the industry to raise tax revenues; he issued an edict in 98 BCE to make alcohol a monopoly, alongside salt and iron. Objections from alcohol producers led to the dismantling of the monopoly in 81 BCE, but it was reinstated again in 10 BCE. Later regimes frequently established monopolies.

Throughout the latter imperial era, alcohol policies continued to reflect state aims and ambitions. Alcohol was at times banned at the beginning of dynasties or in the wake of poor harvests.[72] Monopolies were mainstays of the Tang, Song, Yuan, and Qing Dynasties. During the Song, debate over prohibition raged throughout the court even as alcohol tax revenue became more important to it.[73] Fang Fei has argued that the strictest prohibition in the past millennium was implemented during the fifth year of the Jin Dynasty's Hailingwang reign (1150-61), as alcohol was strictly forbidden, with the death penalty prescribed for violators.[74] Yuan rulers subsequently mandated the use of alcohol only in sacrifices but then loosened restrictions with a monopoly under which production reached new heights, with large-scale facilities centred in present-day Xinjiang and Taiyuan.[75] Toward the end of the imperial period, the production and trade of alcohol scaled new heights.

Over time, certain centres became especially famous for the alcohol that they produced, including *shaoxing jiu* (rice alcohol) in Zhejiang, and *Maotai* in Guizhou. The fame of shaoxing wines was truly remarkable, as they commanded high prices and had been exported since the Ming Dynasty. In the late Qing, it was estimated that there were 2,000 wine shops in the area, with annual production reaching 70,000 tons.[76] Shaoxing wines remain hugely popular to this day and are produced in many areas. Maotai was first made in the Song era, was sold outside of the local area of production from the eighteenth century, and now ranks as one of the most famous wines in China.[77] Frank Dikötter, Lars Laamann, and Zhou Xun have argued that the relatively high price of such liquors made them prized luxury items compared to base-grade opium during the late Qing era.[78] The final years of the imperial period were also marked by German, Polish, and Russian construction of beer-making facilities in the Northeast and in Qingdao, a city now internationally renowned for the beer named after it.

The collapse of the Qing Dynasty in 1912 did not result in markedly different state or societal approaches to alcohol. In 1915 the Beijing-based government of Yuan Shikai (1859-1916) established an alcohol monopoly, and alcohol remained an important source of revenue for administrations throughout the subsequent warlord era. In June 1927 Chiang Kai-shek (1887-1975) apparently modelled the Republic of China's "Temporary Regulations on State Monopoly Sales of Tobacco and Alcoholic Beverages" closely on Yuan Shikai's earlier institution.[79] With the start of the Anti-Japanese War in 1937, taxes on alcohol became an even more significant source for much-needed revenue; taxes were raised by 50 percent and more in many jurisdictions.[80] In the 1930s and 1940s, alcohol was a powerful revenue generator across the mainland, in the Republic and in Manchukuo, as demonstrated in the next chapter.

Opium

Alcohol was a product that many viewed with suspicion but, to date, opium's roles in Chinese history have attracted far more critical and scholarly attention. Received scholarship suggests that opium has been used around the world for 5,000 years, with its origins generally now dated to 3000 BCE, although Dr. Zhang Guochen dated its earliest use by the Swiss to 2,000 BCE and its use by the Chinese to at least 120 BCE, as he argued that a story from the Han Wu Di era featured opium in it.[81] By the Tang Dynasty at the latest, opium had been firmly established in China as an important medical commodity. For centuries, domestically produced opium served medicinal purposes, especially in treating stomach ailments and reducing pain. But it was not opium's application as a medicine that garnered it the most critical attention. Centuries-long medicinal uses were excused as justifiable, but the recreational uses of opium, springing from American, British, Dutch, and Spanish imports dating to 1482, eventually were not.[82] By the nineteenth century, foreign opium and foreign methods of selling and consuming it had spurred crises that touched all corners of the Qing Empire – from the imperial court in Beijing to the farthest borders. The enormous expansion of recreational opium consumption in the nineteenth century dramatically altered social customs, patterns of domestic and international trade, and the very ways that opium itself was understood.

A considerable scholarship exists on opium in Chinese history, especially regarding the Anglo-Chinese Opium Wars (1839-42 and 1856-60) and British dominance of the trade.[83] But the opium trade was not limited to, first, the British and, later, the Japanese alone; Americans, Chinese, Dutch, Koreans, Russians, South Asians, Spanish, and others also engaged in it.[84] But the two mid-nineteenth-century Anglo-Chinese wars, which resulted in unequal treaties, the occupation of the capital, and the disgraceful looting and destruction of the Summer Palace (Yuanming yuan), guaranteed Britain would be most firmly linked in popular memory and scholarship with the opium trade in China. Although scholars continue to argue over whether the wars were instigated by the British pursuit of equality in diplomatic relations and the Qing refusal of it or by the British protection of the drug trade and the Qing ban on it, the wars have left long shadows in Chinese memories and historical narratives that may never be fully reconciled. In short, British traders determined that opium was an ideal commodity; it had a high value and a low weight and was addictive.[85] Opium grown in South Asia was traded in China at first under the auspices of the British East India Company (1600-1874, although its monopoly in the trade ended in 1833). Opium was imported into China to balance payments for the vast amounts of tea, porcelain, and other goods that were exported from it. The demand for opium grew rapidly in the early 1800s as recreational consumption of it grew exponentially. By 1823 more powerful forms of Bengal opium had practically forced domestic opium out of the market and had reversed patterns of trade, causing a heavy flow of silver out of China.[86] The expanding consumption of increasingly strong opium and its socio-economic impacts triggered debate at the highest levels of the Qing court over whether opium should be outlawed.[87] This debate occurred against a backdrop of Qing refusal to recognize the British crown as its diplomatic equal. The latter's requests for equal relations were rejected out of hand by Qing emperors, who believed the empire to be self-sufficient and of self-evident superiority.

Although Qing officials debated the pros and cons of the trade, recreational opium consumption spread throughout the ranks of the imperial court, officialdom, and most other sectors of society. Zheng Yangwen has detailed opium's migration from elite levels of society to a broader mass-based "McDonaldization" that eventuated in its condemnation for its widespread impact and association with foreign imperialism.[88] Opium shed respectability as it shifted from a medicine to a recreational product, becoming at the height of its popularity an everyday part of polite social recreation. Zheng has associated its rapid popularization with similarities between the preparation of opium, meal service, tea ceremonies, and the consumption of tobacco and sugar.[89] Its popularity has also been attributed to its perceived qualities as an aphrodisiac.[90] The Qing "craving for foreign stuff" *(yanghuo re)* included opium, which became an increasingly problematic signifier of the cosmopolitan nature of contemporary culture.[91] Over time, the consumption of opium came to be linked with supposed inherent "Chinese" character traits, such as enjoying indoor activities like writing poetry and luxuries associated with silk, in contrast to Europeans, who seemed to favour alcohol and therefore were believed to excel at outdoor activities, including driving cars, boats, and planes.[92] A similar, yet more negative expression of this ethnic-based consumption has been noted in Miriam Kingsberg's work on Sakai Yoshio (a renowned professor at the medical college of Tokyo Imperial University) who, in the 1930s, associated Japanese alcohol consumption with their "active" ethnicity in contrast to the "lethargic" Chinese who smoked opium.[93]

Opium travelled the breadth of Chinese society via complex trade routes and personal connections. In the Ming palace, the Wan Li emperor (r. 1572-1620) famously absented himself from court for decades, partly because of habitual opium use. Of even greater significance to the society as a whole, however, was opium's movement via the Qing practice of "avoidance" *(huibi)*, through which officials were regularly transferred. As Zheng Yangwen has argued, they took with them their patterns of consumption, spreading across society a recreational product that destabilized the empire.[94] Officials' careers were rooted in Confucian moral responsibility, yet as more of them began to consume, and be consumed by, the intoxicant, they weakened their ability to realize these responsibilities. As opium spread among the lower classes, it was increasingly linked with fatal consequences, ultimately giving rise to arguments that eradication of recreational opium consumption was central to saving the empire and, later, the nation.[95] Latter-day political leaders, such as the Empress Dowager Cixi (1835-1908) and Chairman Mao Zedong (1893-1976), publicly condemned opium yet recognized its value: Cixi is rumoured to have had a propensity for the pipe, and Mao used opium as a revenue source for the Communist Party during the Anti-Japanese Resistance and the civil war.

Qing debate over recreational opium consumption eventually resulted in opium being declared illegal. By the 1830s, mass consumption, heavy silver outflow, and the reliance of farmers on income from growing poppies had outraged critics, who demanded action.[96] Whereas early reformers blamed the importation of opium on individual traders seeking profit, by the 1830s foreign governments were blamed for the opium trade and denounced for their harm to the people of China.[97] In 1838 the Daoguang emperor (r. 1820-50) sent Lin Zexu (1785-1850) to the southern port of Guangzhou to resolve the opium issue once and for all. The incorruptible Lin was met with derision by foreigners, who were soon disabused of their belief that they would be able to manipulate him. Lin ordered them to hand over their stocks of opium and in short order destroyed over 1 million kilograms of opium, enraging the merchants, who demanded British retribution. The Opium War, or First Anglo-Chinese War, ensued. The final reckoning, the Nanjing Treaty (1842), was the first of many "unequal treaties" forced on the Qing Dynasty. It opened ports to British trade, allowed freer access for missionaries, and forfeited Hong Kong and an enormous sum of money, while not mentioning opium. Slow Qing enforcement of the unequal treaty led to the Second Anglo-Chinese War, which resulted in British occupation of the capital, Beijing, as well as the looting and burning of the Summer Palace, the ruins of which remain to this day as a vivid testament to foreign imperialist aggression in China.

By the end of the 1800s, the British had abandoned the opium business, and most opium was being produced and circulated domestically. The opium trade remained lucrative and controversial long after British dominance ended. Locally grown opium competed with more potent forms of opium imported from Persia. Efforts at eradicating recreational opium use continued. David Bello and Joyce Madancy have argued that relatively successful efforts at prohibition were implemented in the period 1906-11, in the final decade of Qing rule, but that administrative dependence on opium revenue was a major long-term impediment.[98] Another anti-opium campaign was launched by the Japanese in Taiwan, from 1895, when they assumed sovereignty over the island.[99] Japanese colonial officials resolved to legalize opium in the colony in order to supervise its growth and distribution with the aim of eventually eliminating recreational opium use. They established an Opium Monopoly to bring dens and dealers under police supervision and to make doctors' exams mandatory for registered addicts; all profits were to be used for public health and education programs.[100] Gotō Shinpei (1857-1929), the first Japanese governor-general of Taiwan, was a leading figure in the Japanese battle against opium addiction who advocated gradual withdrawal for addicts under medical attention rather than outright criminalization.[101] He anticipated that five decades would be required to eradicate opiate addiction in Taiwan.[102] Gotō implemented the system from 1896 until 1906, when he was transferred to oversee Japanese interests in Korea and Manchuria.[103] The policies that Gotō developed in Taiwan provided a model for Manchukuo, the subject of the next chapter.

During the warlord period (1916-27), opium was central to the funding of local armies, which grew exponentially after the end of the Great War (1914-18) as warlords sought money to purchase weapons from the European powers. Links between the Chinese warlords and the drug trade have been well documented. As early as 1924, for example, Huai Yin argued in the *Shengjing shibao (Shengjing Times)* that warlords were self-obsessed hold-overs from the imperial period – and that as long as they held power, no progress could be made to reduce recreational opium consumption.[104] Huai argued that warlords were fatally undermined by their commitment to war and opium, and he advocated a "common people's revolution" *(pingmin geming)* to overthrow them and eradicate opium use. One of the most important warlords, the Northeast's Zhang Zuolin, depended on opium revenues in his quest to rule all of China. The huge sums of money raised from drugs and spent on arms led to a destabilization of society that influenced life in China for much of the rest of the century. During the rule of Zhang's son, Ru Gai argued that although the Japanese had effectively introduced measures to control recreational opium use in Taiwan, similar efforts in China would be impractical because of the nation's enormous size and the heavy presence of the military.[105]

Despite Ru's apprehensions, efforts at prohibition endured, often inflicting, as argued by Frank Dikötter, Lars Laamann, and Zhou Xun, "a cure which was far worse than the disease" – with increasing corruption, a criminal underclass, and the rising popularity of replacements for opium, including heroin and morphine.[106] In the Republic, Chiang Kai-shek officially launched a six-year Plan in 1935 to eliminate recreational opium use. The project was a varied and, as Allan Baumler argues, successful set of programs designed to win him control over opium and the ways that it was understood in Chinese society. Chiang sought "to control both the definition of the opium problem and appropriate solutions to it."[107] Through a combination of control, sales, and suppression – including the execution of addicts – the Nationalists transformed opium from a plague that many believed threatened the very existence of the state into "a social problem like any other."[108] Small-scale pilot projects designed to enhance the sale and control of opium in Nationalist strongholds such as Hankou ultimately had wider application, enabling Chiang to centralize power over an increasingly regulated industry and thereby to lay the foundations for post-1949 Communist drug policies. Recent scholarship demonstrates that the Nationalist regime was a major force in renegotiating the meanings of opium in mid-twentieth-century China, but it was not the only one. The policies implemented by Chiang bear similarities to their counterparts in Manchukuo, although the latter have been so excoriated in popular memory and scholarly studies that they have to date been dismissed as no more than a smokescreen for the nefarious dealings of Japanese imperialists and traitors.[109] Yet as the next chapter makes clear, the recreational consumption of opium inspired reflection throughout society as individuals tried to come to terms with what they believed to be their own, or the state's, best interests.

This chapter has outlined in broad strokes the long-lasting, significant roles that alcohol and opium have played in Chinese society. They were employed for valued purposes – medicinal and recreational – yet they also had more sinister applications through association with foreign imperialism, social decline and, later, addiction. Both are prominent, potentially addictive consumables that for hundreds of years have shaped understandings of Chinese peoples and societies around the globe. Other consumables said to have addiction-forming capabilities, including tea, sugar, coffee, dried fruit, and tobacco, also attracted interest – both positive and negative.[110] Consuming them in excess was known to pose health problems, but moderate usage was seen to be potentially healthful.[111] In terms of the serious health and social issues, especially in the ability to maintain "proper" family function, produce descendants, or keep a job, by the early twentieth century at the latest, the gravity of excessive alcohol and opium consumption overshadowed concerns regarding other hobbies in the Northeast, where smoking tobacco was by some accounts nearly universal.[112]

What the Qing Dynasty, various warlords, the Republic, and the Japanese were unable to accomplish, the Communist Party achieved in rather short order. The Maoist period ended the recreational use of opiates and dampened promotion of alcohol products. But with the opening of China from the 1970s, and the country's increasing connections with the global community, narcotics have again surfaced in China, although this time their consumption is not linked with foreign aggression per se. Alcohol industries, too, have returned with a vengeance in the post-Mao era, as Chinese and foreign companies aggressively advertise their products and consumers demonstrate their capacity for buying them at a rate unequalled since the 1930s. This chapter has argued that the intoxicant industries of China today have important precedents in Chinese history. Chapter 2 examines alcohol and opium in the context of Northeast Chinese society during the turbulent early to mid-twentieth century.

2 Manchurian Context

The Northeast was ruled as the Manchu homeland by the Qing Dynasty to 1912 and then by the Chinese warlords Zhang Zuolin (r. circa 1916-28) and Zhang Xueliang (r. 1928-31) until the Japanese established the state of Manchukuo (1932-45).[1] Each regime attempted to turn intoxicants to its advantage. Alcohol stretched far into the region's past, with commercial alcohol production having thrived in the area since at least the Kangxi era (1661-1722).[2] The importance of alcohol in the Northeast has been stressed by Feng Qi, who argues that alcohol drove regional development and is central to understanding local culture.[3] It was in the Kangxi reign, too, that opium appears to have been first introduced. Eventually, farmers discovered that the soil had an ideal mix of loam and sand for growing opium;[4] it was cultivated from around 1860.[5] Despite an attempted prohibition of opium in 1906, it had become one of the top three agricultural products in the region by the end of the Qing.[6] Throughout the first half of the twentieth century, both intoxicants were mainstays of local economies, supporting many secondary enterprises, including stores, hotels, restaurants, bars, and brothels.[7] Alcohol and opium were prominent features of local social and financial regimes. But decades of militarism, occupation, and war wrought fundamental transformations in how people perceived them and their recreational consumption.[8] This chapter outlines main developments in the Northeast's intoxicant industries from the end of the imperial period through the 1940s to demonstrate their significance to local life and governance.

The latter Qing Dynasty witnessed expansive growth in intoxicant industries. Opium had long been valued for its medicinal properties, especially for the treatment of stomach ailments and pain; in the Northeast, it was also valued for fighting the plague, a recurrent disease.[9] As elsewhere in China, opium became a requirement of polite society that was as routinely offered to guests as tobacco and tea.[10] By the late Qing, opium's growth as a commodity had given it a role "similar to that of gold in the settlement of California," as it lured immigrants from the rest of China to work in a wide range of related industries.[11] The importance of opium was marked in the local dialect, as harvests signalled the beginning of autumn, the "smoke season" *(yan ji)*.[12] Opium was first taxed in 1885 and was subsequently subject to Qing legal restrictions.[13]

The Northeast excelled in the production and distribution of a range of opiates, which were given many names: (1) opium, known by phonetic translation from English as *ahpian* or *yapian* and from Persian as *ahfurong, furong,* or *yarong* and known by description as *dayan* (big smoke), *hei jinzi* (black gold), *yashuang yan* (frosty smoke), *yan tu* (smoke mud), or *yao tu* (medicine mud); (2) heroin, known by phonetic translation as *hailuoyin* or *hailuoying* and by description as *baimian* or *baimianr* (white flour); and (3) morphine, known by phonetic translation as *mafei*.[14] Opium was also referred to according to its colour as *bai tu* (white mud), *hong tu* (red mud), *hong pizi* (red leather), *wu a* (black opium), *gu yan* (wild rice smoke), *hei ya* (black opium), and *wu xiang* (black fragrance); according to its place of production, including *Yun tu* (Yunnan mud), *Jian tu* (Fujian mud), *Chuan tu* (Sichuan mud), *dong tu* (Eastern mud), *xi tu* (Western mud), *yang yao tu* (foreign medicine mud), *yang yao gao* (foreign medicine paste), *yang yao yan* (foreign medicine smoke), and *yang yan* (foreign smoke); and finally, by the 1930s, according to its legal status as *guan tu* (official mud) or *si tu* (private mud). The wide variety of names is suggestive of the extent of usage in the region. Prohibition of such lucrative products that provided the means for rapid economic development and leisurely diversion proved difficult in a vast region with a relatively dispersed population, limited state resources, and officials with disparate priorities. Farmers planted it alongside other crops or began to exclusively cultivate opium (see Figure 1). The use of opium for recreational and medicinal purposes earned it a prominence that could not be dislodged easily. Unless officials were aggressively committed to prohibition, the industry expanded.

Alcohol, too, was a very popular consumable good. Zhang Huinuan has argued that cold winter temperatures, social factors, and traditional herding lifestyles shaped consumption patterns.[15] Zhang argues that alcohol customs contributed to the "tough" *(cuguang),* bold, and generous nature of Northeastern people.[16] The original inhabitants of the region, including peoples now known as Manchus and Mongols, consumed alcohol, especially fermented milk, on social occasions, such as when expressing hospitality while welcoming guests to their homes, and to help pass the cold winters.[17] Manchus were also famed for producing a mountain grape wine, *ahmulu*.[18] Commercial production was long a feature in the region's history, and taxes were first instituted in 1775 during the Qianlong era (1736-96). One of the region's most famous wines, Lao long kou (Old Dragon Mouth), began to be produced commercially by Shanxi native Meng Zijing in 1662; in 1692, on a visit to

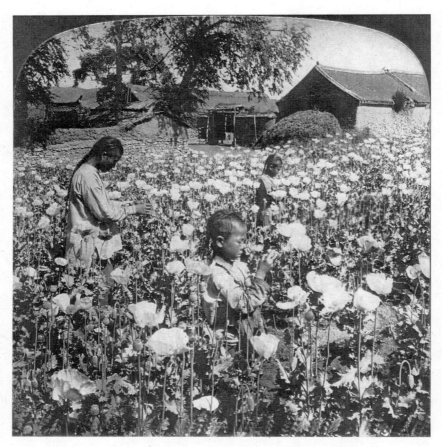

1   Opium field. *Source:* Underwood and Underwood, ceased business in the 1940s, in author's collection.

Fengtian[19] to pay respect to his ancestors, the Kangxi emperor reportedly tasted the wine and mandated its production for the palace, and it was henceforth consumed by his descendants during subsequent pilgrimages.[20] Remarkably, as early as 1663, the Yilong quan (Elan Springs) brand was produced in the range of 175,000 litres annually.[21] Fengtian and Liaoyang emerged as two main centres of alcohol production.[22] The mid- to late-Qing expansion of agriculture and the arrival of Han Chinese and other migrants prompted the development of grain- and other fruit-based alcohol: distilled alcohol, including *baijiu* (locally made from maize) and *gaoliang jiu* (a specialty of the Northeast made primarily from Chinese sorghum);[23] brewed wines such as *shaoxing jiu* (rice alcohol), and *huangjiu* (yellow, especially millet, wine); and *putao jiu* (grape wines), which were popular, with many households producing their own. The remarkable range of alcohol available is demonstrated by Nelson Fairchild (1879-1906), a Harvard graduate who worked in Fengtian in the early 1900s. Fairchild recounted in a letter to his mother on 11 October 1906 the drink menu (in addition to coffee and tea) from a dinner hosted by the local viceroy: "To drink, we had first port, then white wine, then beer, then champagne, and green minthe to finish up with!"[24] Clearly, a wide variety of alcohol existed by at least the early 1900s. By then, Harbin had developed such a vibrant alcohol industry that alcohol production ranked among the city's top three industries, along with oil and flour.[25] Reflecting Harbin's multicultural nature, in the first years of the twentieth century, over twenty factories producing alcohol were opened by Chinese, Czechs, Germans, Greeks, Japanese, Polish, Russians, and other ethnic groups.[26] Migrants, expanding urban centres, and a burgeoning middle class all contributed to growth in the industry.

The regional influence of Russians and Harbin has been underlined in two important works, Blaine Chiasson's *Administering the Colonizer* and David Wolff's *To the Harbin Station*.[27] In Harbin, Russians introduced a drink that has become one of the most popular in China – beer.[28] The first brewery in China, Ulubulevskij Brewery (present-day Harbin Brewery), was established in Harbin in 1900 and named after its Russian founder of Polish origin.[29] Contemporary observers remarked that the Northeast had several advantages for the manufacture of beer – cheap coal and labour and abundant high-quality water. But there were also major drawbacks: although hop cultivation was begun by Russian farmers in 1918, the importation of hops from Czechoslovakia and Germany remained necessary; breweries in Fengtian, for example, used German products exclusively. Severe winters meant that bottles had to be secured with special coverings and stored or transported in heated storages or cars.[30] These factors added to the costs of production. But despite such challenges, Harbin became one of the major centres for the production of alcohol in the Northeast and one of the biggest markets for beer in China. Incredibly, less than ten years after their founding, Harbin's breweries produced over 1 million bottles of beer annually.[31]

Two beverages that were less successful in gaining consumer loyalty were vodka and sake.[32] Vodka was first produced in the Northeast in 1897, but due to a general lack of interest, high taxes, and diminishing Russian influence after the Russo-Japanese War (1904-5), vodka consumption was limited.[33] Still, in December 1903 the American consul at Niuzhuang noted that eight distilleries operated in Harbin "to satisfy a daily consumption of 1,000 Russian buckets of vodka (2,707 gallons)."[34] The Japanese introduced sake, but its attraction, too, was limited because of tastes, costs, and later prohibitions on rice consumption.[35] The high quality of local water was touted as especially favourable for its production, although the main ingredient, rice, was imported from Japan or Korea. Penelope Francks has detailed how from the 1870s sake became one of the most important manufactured goods in Japan.[36] As Japanese migration to the Northeast increased, sake production followed suit.[37] In 1910 sake production began in Dalian and was followed in Fushun in 1916.[38] Unlike beer, however, vodka and sake remained for the most part popular only among the migrant communities within which they had originated.[39]

The late-Qing period witnessed expansive growth of the alcohol and opium industries, despite prohibitions on the latter. As recounted in Chapter 1, recent scholarship stresses the success of campaigns against recreational opium consumption in the final years of Manchu rule. But it was too little too late, and opium flourished in the Northeast. The regime that succeeded the Qing nominally continued to promulgate bans on recreational opium use while encouraging the expansion of alcohol production, consumption, and taxation. Challenges existed for both industries, but they expanded during the Republican period, providing resources for rulers and myriad pleasures and problems for consumers. They were valued for their roles in revenue raising and were important consumer products that came to be identified, for better or worse, as cherished local traditions or as symbols of an oppressive present. Alcohol, like other consumer products, was promoted in a practice that Yu Xuebin has dated to the origins of unified China in the Qin Dynasty – the hanging of signboards outside of drinking shops and establishments.[40] Yu recounts in detail the shapes and colours of such signboards, which ranged from black-, red-, or blue-bordered yellow cloth with writing on them to shapes like gourds or alcohol containers; these often had attractive red streamers hung from them.[41] The signboards informed consumers of, and attracted them to, the establishment's specialities with visuals that compensated for those who might not be able to understand the relevant Chinese characters. They also added considerable colour and local flavour to what were often otherwise drab commercial buildings. In large cities, especially, streets were festooned with signboards for all sorts of businesses, ranging from shoemakers to tobacconists. From the 1910s, such promotional practices moved into print media as well.

Historians have interpreted the Zhang Zuolin regime from various standpoints, but there appears to be a consensus that the prosperity that accompanied his early rule began to falter in the mid-1920s. Ronald Suleski has described how in the early 1920s the region "entered a period of economic vibrancy unlike anything else taking place in China."[42] Tim Wright has argued that the Northeast boasted "greater levels of prosperity and commercialisation" than elsewhere in China.[43] Such vibrancy funded Zhang's aspirations to bring all of China under his control. His compulsion to expand his rule made taxing consumer goods, such as alcohol and opium, highly attractive.[44] Throughout the 1920s, Zhang's military expenditures resulted in increased taxes, the burden of which was made heavier by natural disasters and political uncertainty, and the economy faltered. Wright argues that a small net decline in gross domestic product resulted from long-term structural changes, especially regarding the primary export (soybeans).[45] And in terms of individual standards of living, Suleski stresses that "unchecked warlord rule" from the mid-1920s led to people being "mercilessly stripped of the money and possessions they had."[46] Herbert Bix, too, has calculated that average annual incomes of peasant families dropped from 170 yuan in 1927 to 81 yuan in 1931 and 57 yuan in 1933.[47] The final years of warlord rule appear to have been marked by declining standards of living among the general population.[48]

The Great War (1914-18) and the Russian Revolution (1917) slowed growth in many sectors of the Northeast's alcohol industry, as a slump in business was exacerbated by a brief Russian-imposed ban on alcohol; in 1914, for example, sales of *baijiu* and beer fell one-third below 1913 levels.[49] Some domestic producers – notably the maker of Fengtian's Lao long kou (Old Dragon Mouth) brand – reported growth as foreign competition declined with the departure of Europeans and disruption of supply routes.[50] In 1916 Zhang Zuolin moved to increase revenues from the industry and established an alcohol and tobacco monopoly, which added taxes of approximately 12 percent to sale prices, although no standard taxation rate was achieved for the entire region.[51] That same year, in August, Russian authorities of the China Eastern Railway (CER) in Harbin called for a ban on the production, buying and selling, and consumption of alcohol within an eighty-kilometre radius of CER lines, creating a rift with Chinese retailers and likely not a few consumers.[52] On 12 June 1917 a meeting in Jilin between CER authorities and local Chinese resulted in the latter issuing an appeal to the Foreign Affairs Department to refuse the request. Nonetheless, on 10 July, CER authorities ordered all stores within their sphere of control, including 740 owned by Chinese, to close. Chinese retailers fought the ban until it was repealed in February 1918. Production rebounded in the following three years.[53]

Controversy erupted again in the early 1920s over American demands to guarantee railway loans with alcohol and tobacco tax revenues.[54] Writers in the *Shengjing shibao (Shengjing Times)* denounced the move as a form of imperialism, deemed particularly odious since the United States was in the midst of Prohibition (1920-33). Why, they asked, would Americans seek to profit from a product that was illegal in their own country? Responses to the American demand underline the perceived importance of alcohol. Critics argued that giving Americans control over alcohol and tobacco would threaten local customs and create hardships for the poor since both were considered a part of everyday life and were mostly locally produced. Despite such controversies, rising taxes, and declining incomes, alcohol remained relatively affordable in the 1920s, and there was growth in the industry.[55] By the end of the decade, in Harbin alone, alcohol production had climbed to almost 2 million litres a year, including more than 4.3 million bottles of beer.[56]

Alcohol was an important revenue generator for the Zhang Zuolin regime, but opium was even more valuable. According to Ronald Suleski, "opium was used as a money-grab as Zhang tried to pay for pretensions to rule all of China."[57] Although opium was officially prohibited by the Republican laws that Zhang professed to uphold, he "left his satraps to their own devices to promote or prohibit opium production."[58] In February 1927 Zhang moved to control the opium market and to reap the benefits of it. The General Opium Prohibition Bureau opened in the regional centre of Fengtian, and "local government-run retail shops called, ironically, Opium Prohibition Drugstores" increased rapidly in number in counties bordering railways owned by the South Manchuria Railway conglomerate (Chinese: Nan Man tielu; Japanese: Mantetsu; henceforth SMR).[59] As early as 1918, and again in 1928, the Japanese consul in Fengtian warned authorities that Japanese involvement in the drug trade, which reportedly accounted for half of the Japanese in Northeast China, fomented seriously negative perceptions of Japanese among other populations as recreational opium use expanded.[60] In some jurisdictions – in Rehe province, for example – so much land came to be cultivated with poppies that food had to be imported to make up for shortfalls.[61] In others, serious inspection regimes were implemented. Tang Yulin (1877-1937) imposed such heavy taxes in his jurisdiction that many farmers abandoned cultivation.[62] T. Nagashima noted that when General Zhu Qinglan (1874-1941) assumed command of the CER's Railway Protective Army, he implemented a strict prohibition policy that nearly destroyed the industry along the rail lines.[63] In Andong, inspectors were reported to have visited opium businesses up to four times a day.[64] Andong's government even issued special uniforms for inspectors, featuring dark grey pants and a purple jacket with two words embroidered on the shoulder: "ban smoke" *(jin yan)*. The uniforms were favourably received for providing visual identification even though they inadvertently alerted business owners to the presence of inspectors, as they could no longer blend in with customers. In some jurisdictions, such as Andong, campaigns were launched to encourage people to refrain from smoking opium and tobacco and from drinking alcohol. But despite such efforts, in some areas they were still widely available.[65]

Opium revenues flowed to the state and into private pockets as the Northeast became one of the largest markets for drugs in East Asia. In 1928, after Zhang Zuolin was assassinated by the Japanese, control over the Northeast fell to his son Zhang Xueliang, who in 1929 reasserted opium prohibition to dovetail with Republican law; he similarly outlawed opium cultivation to no avail.[66] According to US estimates, in 1920s Harbin there were approximately 1,000 illegal opium businesses supplied with Persian and Japanese opium and synthetic drugs.[67] With an estimated 10,000 Russian and 50,000 Chinese drug users,[68] Harbin was one of the biggest narcotic markets in East Asia, with its own unique Sino-Russian word for "drug addict" *(damafengr).*[69] The social impact of such widespread drug consumption was considerable. Newspaper reports consistently condemned the scourge of opiate addiction. In 1929 Dr. K. Morinaka, who worked at the Manchuria Medical College in Fengtian, estimated that about one-quarter to one-half of the prisoners in Northeast jails were drug users.[70] In the late 1920s, as opium prices escalated, many consumers switched from opium to cheaper, more powerful morphine; they "abandoned the black for the white" *(qi hei jiu bai).*[71] Physicians and other health specialists began using morphine injections to wean addicts from opium, a procedure that Zhang Xueliang was reportedly undergoing in Beijing when the Japanese invaded Manchuria in 1931. Foreign occupation replaced warlord rule, but opium remained. So did alcohol.

Manchukuo administrators publicly linked intoxicant policies with their "scientific, conscientious, bold experiment"[72] to establish, as Prasenjit Duara has stated, a "visionary modern polity"[73] that would vanquish militarism, communism, and Western imperialism. They also sought to resolve the "English frame-up" *(Yingren de xianhai)* of intoxicant poisoning.[74] Manchukuo was deemed by its defenders to have forged the world's most modern mandate, twinning the best of East Asian tradition, especially the Confucian-based Kingly Way *(Wangdao)* ideology, with Western scientific and material conditions. The founding of Manchukuo in 1932 heralded changes for the economy, including the commercial production and consumption of intoxicants. Chronic underfunding of Japan's imperial project, as demonstrated in studies by Michael Barnhart, Alan Baumler, Miriam Kingsberg, and Yamada Gōichi, made control over intoxicants an attractive source of revenue.[75] In Manchukuo the alcohol industry was amalgamated at first informally and later under state order. In 1932 the Opium Law was established to create a regulatory framework for reform of the trade under Japanese oversight. The Japanese quickly sought control over "traditional industries in which the Chinese interest was heavy. By bringing them under control, the Japanese hold over the economy was strengthened."[76] The government implemented policies that encouraged growth in certain sectors of the economy, especially construction, which led to economic recovery within a few years. Kang Chao has argued that in the 1930s manufacturing "under Japanese tutelage" was "a most dynamic sector."[77] In the mid-1930s the British consul even reported "an increase in the prosperity of the population in general."[78] However, Herbert Bix has noted that it was not the local population or even Japanese settlers who tended to prosper in Manchukuo but rather large state enterprises such as the SMR.[79]

With the Japanese invasion, the Guandong Army seized control over a region that was difficult to rule and that fostered extensive intoxicant industries. Manchukuo officials attempted to justify the state's existence in terms of rescuing the people from various dangers, including addiction. In October 1931 SMR staff estimated that "roughly 5 percent of [the region's] total population of 30 million were opium and narcotic addicts – 1.5 million people."[80] More recent estimates suggest that there were far fewer addicts in the early days of Manchukuo: Lü Yonghua suggests that there were 200,000, whereas Jiao Runming places the number closer to 30,000 addicts.[81] Regardless of such discrepancies, the editors of the 1941 *Manchukuo Yearbook* argued that the Japanese had to intervene in the region to save the indigenous population: "With the Manchu and Mongol races opium-smoking is, so to speak, a historically hereditary disease," which was exacerbated by inhumane Han rule.[82] Manchukuo officials condemned the decadence of local society, decrying "the whole body of public servants [who], in fact, seemed to be devotees of Morpheus."[83] Officials and anti-opiate reformists in the new state publicly attacked opium as the "archenemy of mankind," advocating restricted cultivation and an end to imports.[84] Officials were encouraged to travel to Korea and Taiwan in order to examine Japanese successes there. Work immediately began on drafting Manchukuo's Opium Law, which was promulgated in November 1932. It advocated control over the production and distribution of opium so that recreational consumption "can be gradually lessened, and the evil eventually exterminated."[85] According to the Opium Law, permits for smoking opium would be granted to adult, non-Japanese addicts, who were to commit to rehabilitation.[86] Manchukuo's Opium Monopoly (Yapian zhuanmai gongshu; henceforth Monopoly) began to oversee implementation of the Opium Law at the beginning of 1933.

The Monopoly was launched amid much fanfare as an anchor of Japan's East Asian modernity project and to demonstrate the benevolent nature of Manchukuo rule. Reflecting state policies, recreational opium consumption was denounced, as was long the custom in the *Shengjing shibao,* the region's largest Chinese-language newspaper. Rana Mitter has noted that despite all official efforts to control such media, the *Shengjing shibao* was "by no means a crude propaganda organ for the Japanese presence in the region."[87] To promote awareness of the harm of opiates, reports on their use and accounts of recovered addicts regularly shared headlines with top news stories of the day; representative titles included "Yinzhe de xin" (An Addict's Letter) and "Jin yan lun" (Discussion of Opium Prohibition).[88] Private dealers and licensed businesses were constantly criticized for disobeying the law. The prominent space devoted to raising public awareness of the costs of addiction underlines the earnest position of anti-opium reformists, who sought aggressive eradication policies to relieve the suffering of the masses. Many advocated harm reduction for users. Prime Minister Zheng Xiaoxu (1860-1938), for example, reasoned that "to impose prohibition while ignoring the treatment of addicts ... [is like] 'damming a lower stream without adjusting the source.'"[89] In 1939 T. Nakashima argued that those who advocated for an immediate ban did "nothing but publicize his [sic] ignorance of the problem and its nature."[90] But anti-opium reformers, both men and women, faced an uphill battle against long-entrenched opiate usage, popular and official noncompliance, insufficient resources, and, not least of all, the greed that drove the industry.

In Manchukuo an environment was created in which sales of opiates were facilitated by officials who were supposed to implement the Opium Law. Kathryn Meyer has shown how they "employ[ed] the rhetoric of opium control to destroy independent competitors, not opium use."[91] At the high end of the industry, Japanese were chemists, wholesalers, and importers, whereas Koreans or Chinese tended to run street-level opium retail outlets and dens; Miriam Kingsberg cites a study by Eguchi Keiichi that "finds that up to ninety percent of urban Koreans in Manchuria – approximately 600,000 individuals – served as opium dealers."[92] The manufacture of heroin and morphine was brought under the control of the Kempeitai (the military police) and the Special Service Section (army intelligence), driving out the last European firms; private local heroin manufacturers who survived came to terms with the army.[93] In 1933 the Japanese general Doihara Kenji (1883-1948), the so-called "Lawrence of Manchuria," who was subsequently convicted of war crimes by the International Military Tribunal for the Far East and executed in 1948, argued that Japanese success in Manchuria had been won through the lucrative trade in opium, weapons, and women.[94] Aggressive Japanese moves to control the industry in conjunction with extensive media condemnation of the recreational use of opiates stigmatized addiction to the extent that efforts to identify and license users failed; by 1935 only 217,060 had been registered.[95] Officials conceded that addicts were reluctant to register out of fear of taxes, compulsory labour, or other punishment.[96] Despite all of the publicity generated for the Monopoly's agenda, the illicit drug trade and the inconsistent application of the law cast suspicion over the entire industry.

Considerable challenges also arose for the local alcohol industry as individual Japanese and the Manchukuo state increased their presence in it. In the early occupation, many local producers were driven out of the market by Japanese domination, rising costs, declining revenues, and difficulty with grain procurement. Despite these difficulties, alcohol sales grew, as did tax revenues: in 1933-34 tax revenues were cited as 7.96 million yuan and in 1935-36 as 11.45 million yuan.[97] In both of these years, taxes collected from alcohol were higher than those cited from other sectors, including land, manufacturing, mining, cattle, and tobacco.[98] These substantial numbers underline the significance of the industry, as do amendments to the laws governing alcohol. On 1 July 1935 the Manchukuo alcohol law was enacted; it was subsequently reformed in August 1937, December 1937, March 1939, and December 1940, and a fifth revision was promulgated on 30 August 1941. These laws focused mainly on taxation and the issuing of permits. In the midst of these amendments, in January 1938, an Alcohol Monopoly was established.[99] Alcohol was prominent not just in policy but also at official functions. Figure 2 demonstrates the importance of alcohol at an official function on 15 September 1934 celebrating the second anniversary of the military actions that led to the founding of Manchukuo, which was hosted by Foreign Minister Xie Jieshi (1878-1946) and attended by Japanese and Manchukuo officials and by Prime Minister Zheng Xiaoxu.

Japanese changes to the alcohol industry are well illustrated by the beer sector.[100] In the early occupation, beer sales rebounded.[101] Fengtian and Harbin emerged as important centres of production, which was increasingly brought under Japanese management.[102] In 1934 a number of small breweries in Harbin were combined into four large ones: the Manchuria Hop and Beer Company, Taxing Ltd. Brewery, Oriental Brewery, and Wanson Company.[103] In 1936 the Japanese-owned Harbin Brewing Company annexed the Manchuria Hop and Beer Company and Taxing Ltd. Brewery.[104] The following year, the beer industry was included in the Important Industries Control Law of May 1937 (Imperial Ordinance No. 66).[105] From 1931 to 1939 beer production increased more than eightfold, from 80,000 cases in 1931 to 200,000 cases in 1936, 500,000 cases in 1938, and 670,000 cases in 1939.[106] These numbers were in

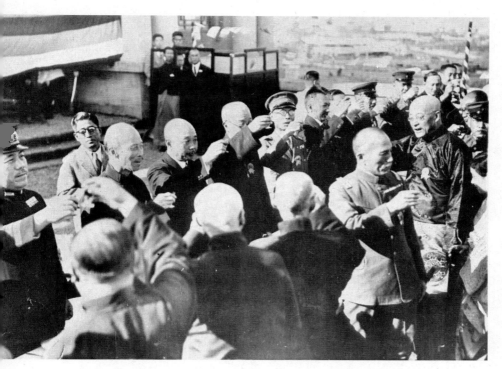

2 Ceremony hosted by Foreign Minister Xie Jieshi, third from left in back row, and attended by Prime Minister Zheng Xiaoxu, second from left in back row. *Source:* Courtesy of Associated Press.

addition to imports from Japan, which before 1931 averaged 300,000 cases and by 1938 had reached 800,000 cases.[107] In Fengtian, especially, breweries were established with Japanese capital. In April 1936 the Manchuria Ale Company, producer of Red Star Label *(Hong xing)* (founded in Japan in 1935),[108] established a branch in Fengtian, the opening of which was reported to have been attended by the American ambassador.[109] Jin he (Golden Crane), another major brand, began production in Fengtian in 1936 in an 80,000-square-metre factory.[110] The popularity of beer was enhanced by articles in the *Shengjing shibao* detailing the latest production methods. In its pages, too, Jun Qing pronounced beer a "fashionable beverage" *(liuxing de yinliao)*.[111] The beer industry grew under Japanese control, and the more that it did, the greater the control that was exerted over it.

The main competition for beer was Chinese wine *(gaoliang, shaoxing,* and *huang)*, which was considered the "most favorite alcoholic beverage of the Manchurian population."[112] The most favoured of these appears to have been gaoliang. By the late 1930s, there were approximately 1,000 commercial gaoliang producers in Manchukuo, and annual consumption was in the range of 200 million litres.[113] The ongoing popularity of gaoliang was noted with dismay by Japanese producers, who sought to popularize other alcohol. Shaoxing, for example, despite its prohibitive price, was regarded by the author of "The Brewery Industry in Manchoukuo" as "agreeable to the taste of practically anyone and is best suited to Chinese dinners."[114] Although local annual consumption of shaoxing ranged from approximately 500,000 to 700,000 litres, it, like sake, was consumed mostly by Japanese, who maintained strict control over rice consumption, which was banned for Manchukuo's Chinese subjects.[115] Shaoxing originated in south China and was difficult to produce in the Northeast because winter conditions could destroy the fermentation bacteria. But Dr. Yamazaki Hyakuji overcame this obstacle through experimentation with the use of heated rooms, leading to the establishment in 1933 of the Manchuria Distilling Company, run by Suzuki Saburōsuke and Nakatsukasa Hatsutarō, to produce shaoxing.[116] Unfortunately for them, their efforts did not result in greater attraction to their product. Sake did grow in popularity but only among Japanese consumers. By the late 1930s, Japanese sake manufacturers had established seventy-three factories in the Northeast, with thirteen in Fengtian, making it the regional centre of sake manufacturing. In 1939 sake sales reached 16.7 million litres, of which 12.5 million litres were produced in Manchukuo, and Fengtian produced over half of that.[117] Other types of alcohol also vied for consumer interest. In 1937 Feng Sen argued that local *baigan jiu* (white dry liquor) was the best alcohol, perhaps matched by brandy but not equalled by the grape or yellow wines.[118] Another noteworthy wine, called Dongbei fang (Northeast Mill) and first produced in 1930, became Manchukuo's official wine: it was served at the enthronement of Manchukuo's Kangde emperor (r. 1934-45), Henry Aisin-Gioro Puyi (1906-67), on 26 March 1934 and was subsequently featured at state banquets.[119]

Besides commercial production, homemade wine was very popular, and articles instructing readers on how to produce it appeared with some regularity in newspapers.[120] Homemade wine was praised for being economical, of guaranteed quality, and pleasurable: "Put a glass of self-made wine to your lips and your spirit will be full of joy."[121] Homemade wine let consumers avoid the high prices, poor quality, and fake alcohol for which critics constantly denounced retailers.[122] Feng Sen, for example, noted that small stores sold alcohol that made consumers ill because it was mixed with unboiled water or pigeon excrement (which was said to make the alcohol spicier and bitter).[123] He warned shoppers not to be hoodwinked by the fake alcohol's allure: one must not "smell the fragrance and get down from the horse" *(wen xiang xia ma)*.[124] Retailers were also accused of dressing up used bottles to appear to be foreign-produced three-star brandies or five-star wines, thereby selling questionable products that cost around 0.25 yuan to produce for 2 or 3 yuan.[125] Average consumers were said to be vulnerable due to a general lack of education concerning alcohol and their desire to entertain and gift well. In 1931 Leng Fo argued that consuming the fake wines might not be harmful but that they had the potential to poison and cause serious damage.[126] Such criticism of retailers, in addition to declining domestic incomes, encouraged home-made production, which certainly did not go unnoticed by the government. On 1 August 1935 laws governing homemade alcohol production were promulgated. The payment of taxes for relevant licences allowed for self-use or for consumption by one's own family while explicitly excluding members of the household who were not related.[127] Additionally, individual families were allowed to produce no more than 12.7 litres of alcohol per year, the permit for which was 5 yuan; penalties for violating permit terms ranged from 10 yuan to 500 yuan.[128]

As with opium, facilities for the sale and consumption of alcohol grew in number during the early 1930s. Four postcards demonstrate contemporary bar culture. Two postcards of the Sapporo Bar in the Yamagata-dori district in Dalian picture the bar from outside and inside.[129] Outside, on the top of the building, is the sign "Sapporo Bar" (see Figure 3). Above the entrance, the words "restaurant," "bar," and "cafe" suggest the various names that businesses invoked to attract customers. The foreign nature of the establishment is underlined not only by these words but also by stained-glass windows above the door and an English-language sign on the right side of the building proclaiming that the business sells the "Best Foreign Wines and Liquors." The international nature of the Yamagata-dori district is highlighted by the Sapporo Bar and its neighbours – the York Bar and Restaurant and a "money exchange." Three hostesses pose to the left of the bar, and three rickshaws are parked on the right. Inside, the room features a fully stocked bar with an impressive array of bottles of various shapes and sizes (see Figure 4). The tables are outfitted with tablecloths and glass containers with sauces for food. The hostesses are dressed in Japanese-style clothing and white aprons, stressing the women's presence to serve, in a domestic fashion, the Caucasian men who pose in Western-style formal wear. The image that the establishment sought to evoke was formal, exotic, and tasteful.

A Russian postcard, "Former Friends," by Russian painter Nikolay Bogdanov-Belsky (1868-1945), depicts two Caucasian men in a bar drinking alcohol while engaged in thoughtful conversation over a book (see Figure 5).[130] They

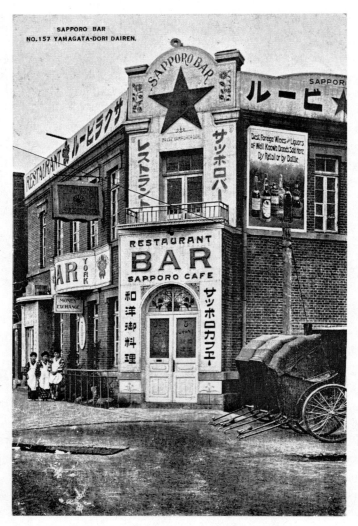

3   Sapporo Bar postcard, exterior. *Source:* Author's collection.

appear to be middle-class, educated consumers. They are surrounded by posters on the walls and newspapers on tables in a room that is not luxurious but clean. Li Zhengping, who dates Harbin's bar culture to the White Russian era, has argued that such bars created a classless environment that stressed sociability, drinking, and the respectful exchange of ideas rather than the meals and rituals that tended to be central to earlier patterns of consumption.[131] The popular writer and entertainer Yang Xu (1918-2004) noted that writers in the capital, Xinjing, would frequently meet in such bars to discuss

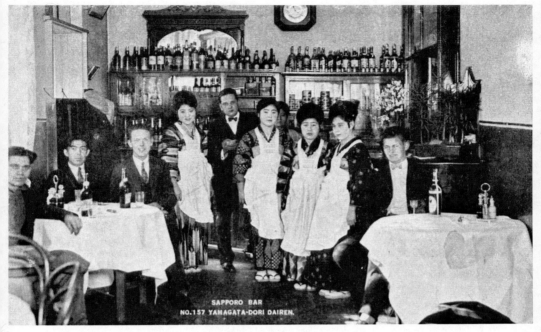

4 Sapporo Bar postcard, interior. *Source:* Author's collection.

the latest publications and to commend each other's achievements.[132] Her description parallels this image of a respectable social space. But these foreign-style bars were not the first in the region (as evidenced by the long-term use of alcohol signboards), nor were bars universally understood to be proper, upstanding businesses or social spaces. As a late-Qing postcard of a local tavern illustrates, places for the consumption of alcohol varied widely, from the "ultramodern" to the more traditional (see Figure 6). The postcard illustrates how the makeshift business and photographer caught the attention of passersby. The lure of such places was regularly debated throughout the 1930s and 1940s in media and popular literature, as bars and restaurants, just like opium retail outlets and dens, were criticized for being spaces of social disruption and for enticing innocent youth to enter at their peril.[133] The growing number and types of drinking, eating, and smoking establishments was cause for concern among social reformers and, eventually, among officials as war spread across Asia and as dominant social narratives shifted from the promotion of alcohol consumption as a mark of civilization to its denigration, alongside opium, as a social scourge.

Throughout the mid-1930s, commercial alcohol production increased, as did criticism of alcohol consumption. The *Ha'erbin shi zhi (Harbin City*

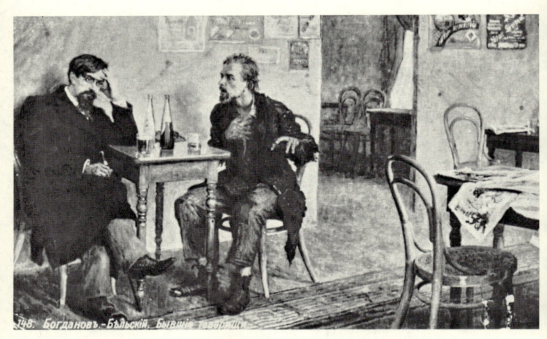

5   "Former Friends" Russian postcard. *Source:* Author's collection.

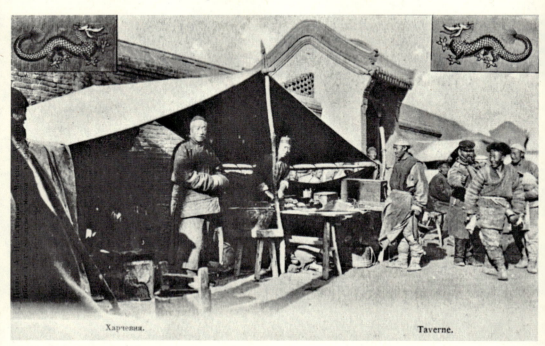

6   Qing-era tavern. *Source:* Author's collection.

Records) cite local commercial production in 1932 of approximately 2,155 tons; in 1935 this number climbed to over 6,090 tons, and in 1937 over 9,000 tons were produced.[134] Domestic production for Manchukuo appears to have peaked in 1937, as a bountiful harvest in the fall of 1936 allowed grain to be diverted for alcohol production; commercial alcohol production reportedly increased by 50 percent.[135] Imports also rose. To meet demand from Japanese soldiers in Harbin, for example, imports from Japan were increased: in 1938 approximately 3 million litres of Japanese spirits were imported, and by 1939 this number had increased to 4.5 million litres, although in 1940 it declined to just over 2 million litres.[136] These numbers did not guarantee profit across the industry. In October 1934 crops rose in cost by about 20 percent as prices for alcohol declined a similar amount, forcing producers in Liaoyang, for example, into the precarious position of seeking compensation from the state.[137] In the following years, prices increased. In 1935, 500 grams of *baijiu* sold for at least 0.2 yuan; four years later, this cost rose to 0.3 yuan.[138]

With the expansion of hostilities in China from 1937, the alcohol industry was subject to even greater state control. The availability of ingredients for the production of alcohol declined, and so, too, did the importation of alcoholic beverages, except for those from Japan. On 4 February 1938 rations were introduced. Specific amounts were allocated to various sectors of society, including families, the army, and retailers, such as stores, restaurants, and bars. Average tax rates doubled to 80 percent.[139] Commercial alcohol producers were ordered to purchase ingredients only from state-controlled suppliers. Alcohol retailers faced difficulties as increasing costs and heavier taxes forced closures in 1938.[140] A 4 October 1938 *Shengjing shibao* article reported that restaurants and bars were netting increased profits but noted that often the alcohol was tainted by a strange smell and that drinkers reported feeling sick, pointing to the sale of fake alcohol that plagued the marketplace.[141] Private production was officially prohibited but continued nonetheless for domestic use and illegal sales.

Japanese control over the alcohol industry created concern and anger among those who were being cheated or excluded and among those who advocated prohibition, but criticism of the alcohol industry never reached the level attained by its opium counterpart. The Japanese were criticized for launching the Opium Monopoly as "a legitimate, bureaucratically controlled opium monopoly to cover their covert schemes" since dealing in opiates was apparently a lucrative and legitimacy-producing venture.[142] Nitan'osa Otozō rose from obscurity to reign as a regional opium king. Yamauchi Saburō founded the South Manchuria Pharmaceutical Company, through which he and other producers donated as much as 50,000 yuan to the Japanese imperial army in exchange for decorations in formal military ceremonies; Yamauchi even claimed that Fujita Osamu, who built his fortune in the drug trade, had financed the establishment of Manchukuo.[143] Under Japanese rule, the neighbouring port of Dalian was transformed into "an opium smuggling centre," with the highest annual consumption rates of morphine and cocaine in the world.[144] Chinese critics condemned the Opium Law as "a bloodless means of killing the people" *(sha ren bu jian xue)* that destroyed morality.[145] Newspaper articles often criticized the sale of women to support opiate addictions.[146] In Harbin in December 1933, for example, morphine addict Han Wenming reportedly sold his wife, surnamed Li, to Sun Hanzhong for 110 silver dollars, despite the fact that she had borne him a son and a daughter.[147] Han was noted to have been disfigured by needle marks and to have emitted an unbearable odour; he spent all the money he received for her in a morphine shop. Most dramatically, the "ash heap of Mukden" outside of the city's west gate was an entirely unceremonious dumping ground for dead and dying addicts and was the most visible manifestation of the failings of Manchukuo's drug policies (see Figure 7).[148]

In Manchukuo, from remote farmlands to the highest level of the court, opium played a role that was attested to by Manchukuo's rulers. In his autobiography, *From Emperor to Citizen* (1964), Puyi later claimed that one-sixth of Manchukuo's revenue was derived from opium.[149] Opium propped up a court that it decimated. By 1943 Puyi's empress, born of noble Manchu parentage, Elizabeth Guobuluo Wanrong (1906-46; r. 1934-45), was reputedly so struck by drug addiction that she was incapable of standing unaided;[150] her smoking room in the palace in Changchun has even been recreated for visitors to view today. Empress Wanrong symbolized Manchukuo's subject position in the Japanese Empire and the extent of the regime's opium industry. Demand was reputedly so high that opium had to be imported, including roughly 75 percent of Korea's production from 1933 to 1941.[151] Researchers strove to increase levels of morphia in poppies and to bolster production of morphine for export to Japan in order to reduce reliance on German sources.[152] As opium spread throughout society, it became cheaper and more potent, an ominous combination.

In response to criticism, in 1936 the director of the Manchukuo General Affairs Board, Hoshino Naoki, acutely aware of the negative publicity generated by the Monopoly, argued that his government recognized that the losses of opiate addiction outweighed its benefits.[153] Officials vigorously denied that the state benefited from the Monopoly, insisting that its highest annual profits were less than 10 million yuan.[154] This was an insignificant figure because, they contended, annual opiate sales in Manchukuo were worth approximately

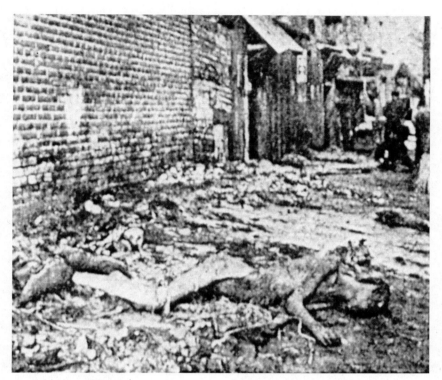

7 Ash heap of Mukden. *Source:* Assemblies of God, Foreign Missions Department, *Gospel Rays in Manchoukuo* (Springfield, MO: Assemblies of God, 1937), 19.

180 million yuan;[155] this number was also less than published earnings from alcohol taxes. Officials calculated that the eradication of opiate addiction could free up to 300 million yuan annually for industrial development and loudly voiced their intention to achieve this goal. Undeterred, critics charged that the perpetuation of the lucrative industry under the auspices of the Japanese was evidence of the genocidal nature of their rule; opiates were politicized as never before.

Western critics joined the chorus condemning Manchukuo's opiate industry. In 1934 famed sinologist Edgar Snow recounted his impressions of Manchukuo for the *Saturday Evening Post*. Snow argued that the Monopoly "vastly stimulated both production and consumption" of opiates.[156] He blamed the Japanese for turning "once delightful" Harbin into "a place of living death."[157] In 1938 Vespa Amleto contended that in Harbin "one cannot find a street where there are no opium-smoking dens or narcotic shops."[158] He noted that Harbin had 56 "opium dens" and 194 "licensed narcotics shops."[159] Although 250 businesses is not an insignificant number, in a city of over a half-million people, it is doubtful that it allowed for every street to have had a den or shop. In order to support his argument that the Japanese sought "to poison the whole world," Amleto cited a Japanese Military Command booklet: "The use of narcotics is unworthy of a superior race like the Japanese. Only inferior races, races that are decadent like the Chinese, the Europeans, and the East Indians, are addicted to the use of narcotics. This is why they are destined to become our servants and eventually disappear."[160] This racist rhetoric parallels assertions in the Japanese-produced *Manchukuo Yearbook* that Manchus and Mongols shared a "historically hereditary" addiction to opium smoking. In 1943 Alexandre Pernikoff argued that the Japanese sought the "moral destruction" of Manchuria by disseminating free or artificially cheap narcotics among peasants (including "trial offers" for property owners and "junior doses" for children that were cheaper than bread), by promoting cheap prostitution, and by breaking up families.[161] Pernikoff maintained that such tactics were "more subtle and more effective" than jail, torture, or murder.[162] In 1949 F.C. Jones contended that profits from opium were the "principal consideration" for Monopoly officials, in contrast to their "glib professions of concern for the welfare and improvement of the peoples whom their armies subjugated."[163] Jones argued that "widespread evasions of the Monopoly by illicit growers and traders, the need for revenue and the opportunities for private profit on the part of the 'Manchukuo' officials resulted in opium being at least as widely sown and as easily obtainable as it had ever been."[164] These critics argued that "Manchuria was being slowly poisoned to death, while the Japanese army supervised and encouraged it, reaping huge financial benefits."[165] Amid claims that Japan was producing 90 percent of the world's illicit drugs, the majority of the League of Nations' Opium Advisory Committee were persuaded that the Manchukuo Monopoly was designed "to encourage, rather than control, drug abuse."[166]

Some officials, however, were lauded in the press for strict implementation of the Opium Law. In 1936 in Fengcheng city, for example, Sun Ying was praised for insisting that all opium retail outlets be treated equally, with no interference.[167] Sun ordered lawbreakers to be immediately investigated and sent to trial. Registered opium merchants expressed gratitude to Sun for ensuring that operators who worked under the table or used personal connections to circumvent the law were dealt with promptly. In September 1936, in Xifeng, director Liu Yu'an and his security chief, Ai Jingpu, met with retail operators and outlined strict rules for opium establishments, which were required to provide hygienic facilities for men and women to consume separately but were absolutely forbidden to engage in open sales of opium, side sales, overselling, and the provision of instruments.[168] Monthly reports of sales had to be submitted on time, and those who circumvented the law were to be prosecuted. In August 1938, in a dramatic enforcement of regulations, eighty officials from the Harbin Police Office were discharged for opium use.[169] The earnest actions of officials such as Sun, Liu, and Ai and the concerns expressed by health professionals (the focus of following chapters) have since been dismissed out of hand for their glibness by critics who have focused on the failings of the Monopoly, which they contend was no more than an appendage of the Japanese military and those Japanese who profited from the trade.

The negative atmosphere surrounding the Monopoly enabled reformists and officials who sought a reduction of the opium industry, and those who sought greater control over the industry, to secure revisions of the Opium Law. The revisions expanded state control, placing the industry even more firmly under Japanese dominion. In December 1937, Imperial Ordinance No. 487 established a State Retail Sale System to eradicate the "undue profiteering" of private trade; control over opium, cocaine, heroin, and morphine was to be transferred to municipalities, counties, and banners. Land designated for poppy growth was to be reduced in conjunction with declining numbers of addicts.[170] The anchor of the revised, state-run program was a ten-year prohibition act that would identify addicts in 1938 and 1939, immediately begin rehabilitation, and completely end recreational opium use by 1947. Fengtian was argued to be central to the entire operation: "Government policies of opium prohibition – their success or failure – all depend on Fengtian."[171] And it was in this most important city that the *Shengjing shibao* continued to publish critical reports on the opium industry. On 1 January 1938 the new State Retail Sale System was enforced, and 1,867 private establishments were co-opted or dissolved, leaving 1,363 licensed opium retail outlets in their stead.[172] Government-run opium retail outlets opened but often with insufficient stocks of questionable quality, which encouraged the underground market.[173] Low levels of compensation to farmers for their crops also resulted in bootleg sales; the opium produced and sold to the state appears to have dropped from 50 percent to 25 percent between 1938 and 1941.[174] Difficulties plagued the industry, yet in 1939 the Monopoly's director, Lo Cheng-Pang, still insisted that the Manchukuo government had established the Monopoly in good faith to achieve "the eventual eradication of the noxious habit permeating the whole of society."[175]

Demands for rigorous compliance with the Opium Law and the registration of addicts were not successful. An article in the *Shengjing shibao* on 11 June 1938 noted that only approximately 10 percent, or around 3,000, of the addicts in Harbin (the city alleged to have the most addicts) had registered; of these, more than 10 percent were Japanese, a rare acknowledgment of Japanese addicts in Manchukuo.[176] In 1941 colonial officials maintained that for the whole country the "number of addicts is roughly estimated at one million, although no thorough surveys have as yet been made."[177] Resources were insufficient, and even the most dedicated reformers faced resistance from those who profited from the trade and those who suffered it. In the press, "opium fiends" were condemned as immoral, physically weak, and in pursuit of a "dope habit" that was ruinous to the labour pool.[178] Addicts were maligned for consuming, rather than producing, resources: they were "fond of eating, but dislike work."[179] Crime rates were alleged to increase in direct proportion to their number; studies from Taiwan were used to argue that crime rates for users were more than two to three times those for abstainers. Crimes regularly associated with users ranged from theft to murder, and dealers were accused of tax evasion, gambling, and rape.[180] Intensified anti-addict, anti-dealer sentiment attests to the ongoing, at least rhetorical, battle against opiates and the imperialism on which their presence was blamed.

Efforts to rehabilitate Japanese involvement in the opium trade came in many forms, notably through essays, personal accounts, crime reporting, and songs. In this "Jie yan ge" (Quit Smoking Song) from 1941, the writer Jing Chun explicitly linked the region's opium problem with England:

> Opium smoke
> Has come from England
> It has weakened our various races and burned up our wealth
> The poison has been flowing for 100 years
> Its yellow smoke is destructive
> Thinking of it is indeed very sad.
> The opium smoke
> Came to Asia
> It has harmed the country and damaged the people for several hundred autumns
> Soldiers cannot be deployed
> Taxes cannot be collected
> Hateful England is the origin of this disaster.[181]

Not to be confused with Li Xianglan's famous song of the same name, this "Jie yan ge" blames the English for opium's devastating harm to people across Asia, linking the drug with more than 100 years of foreign-induced disaster while implicitly tying Manchukuo to the rest of "the country." Similarly, in the "Jie yan si ji ge" (Four Seasons of Quitting Smoking Song), published ten days later, Zhang Nianhui condemned the English for the opium trade:

> England transported opium smoke.
> Lin Zexu, the governor of the two Guangs,
> Burned the opium and used the army, swords, and guns
> ... England willingly was the first to bring disaster.[182]

Zhang, too, blamed England for the opium trade and praised the Qing patriot Lin Zexu for fighting the foreign oppressors. Both Zhang and Jing condemned the English while not explicitly defining roles that other foreigners and local Chinese played – Zhang simply noted that England was "the first." The authors also did not account for the fact that by the time of these songs' publication, the English had long left the trade, which then moved to Japanese, Korean, and Chinese dominance.

In the early 1940s, the necessity of a reasoned approach to the banning of opium was relentlessly recounted in the *Shengjing shibao*. In 1940 the director of the Opium Administration in the Opium Prohibition Department, Yong Shanqi, reasoned that if the state cracked down too hard on the selling of opium, private sellers would increase.[183] He called on those who continued to sell and consume opium to desist since increasing ties between the mainland and Japan could spread the problem throughout the empire.[184] Additionally, Yong asserted, if opium consumers were punished like criminals, they would go into hiding or would be vulnerable to blackmail from others, neither of which would improve society. Such difficulties problematized opium law enforcement and necessitated a project of over ten years to achieve completion. In October 1940 the Health Department in Qiqihaer called for increasing public campaigns against opium use, involving conferences, dramas, and student movements to raise awareness of the dangers of drugs and to improve compliance.[185] Wang Dashan, the local chief of police, argued that banning opiates was not easy but that it had to be done to ensure the health of individuals, the sustainability of the nation, and the peace of Asia.[186] The director of the Xinjing Healthy Life Institute, Dr. Kudō Fumio, argued that efforts to implement the law and successfully rehabilitate addicts had to be redoubled because every addict meant one less producer for the country, an intolerable burden on the national economy.[187]

Although most of the above literature was directed at men, women consumers were also addressed, often in starkly patriarchal terms. For example, on 5 September 1941 the article "Nü yinzhi: Xing xing ba!" (Female Addicts:

Wake Up!) argued that a significant number of addicted women weakened society.[188] The article described women addicts as staying in their homes with dirty faces and hair, ignoring household responsibilities, and using makeup to "pancake their faces" before going to dens to lie on the bed "enjoying the addiction" *(da guo qi yin)*. The women were described as "degenerate" *(duoluo)* and shameless for happily being "garbage at home." The article criticized women addicts for wasting their husbands' hard-earned money; women were cautioned that their behaviour pained their fathers, brothers, and husbands. An investigation of women addicts was cited for noting that most were young and either indiscriminately spent money or, if they were married and their husbands were strict, secretly visited pawn shops or sold rations. Further, women were criticized for mingling with men in dens. Whereas at home they might behave respectably, once in the dens, they were said to lose their self-respect. But the women were not to be completely blamed, for they were described as "inherently weak" *(tiansheng rouruo)* and unable to stop on their own; they needed men to wake them up from their smoke-induced debauchery. The writer argued that men had to be firm even when women started crying and making a nuisance in order to return to opium. Men were advised to use their rights as husbands and send their wives for rehabilitation. As shown in Chapter 5, this type of narrative was countered by women writers who depicted fictional female characters that recognized or overcame their addictions on their own initiative. Both fictional and nonfictional accounts stressed the difficulties of treating addiction because of societal, physical, and spiritual conditions.

In March 1941 Wang Shaoxian, the director of the Anti-Opium Bureau in Rehe province, argued that the most important problem facing anti-opium activists was the social environment that encouraged addiction.[189] Wang cited research showing that 48 percent of smokers were under the age of 39, 27 percent were between 39 and 49, 17 percent were between 40 and 59, and 8 percent were over 60. According to Wang, at least half were middle-aged, a factor that hindered Manchukuo's economic and cultural potential. Wang argued that the state had to allow opium cultivation so that foreign powers could not benefit from sales needed for medical and other uses, but he mourned the negative uses to which the product was being put. That same year, the article "Qudi de juewu" (Understanding the Ban) argued that if people could abandon practices such as foot binding and the queue, then opium should also be discarded lest foreigners continue to view Manchukuo subjects as savages and peasants; Chinese needed to stop treating "cruelty as pleasure and ugliness as beauty."[190] Also in 1941 Li Shixun, a department head in the Central Distribution Department, gave a speech criticizing the

Republic's New Life Movement and its focus on banning opium in only six years.[191] Li argued that applying torture or the death penalty to opium users was bound to end in failure – that the government and the citizens in Manchukuo, both Chinese and Japanese, had to work together to find a more reasonable solution. Li also warned that bureaucratic infighting and divisions between anti-smoking officials and police were counterproductive.

Calls for the eradication of recreational opium use got louder. The June 1941 New Citizens' Forum focused on the development of a morality movement and its role in reducing drug use.[192] Chairperson Murakami argued that the fight against opium was a type of war, with two factors influencing its progress.[193] First, the state was clearly incapable of controlling the hearts of Manchukuo citizens, and second, as Li Shixun argued, prohibition could not be accomplished quickly. Murakami blamed Japanese for not pursuing the issue with sufficient force because they did not believe that the issue directly affected them and their health; he also recognized that they had failed to inspire popular loyalty to the Manchukuo regime. Murakami noted that the Manchukuo context differed from that in Taiwan because, he argued, the Taiwanese initially did not believe that opium was hurting them and thus objected to bans. Manchukuo's subjects, in contrast, were under no such delusion but required serious, sustained assistance to reach the required goal. Zhuang Kaishui added that people needed to view those who illegally transported and sold opium as guilty of a crime even more serious than rape, which he argued was only one person's loss, whereas the opium trade impacted the whole society.[194] Zhuang also criticized anti-opium advertising in media such as the *Shengjing shibao* for what he saw as a misguided focus on individual use of opium and its impact on the family.[195] Zhuang called for an end to such advertising because it piqued youth's curiosity about trying drugs rather than depicting a business that was a danger to society, a stance that he believed would be more effective if the secret transport and sale of opium were described as a form of murder. Kudō Fumio argued that love for society should be fostered in the fight against intoxicants rather than what he believed was the main reason for reporting violations of the law – vengeance against secret dealers.[196]

In the final years of Manchukuo, both the opium and alcohol industries were subject to the pressures of Holy War demands. Statistics cited in the *Shengjing shibao* suggest that the number of addicts declined after the start of Holy War, despite rising population numbers.[197] More recently, Mark Driscoll has argued that the numbers of addicts (to opium, heroin, and morphine) increased to truly shocking levels – to 5 million people, or 20 percent of the Chinese population.[198] Whether the numbers of the "addicted" declined, stayed steady, or rose, condemnation of recreational intoxicant consumption increased in tone and volume. Alcohol production was structured by state policies that prioritized large-scale industry directed at the war effort, such that by 1943 "very little, if anything, produced in [the] modern enclave economy benefited ordinary consumers."[199] From 1939, inflation and rations eroded the general population's standard of living; by 1941, costs were double those of 1937, yet wages did not keep pace.[200] From 1940, commercial alcohol production declined while illegal sales reportedly rose. Rising alcohol taxes were accompanied by official warnings that "wicked merchants" were not to raise prices on existing stock.[201] Special forms from relevant tax departments were mandated for alcohol containers to prevent the underground selling of alcohol and to ensure quantities did not exceed mandated quotas.[202] In Harbin alone, commercial producers reduced in number from twenty to ten, fewer than at the start of the occupation.[203] But despite pressures on the industry, in 1941 taxes collected from alcohol were still expected to rank fourth in importance to the Treasury.[204] Taxes on alcohol production were extensive: they were levied on the manufacturing plant and on the product both when it was bottled and when it was shipped out of the factory.[205] In 1939 taxes had risen 50 percent, resulting in expected revenues of 25.5 million yuan, double the previous year's levels.[206] Tax hikes were implemented alongside rations. In Jilin in 1941, for example, beer rations were fixed by the police and government officials, who argued that equitable distribution of beer was essential, especially in the hot summer: 48 percent was put aside for domestic consumption, restaurants and hotels were allotted 32 percent, and 20 percent was allocated for "other" uses.[207] Jilin regulators, among others, also placed controls over alcohol that was not locally produced. Imports were decried for flooding the market, lowering prices, and causing unstable local conditions. Officials in several jurisdictions forced the return of imports – for example, to Fushan, where prices of distilled alcohol then fell from 0.96 yuan to 0.86 yuan.[208] In Zhizhong, too, producers had their alcohol returned because markets were flooded with cheaper products from Shanhaiguan.[209] Instability increasingly characterized the alcohol industry during the final years of Japanese rule.

Scholarly accounts of alcohol history in Japan stress that, for the most part, official efforts to control the industry were influenced by crop shortages and austerity measures, not by the political or health concerns that seemed uppermost to Chinese policy makers.[210] All of these concerns, as well as profit making, structured Manchukuo alcohol policy in the early 1940s. As the 1940s wore on, prices for alcohol skyrocketed as alcohol grew increasingly scarce. In 1942 the average price for *baijiu* was 1.59 yuan for 500 grams; by 1945, the price was 10.45 yuan. By 1943, reports regularly noted that supplies of alcohol were severely limited and of questionable quality.[211] From 1943 to 1944, in response to grain reallocations and other wartime policies, beer production fell by half.[212] Red Star and Kirin were argued to still be of reasonable value, but foreign wines, like champagne, all but disappeared.[213] Russian brandy and whiskey became difficult to acquire. Medicinal wines were available but held little appeal. Fake products reputedly dominated the market, and consumers were constantly warned to be vigilant when dealing with retailers.

The alcohol industry faced pressures not only from the state and from declining consumer incomes but also from prohibitionists, who argued that, like opium, alcohol should be prohibited. Japanese activists travelled to Manchukuo to advocate for a ban on alcohol production and consumption. In 1933, for example, members of the Prohibit Alcohol Alliance of Japan (Chinese: Riben guomin jinjiu tongmeng; Japanese: Nihon kokumin kinshu dōmei) travelled to Manchukuo.[214] The group was led by Koshio Kanji, with students and representatives of the alliance travelling to Xinjing in order to meet with the prime minister, the finance minister, and the local Xinjing representative, Nakajima Morinobu. Local activists also advocated for prohibition. Every year on 1 September, for instance, to commemorate the 1923 Great Kantō Earthquake in Japan, local activists used the example of the Prohibit Alcohol Alliance to hold a day-long ban on alcohol consumption.[215] On 1 September 1935 the Harbin branch of the Married Women's Rectify Customs Society (Furen jiao feng hui) launched a ban-alcohol movement with 5,000 flyers produced to hang in households.[216] Similarly, in 1938 in Binjiang province an architecture firm held a 100-day ban on employee alcohol consumption, from 15 February to 15 May, with the aim of increasing patriotism and promoting Japanese-style laws that forbade consumption by those under the age of twenty-five.[217] In 1940 Fengtian's Concordia Association criticized New Year celebrations, when most people would drink alcohol and gamble, hobbies claimed to be their favourite.[218] The association urged citizens to become conscious of the negative effects of such activities and called on people to treat the 13th and 14th of the month as two days of "self-respect" *(zi su)* during which there would be no drinking, smoking, or gambling. Ultimately, these prohibition movements appear to have had little effect on the industry, which endured the final days of Manchukuo, impacted more by declining incomes, market instability, and wartime dislocation than by any morality movement.

Manchukuo collapsed in 1945, and in its wake came Russian occupation, civil war, and revolution. Amid the turmoil, commercial alcohol production carried on; by some accounts, it thrived.[219] As the Chinese Communist Party

(CCP) scored victory after victory, it established control over alcohol production, initially disallowing the importation of alcohol and private production. Opium was banned outright. Although sales of opium may have helped to fund the People's Liberation Army during the war, with the founding of the People's Republic of China in 1949, the state moved quickly on intoxicant industries, disbanding the opium industry and regulating alcohol production. Recreational opium use was condemned as a symbol of the old order, a root cause of China's national weakness that had to be eradicated. And it was. The movement of the early 1950s to ban opium succeeded where the Qing Dynasty, warlord regimes, the Republic, and the Japanese had failed. Alcohol production, too, was transformed under the dictatorship of the proletariat, decreasing the aggressive advertising and product promotion of the 1920s and 1930s, which are the subject of Chapter 4. But although the CCP discouraged "excessive" consumption of alcohol, echoing narratives of the latter Manchukuo era and more longstanding beliefs, no outright ban was implemented. Alcohol continued to serve a wide variety of purposes, whereas opium connoted a negativity that has linked it to this day with foreign aggression.

The Manchukuo regime and the Japanese have long been denounced for their roles in the region's intoxicant industries, especially for using opium as a "secret weapon" *(mimi wuqi)* to destroy the Chinese people.[220] Without doubt, Japanese were involved in the alcohol and opium industries, in both official and illegal capacities. So, too, were Chinese, Koreans, and other peoples. By any count, these intoxicant industries were immense – and immensely lucrative – and at the time they attracted a great deal of critical attention. The brutal nature of Japanese rule, expansion of the intoxicant industries, creation of institutions that were flawed and unable to fully implement the law or to procure truly effective rehabilitation, and a popular media and cultural producers committed to exposing the system's failings all conspired to eviscerate any accomplishments of those in Manchukuo who sought to reduce or eradicate intoxicants. Those who were at the forefront of questioning recreational intoxicant consumption in Manchukuo are the focus of the following chapters.

3 Evaluating Alcohol

One cup: the person drinks the alcohol.
Two cups: the alcohol drinks the alcohol.
Three cups: the alcohol drinks the person.

CHINESE FOLK ADAGE

Today, alcohol consumption in China's Northeast is often discussed in terms of its constant presence and influences on health and culture. Feng Qi argues that Northeasterners "drink alcohol to resist the cold" *(he jiu yu han)* and have created a "unique alcohol culture" *(dute de jiu wenhua)* that has driven regional industrial development.[1] In "Dongbeiren yu Dongbei jiu wenhua" (Northeasterners and Northeast Alcohol Culture), Yang Jun argues that Northeasterners' drinking capacity is a frightening reflection of their will-power.[2] Yang cautions that to view their alcohol use as either an "addiction" or "hobby" *(shihao)* or a "pastime" *(xiaoqian)* is mistaken: "Drinking alcohol is Northeasterners' most important means of connecting" *(he jiu shi Dongbei ren zui zhongyao de goutong fangshi)*. These assertions reflect mid-twentieth-century beliefs regarding alcohol consumption; in 1941 Dr. Shao Guanzhi, for example, wrote that alcohol had become an "essential article" *(bixu de wupin)* of life in Manchukuo.[3] This chapter interrogates dominant alcohol narratives in the region's most popular 1930s and 1940s media. At first, alcohol consumption was generally depicted as a positive support for the regime's modernity claims, which reflected lengthy traditions of alcohol use in the Manchu, Mongol, and growing Han Chinese, Japanese, and Russian communities. But by the late 1930s, health concerns and socio-economic instability resulting from occupation, war, and poverty had inspired increasing condemnation of alcohol.

Alcohol consumption in the 1930s and 1940s was extensive, and views toward it are reflected in the variety of terms that described it in local media. The most common term was to "drink alcohol" *(he jiu* or *yin jiu)*. To "drink alcohol" was less value-laden than to be a "big drinker" *(da jiujiazhe).*[4]

Similarly, to have a drinking "habit" *(xiguan)*,[5] to be "fond of drinking alcohol" *(hao yin jiu)*,[6] and to be a "person who is fond of alcohol" *(hao jiu de ren)*[7] were less freighted than to have a "loathsome habit" *(wu xi)*[8] or to have the "tendency to get drunk when coming upon alcohol" *(feng jiu ze zui de qing-xiang)*.[9] All of the above pale in comparison to references to addictions, such as "alcohol addiction" *(jiu yin)*[10] or a "loathsome addiction" *(e pi)*.[11] References to addiction had become commonplace by the late 1930s, although there was, and remains, no singular definition of, or even word for, the term; addiction was variously referred to as *yin* (addiction, habitual craving, or strong inter-est), *pi* (addiction, weakness for) or *shi* (have a liking for, be addicted to).[12] A person's "capacity for alcohol" *(jiu liang)*[13] could also be measured by one's "alcohol intestines" *(jiu chang)*, which Zhang Feng argued varied in width between individuals and could be influenced by the environment.[14]

As the above terms suggest, the extent of local alcohol consumption evoked earnest reflection on alcohol's roles in society. As early as 1923, Pei Ru had argued that "humans are not born to drink alcohol" *(ren fei sheng er hao jiu)* but that it had become "a special habit" *(te xi)* that had spread throughout society.[15] In 1933 Yi Mei noted favourably that 50-60 percent of the general population regularly enjoyed drinking alcohol.[16] In the 1935 article "Tan yin jiu" (Discussion of Drinking Alcohol), Zhong Xin named alcohol the best of the three most popular "stimulants" *(xingfen)*, which also included tea and tobacco.[17] Zhong praised alcohol for its roles in celebrations and cultural production but criticized an overly close relationship people traditionally had with alcohol, urging consumers to respect the limitations advised by modern medical science. In 1938 Yin described alcohol as a stimulant popu-larly used for medicinal purposes, namely to improve circulation and mental well-being.[18] That same year, Hong Nian estimated that at least one-third of the population regularly consumed alcohol and noted that at banquets it was unavoidable.[19] In 1941 Shao Guanzhi argued that in urban centres virtually everyone smoked tobacco and that drinking was even more popular.[20]

Descriptions of drinking practices delineate a wide variety of alcohol prac-tices. In 1935 Zhang Feng noted two major types of drinking: "scholarly drinking" *(ru yin)* and "ferocious drinking" *(xiong yin)*.[21] "Scholarly drinking" involved two or three friends composing poetry and singing; an ideal way, according to Zhang, to pass the night. Far less enjoyable or cultured, to him, was "ferocious drinking," which occurred at weddings and banquets, when people were subject to unanticipated, often conflicting emotions. Zhang compared the endless rounds of required drinks to being in prison and blamed "ferocious drinking" for negative perceptions of alcohol. In 1938 Yin further differentiated between urban and rural drinking.[22] Yin noted that city dwellers regularly socialized while eating and drinking, that a host was responsible for pouring alcohol for guests, and that everyone drank from glasses. Yin contrasted this behaviour with that of rural people, who, he argued, tended to drink in larger quantities from bowls, to frequent alcohol shops or taverns, and not necessarily to combine drinking with the consumption of food or with the leisured socializing of urbanites. Yin also cited several specific categories of people who frequently drank – among them scholars and merchants with big bellies – noting that they, too, drank with bowls and talked for a long time. Yin wrote that it was also commonplace for average people to drink as they discussed important matters or signed agreements. To Yin, farmers were another case altogether: they would drink whatever they could and whenever they could, until all their money was gone.

Discussion of such drinking practices was often framed with reference to Chinese customs and personalities. The famed writer Zhou Zuoren, for example, was quoted by Lian, in "Tan jiu" (Discussion of Alcohol), for his assertion that it did not matter whether one drank from bowls or glasses because a vast array of drinking vessels had been used throughout Chinese history and stood as proof of China's long-lived and inspiring culture, notwithstanding Japan's contemporary occupation of much of the nation. Zhou argued that "it could be said that in ancient China the anaesthesia method that was the quintessence of Chinese culture was drinking alcohol" *(Zhongguo gu yi you zhi guocui de mazuifa, dayue keyi shuo shi yin jiu).*[23] Zhou approved of drinking but warned that it was not to be done in an addictive manner, which to him was to "pour it gurgling in, in one breath" *(gulu gulu de guan yi qi);* his personal preference was to use a small cup while leisurely talking with friends.[24] Zhou suggested that if one were anxious to get intoxicated, injecting a drug would be faster than drinking alcohol. Expanding on Zhou's generally positive views of alcohol, Lian wrote that to forget anxieties by drinking all day was a "pleasure" *(leshi)* yet warned that some people embarrassed themselves by getting loud or overly emotional when drunk, so he advised that it was best to drink only until happy.[25] Lian cited a Chinese folk adage: "When people have alcohol they 'must get intoxicated' *(xu dang zui),* a drop will not take you down to hell."[26] Both Lian and Zhou praised moderate alcohol consumption and the form of intoxication it provided.

Some writers were even more effusive in their celebration of alcohol. Yi Mei called alcohol a "wonderful pharmaceutical" *(miao ji)* that, no matter how depressed one was, made being intoxicated "a pleasure in life" *(rensheng yi chun leshi).*[27] In 1937 Zhi Xing argued that drinking was most rewarding when one was really intoxicated, not slowly sipping and relaxing. Zhi explicitly stated that his fondness for being intoxicated was not an addiction, beginning his essay "Jiu yu tianzhen" (Alcohol and Innocence) with, "I really like drinking alcohol. But I do not have an alcohol addiction *(jiu yin)*."[28] Zhi wrote that he drank to regain the lost innocence of youth, which he believed was possible when one was drunk with friends. He quoted an observation by the Japanese writer Kuriyagawa Hakuson (1880-1923): "In Roman times there was a famous saying, the so-called 'in wine there is truth' *(jiu zhong you zhen)*."[29] Yin argued that those who criticized drinking did so only because they feared showing their own true character when intoxicated.[30] Yin accorded alcohol the power to restore his youth and unmask the truth, which provided an escape from the reality of daily life.

In the early 1930s, alcohol was promoted as an element of healthful living, as demonstrated in traditional and foreign medical knowledge; optimum health and intelligence were often argued to rely on limited consumption of alcohol.[31] Medical studies from France, Germany, Japan, and the United States were referenced to argue the benefits of drinking five ounces of alcohol per day, with a few ounces at every meal. Regular, limited consumption was deemed especially beneficial to people with poor nutrition, pale complexions, and a lack of appetite. But consumers were consistently warned to keep consumption within prescribed bounds to optimize mental and physical health.[32] Many rejected arguments that alcohol was dangerous: "Chinese people do not use alcohol to cast off their soul, they conquer alcohol" *(Zhongguo ren bu shi jiu tuo hun, er zhengfu jiu)*.[33] This nationality-based conquering of alcohol was to be achieved through limited intake, an achievement that the author noted eluded the Japanese.[34] Drinkers were urged to restrict daily drinking to "one pint" *(yi paiyintuo)* for professionals and office workers and to three pints for labourers and outside workers.[35] Abstainers over the age of forty-five were encouraged to begin drinking or risk not achieving their full potential. Citing a French saying, "alcohol is milk for the elderly" *(jiu wei laonianren zhi niuru)*, an article in the *Shengjing shibao (Shengjing Times)* argued that as one aged, alcohol became increasingly beneficial.[36] Throughout the early 1930s, at least, limited alcohol consumption was frequently prescribed for health reasons.[37]

The end of American Prohibition (1920-33) encouraged local writers to reflect on alcohol's place in society. "Jiu lun" (Discussion of Alcohol), belittled the Chinese translation of the American slogan "Drinking water makes people healthy," arguing that it should be altered to, "If you want to be healthy and intelligent, you must drink alcohol."[38] French doctors were cited for their opposition to Prohibition, arguing that it increased the death rate. Ao Shuang'an wrote that Prohibition was worth no more than the paper it was written on because sales still continued, to the profit of criminals and without benefit to society or the state.[39] Other reporters noted that the end of Prohibition caused celebrations in New York, as it spelled the decline of criminal elements.[40] The Democratic Party was argued to have pushed for an end to Prohibition in order to increase employment and restore tax revenues to the state.[41] Before Prohibition, in 1918, taxes collected from beer sales alone were estimated at $300 million, reputedly one-fifth of annual taxes.[42] In terms of health, social stability, and state finances, American Prohibition was pronounced a failure from which Chinese should learn. Prohibition was criticized as having no suitable application in the West or in Asia. Ao granted that Prohibition may be progressive in theory but argued that in practice it was an utter failure.[43] The major beneficiaries of Prohibition were criminals and bordering states that profited from alcohol production; the Canadian city of Montreal was noted to be a major producer of alcohol, and the Mexican city of Tijuana was described as a magnet for those drawn to alcohol and prostitution.[44] American Prohibition was compared to Chinese bans on prostitution: both created a swathe of problems for law enforcement through their questionable application of legal restrictions to millennia-old customs. In the 1920s these writers did not view Prohibition as a model for China.

One long-held belief in the Northeast is that alcohol can be used to "resist the cold" *(yu han)* because alcohol increases one's body temperature.[45] In the 1930s commentators argued that seasonal aspects of alcohol consumption were important to observe, but most wrote that alcohol was not as effective in combating the cold as was widely believed; in fact, many deemed it detrimental, especially for people who were suffering from an illness. In "Jiu lun" (Discussion of Alcohol), readers were advised that ideal consumption practices should vary with the seasons and with respect to one's age and blood pressure.[46] In winter, one should relax while drinking, sitting by a warm fireplace or on a rocking chair; sparing amounts of alcohol could improve circulation, enabling one to more comfortably pass the cold weather. In the summer, drinking in swimwear was suggested, although one was advised to avoid drinking distilled liquors, such as *baigan jiu* (white dry liquor), in the heat.[47] Proponents of moderate alcohol consumption argued that limited amounts of alcohol could reduce the physical impact of seasonal extremes, perhaps even more effectively than medicine. Almost as significant as the social and health dimensions of alcohol consumption were its supposed roles in cultural production.

Alcohol's long association with Chinese culture and history was featured in alcohol narratives throughout the Manchukuo era. In 1933 Yi Xi wrote that there were "three special factors for [the production of] literature – drinking, smoking, and women."[48] Yi cited the examples of Li Bai, Du Fu, and other Chinese classical literati, as discussed in Chapter 1, in support of his argument that artistic inspiration was enhanced by alcohol, tobacco, and sex.[49] In 1935, in "Tan yin jiu" (Discussion of Drinking Alcohol), Zhong Xin argued that drinking increased scholars' courage and assertiveness, especially if they nursed a grievance.[50] In 1938 Hong Nian mused that "since ancient times, literati have greatly loved alcohol" *(zi gu wenren duo'ai jiu).*[51] Hong reasoned that scholars drank more than average people because

> they are full of a sensitive talent. They have anger inside, a firm sad melancholy. Usually when they are sober, if they don't talk, things are peaceful. But as days and nights go by, their anger will on occasion explode. Sometimes it is sadness that will boil up. The spark for this is so-called alcohol. This is the original reason for drinking so much. When they cannot bear to see things, and cannot take it anymore, they use alcohol to intoxicate themselves. They forget everything, but then after they get drunk, whatever their intentions were, the opposite comes.[52]

Hong described the use of alcohol among literati as a mechanism to cope with the negativity, anger, and sadness that haunted them. Intoxication enabled them to overcome their sensitive natures and express grievances, even if their intoxication produced "the opposite." Hong recalled Kong Rong's (153-208) criticism of his political opponent Cao Cao for not drinking, noting that Cao himself had once written that "to relieve worries, only Du Kang will do."[53] Alcohol's potential to relieve worries was described positively by Hong as he recounted Li Bai's boast that he was "drunk as mud" *(zui ru ni)* every day of the year, Du Fu's assertion that "alcohol should bring relief" *(kuanxin ying shi jiu),* and Liu Ling's love of intoxication. Hong also cited Song Jiang's drinking in the *Shui hu zhuan (Water Margin)* as an aid to help Song overcome his grief and inspire a poem instigating rebellion.[54] Hong suggested that although optimal drinking conditions included two or three good friends, drinking alone could also reduce stress. Readers in Manchukuo could not have failed to grasp the parallels being exemplified by Hong through his reference to Chinese icons who had survived personal challenges and political instability by turning to alcohol for inspiration or support.

In the early 1940s, discussion of alcohol consumption became more circumspect as officials sought to stress what they believed were more positive aspects of Manchukuo's independent (i.e., not Chinese) culture. Like Hong Nian and Yi Xi above, some writers continued to defend and celebrate alcohol use, often with explicit Chinese cultural references. In 1942 Jia Xiao mused,

"If in this life I had no smoke or alcohol, I do not know how lonely I would be!"[55] Jia recalled that in primary school he had written an essay that echoed the opinions of teachers and newspaper articles he had read that condemned smoking and drinking. Jia wrote that life experiences and Manchukuo's socio-economic environment had made him come to view alcohol as "my spiritual beauty, my thoughts' good partner, the comfort for my boredom, the stimulant to my happiness."[56] Writing defensively against those whom he believed would judge him to be "weak," he recounted his enjoyment of drinking with friends and smoking alone in bed when intoxicated. He claimed a "Li Bai style," boasting that he once even pawned his spring clothes to buy alcohol, replicating the poet's famed experience. In a similar vein, in 1943 Han Hu argued that alcohol had a history of hundreds of years and that it was therefore entitled to a cultural status that other popular consumables, like tobacco, did not deserve. Evoking Zhou Zuoren's celebration of China's historic alcohol culture, Han attributed the main attraction of alcohol to the customs surrounding it.[57] Han noted that "people of exceptional ability are fond of alcohol" *(haojie zhi hao jiu)* for the same reason that heroes womanize: to enhance their abilities. Further, Han argued that drinkers were generally more talented than teetotallers, describing the drinking of literati as a "refined matter" *(wenya de goudang)*.[58] In 1943 the prominent Japanese writer and translator Ōuchi Takao noted in the journal *Xin Manzhou (New Manchuria)* that Du Fu, Li Bai, and Tao Yuanming were literary icons whose drinking was an inherent element of their successful literary careers, and he commiserated with his Chinese friend, fellow writer Xin Jiajun, who wrote that life without alcohol was lonely.[59] In the early 1940s Jia Xiao, Han Hu, and Ōuchi Takao defended drinking alcohol as a valued cultural practice made defensible by the Chinese past and Manchukuo present.

Not surprisingly, views regarding the health and social benefits of alcohol consumption for women were often expressed in distinctly gendered ways. In 1937 Zhi Jing observed, approvingly, that women were gradually drinking more and, as a result, were becoming increasingly sociable, with the additional benefit of boosting alcohol sales.[60] Zhi argued that when women drank, at banquets especially, the alcohol made them more talkative and beautiful:

> They raise a glass to their red lips and swallow the contents down to their stomach. The alcohol goes right to their cheeks, both turn purple like clouds, increasing their prettiness. Being drunk could be advocated as a method of beautifying themselves. Indeed, alcohol can connect people's feelings.[61]

Zhi praised alcohol for enhancing women's beauty and for lubricating personal relations. Whereas the latter was noted to be positive for men and women, discussion of alcohol's enhancement of physical attractions was limited to women, or more precisely, men's appreciation of them. Occasionally, women wrote of their experiences with alcohol. The writer and singer Yang Xu, one of the most famous celebrities in Manchukuo, praised getting drunk: "What luck, who would have thought I would get intoxicated again! ... When can I get intoxicated again? These days, my mood is making me think again of drinking alcohol."[62] Yang overtly challenged conservative ideals of womanhood, and her Islamic upbringing, to assert her delight in intoxication. Yang's public defence of drunkenness in 1943, in the midst of Holy War and official campaigns to limit alcohol consumption, demonstrated the bravado for which she was known.

The above, generally positive narratives of alcohol's health and social benefits share similarities with their Japanese counterparts, especially in terms of sake, the esteem for which is expressed in the traditional saying, sake is "the best of all medicines" *(hyakuyaku ni masaru).*[63] In Japan the potential health benefits of alcohol consumption were clearly spelled out in the Edo-era (1603-1868) book *Hyakka Seturin (One Hundred Teachers Preach)*: sake could help to dispel depression, prevent ill health, clean poisons from the body, and extend lifespan.[64] Japanese migrants, like others, arrived in Manchuria with their own attitudes toward alcohol, which influenced consumption and the creation of state policies.[65] The popularity of alcohol consumption to mark celebratory occasions is exemplified by a photograph of General Nogi Maresuke (1849-1912) and colleagues (see Figure 8). Celebrating a victory in the Russo-Japanese War, they stand around a table loaded with food, bottles of alcohol, and a large, menacing missile.

Penelope Francks has noted that before Japanese migration to Manchuria began, in the late 1800s, Japan's urban middle classes had begun gathering more often in small or private groups to consume stronger, more refined products than previously; they also had begun to frown on rural customs such as drinking in the morning.[66] New peak levels of per capita consumption were reached in Japan in the late nineteenth and early twentieth centuries.[67] Whereas in the 1890s beer was seen as foreign and expensive, within two decades it was considered the drink for "modern" public occasions, boosting beer's profile in Manchuria as well. Even as late as March 1945, in "Kessenka no sake to tabako" (Sake and Tobacco under the Condition of Total War), Nakamura Kōjirō argued that sake inspired soldiers and that other forms of alcohol had great value, especially for men: factory workers, for example, could be better served by their wives with a beer in their home than with

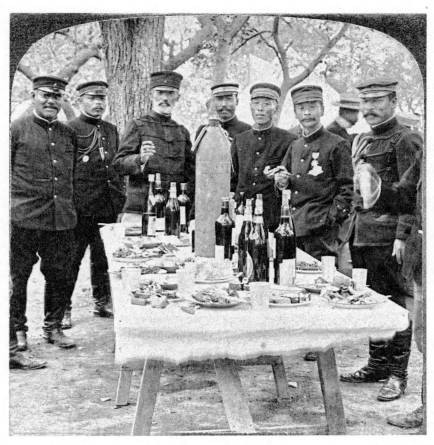

8 General Nogi Maresuke, Russo-Japanese War celebration. *Source:* Underwood and Underwood, ceased business in the 1940s, in author's collection.

"hundreds of medicines."[68] Nakamura, who came from a line of wholesale dealers of sake, asserted that long-cherished, positive views of sake were supported by the modern science of nutrition since it was "commonly recognized scientific knowledge" that sake consumed in moderation was nutritious.[69] Nakamura cited several former presidents of the Institute of Science in China (Tairiku kagakuin), among them Naoki Rintarō and Suzuki Umetarō (who held doctorates in engineering and agriculture, respectively), for their enthusiastic support of sake.[70] Through reference to China-centred scientific knowledge in support of popular Japanese beliefs, Nakamura argued the beneficial nature of men's alcohol consumption with an assertiveness that reflected his support for an industry under increasing pressure.

Such positive evaluation began to wane in the mid-1930s as war spread across Asia and the dangers of intoxicants increasingly dominated discussion of alcohol. In 1933 Mei Shan cautioned that newly established, and seemingly already authoritative, life insurance companies were reporting that drinking alcohol shortened lifespans.[71] In 1934 Ren Ji warranted that in the past people had believed alcohol to be an "all-purpose medicine" *(wanneng zhi yao)*, but he advised that modern science had demonstrated that "alcohol is the mother of all disease" *(jiu wei wan bing zhi mu).*[72] Alcohol may not have been considered a poison per se, but it was linked with damage to vital organs, especially the liver, heart, and kidneys, which consumption made susceptible to various "diseases of an alcohol nature" *(jiu xing zhi bing).*[73] The stimulants claimed to be in alcohol (as well as tea and tobacco) were deemed especially dangerous for those with high blood pressure and at risk of stroke. In July 1937 Feng Sen decried the popularity of alcohol intoxication, arguing that "fashionable people suffer a fashionable disease" *(shimaoren hai shimaobing),* and he warned especially people with high blood pressure against consuming alcohol.[74] Alcohol was denounced for causing consumers to live "opposite to physiological conditions" *(shengli tiaojian xiangbei).*[75] In 1942 Xiao Ling went so far as to condemn alcohol as an "archenemy" *(dadi)* of humanity.[76]

By the late 1930s, the two primary reasons for the previous promotion of alcohol – health and sociability – were regularly inverted, as alcohol was increasingly linked with disease and disorder. Many were argued to be physically incapable of consuming alcohol because their stomachs were unable to adequately absorb it, leading to excessive acidity in the digestive system.[77] This acid destroyed beneficial proteins and reduced the body's ability to kill germs; Nobel Prize winner Ilya Mechnikov's (1845-1916) research on intestinal bacteria was cited for demonstrating that alcohol diminished the body's ability to defend itself.[78] Whereas limited amounts of alcohol had once been believed to aid digestion, drinking before dinner was now decried for creating exceptional hungers that led drinkers to eat too much, a problem both despite and because of war rations.[79] Warnings that were relatively rare in the early 1930s, including Ren Ji's argument that any supposed medicinal qualities of drinking alcohol in the evening were false, increased in number and tone as alcohol was blamed for stemming the appropriate development of physical and mental abilities. The 1941 article "Jiu yu shensi" (Alcohol and Development of the State of Mind) argued that alcohol reduced physical and mental strength.[80] Actors, scholars, and others who drank alcohol to enhance their work were warned that they were inflicting serious harm on themselves. Those who consumed alcohol for its stimulant qualities were informed that research from Columbia University revealed that alcohol was actually a depressant.[81] Thus, in addition to being warned of the dangerous physical ramifications of alcohol use, those who were depressed, worried, or felt "defeated" *(zhanbai)* by life were advised not to drink, as the depressant would compound their problems.[82] Yin even quoted a Li Bai poem to suggest that if one "raises the glass to decrease sorrows, more sorrows will come."[83]

In 1941 the physician Shao Guanzhi raised concerns also expressed in ads for the health supplement Ruosu (Basic Element) by urging consumers to avoid excessive consumption of alcohol, which could lead to excessive "stimulation" *(xingfen)* or, even worse, a "habit" *(xiguan)*.[84] Shao argued that whereas smoking cigarettes cost consumers over 100 yuan a year in wasted money, the costs of drinking alcohol were far heavier. More regrettable even than the financial burden was the toll on one's health: he argued that alcohol impaired critical thinking abilities; caused damage to the intestines, liver, heart, kidneys, veins, and skin; and problematized recovery from surgery.[85] Shao cautioned that although moderate consumption of alcohol could enhance health, it was far too dangerous a source of nutrition since, unlike other liquids, it did not satiate thirst but rather created an even greater "urge to drink" *(he yu)*, leading to excessive damage to the human body.[86] Shao especially noted the dangers of consuming furfural, a toxic organic compound in alcohol.[87] Finally, Shao cautioned that alcohol consumption led to illegal activities, social disorder, and calamity for one's descendants, such that true happiness could be attained only by total abstinence.[88] Shao warned that although drinkers were generally conscious of the damage alcohol caused, they were unable to stop drinking because of reluctance to fully incorporate into their personal lives the most modern medical knowledge of the body.

Shao Guanzhi's warning represents dominant criticisms of alcohol in the latter half of the Manchukuo era. Consumers were consistently warned that alcohol led to diminished mental and physical capabilities. Breathing was impacted by reduced energy and increased susceptibility to tuberculosis and other lung diseases. Circulation was disrupted by changes in blood pressure and reduced oxygen levels and body temperatures; the latter threatened especially those suffering from other ailments.[89] The excretory system was harmed by weakened abdominal muscles and kidneys, leading to proteinuria. Heart muscles became fatty. Belly size increased. Whereas the bones of adults who drank alcohol generally did not suffer harm, the bones of children who drank alcohol would not develop adequately. Alcohol's potential to damage the body was compared to sugar, the danger of which was argued to be equivalent, despite the refusal of average people to believe it; the effect of consuming sugar was compared to alcohol intoxication. Dr. Lin of the Physiology School at Japan's Keio University was cited for reporting that excessive sugar levels in the bloodstream resulted in side effects similar to intoxication, including dizziness, vomiting, and nerve damage.[90]

Alcohol was blamed for harming not only consumers' bodies but also those of their descendants. In 1923 Pei Ru had argued that "for my own body's sake, for my family's sake, for my descendants' sake, and for society's sake, I must forbid drinking alcohol. Humans are not born to drink alcohol, but it has become a special habit. Once you get poisoned, if you want to quit, it will be very difficult."[91] Pei warned that alcohol could inflict long-lasting damage across generations, inflicting long-term damage on society in general.[92] The article "Funü yin jiu yingxiang ertong jiankang" (Women Drinking Alcohol Influence Children's Health) referenced medical research on children of drinkers, finding that they suffered mental and physical "shortcomings" (quedian), including headaches, ear problems, numbness in the limbs, and pain in the shoulders, waist, and legs.[93] Strong criticism and expressions of concern were directed at women and at their impact on the health of children before and after they were born. Children were argued to have inherent "rights" (quanli), including a healthy birth and a proper upbringing.[94] If the parents (especially the mother) drank, these rights were violated because "alcohol harms the body" (jiujing hai shen).[95] A study of 180 families in which both parents drank alcohol found that a majority of the 200 babies produced were physically and/or mentally challenged.[96] In 1935 Yao Jibin warned of genetic problems caused by drinkers: children of drinkers were argued to be more violent and prone to drinking problems of their own.[97] Third-generation drinkers suffered increased cases of epilepsy, mental challenges, and criminal behaviour. Procreation was greatly reduced for the fourth generation; if they could have children, they would face severe challenges. Yao also reported on a French study of eighty-three patients with mental challenges, revealing that six of their fathers had died of alcohol poisoning and that the others had been negatively impacted in some way by long-term alcohol use. The 1943 article "Jiu yu yousheng zhi guanxi" (The Relationship between Alcohol and Eugenics) recounted the example of a family of drinkers in which all the men had died prematurely, before the age of sixty.[98] Their "degenerate" (bianzhi) drinking practices were blamed for an irreversible decline in family health, which impacted generation after generation. Alcohol was criticized for damaging reproductive cells and leaving children "mentally deficient" (dineng).[99]

The denunciation of the physical costs of alcohol consumption was paralleled by complaints of social costs. In the 1941 essay "Jiu yu nüren" (Wine and Women), Ye Xing characterized writings that lauded alcohol and women as a superb yet "decadent" *(tuifei)* literature, symbolic of the "depressed" *(kumen)* nature of writers, a condition he dated in China to the May Fourth era.[100] Ye praised Kuriyagawa Hakuson's observation that "wine, women, and song" were three types of pleasures enjoyed in Europe to relieve life pressures and to provide feelings of liberation and joy. But Ye decried writers of decadent literature, comparing them to China's classical "romantic poets," like Li Bai, whom he criticized for being alienated from politics and for getting "dead drunk, as mud" *(lan zui ru ni)* in the belief that "one intoxication solves 1,000 worries" *(yi zui jie qian chou)*.[101] Ye criticized depressed literati for drinking and cavorting with dancing girls instead of raising consciousness about "national enemies" or "family difficulties."[102] Ye argued that their obsession with individual pleasure had led to the creation of a moving yet, considering the subjugated state of the nation, inappropriate literature. Ye criticized writers in Manchukuo like Yi Chi (1913-?), who openly self-identified as a depressed writer and produced literature lauding alcohol and women.[103] Ye Xing advocated more socially responsible, explicitly negative representations of alcohol consumption for the sake of the nation.

The social costs of alcohol consumption were not restricted to individual physical harm or cultural production. Mei Shan and Shao Guanzhi, among others, cautioned that alcohol intoxication led to addiction, which resulted in social disorder, illegal activities, and calamity for one's descendants, such that true happiness could be attained only through abstinence.[104] In "Jie yan jiu lun" (Discussion of Quitting Smoking and Drinking), Qi Jinchang argued that alcohol and opium were both poisonous but that whereas opium damaged the brain, alcohol led to more dangerous disorderly conduct.[105] Alcohol addiction was linked with reckless behaviour, including wasting money to buy alcohol in the effort to make friends. These arguments were not new. In 1923 Pei Ru had written of his fondness, and enormous capacity, for alcohol consumption; he described getting as drunk as Tao Yuanming in his youth.[106] He placed himself in the troubled category of users who after one drink would have to get drunk, which caused many problems in his life. Pei argued that he engaged in such destructive behaviour because alcohol stimulated his brain cells while reducing his ability to reason.[107] From the late 1930s, reports of immoral behaviour blamed on alcohol consumption were regularly featured in newspapers. For example, on 31 May 1937 the case of the "dissolute" *(fangdang)* carpenter Cai Weijian appeared in the *Shengjing shibao*. Cai was a thirty-nine-year-old migrant from Shandong who lived in Dalian and was married to Ms. Li, a reportedly good wife and mother.[108] Cai was employed by Japanese and earned a good income, but because of his "opium addiction" *(yapian zhi pi)* and "addiction to the thing in the cup" *(shi bei zhong wu)*, he planned to sell his wife.[109] One night in February 1937, he returned home drunk, beat Li, and drove her and their five-year-old daughter out of their house. The reader was led to infer that the mother and daughter had died as a result of their treatment. This type of short story began to be published on an almost daily basis in the late 1930s, constantly reinforcing negative perceptions of alcohol and perceptions of general social decline.

Alcohol was depicted as a major instigator not only of disorderly conduct but also of criminal behaviour.[110] Commentators argued that most, if not all, criminal activities were directly related to alcohol consumption.[111] Intoxicated people "lost virtue" *(shi de)* and then committed a wide range of crimes, including robbery and murder.[112] In a warning of the risks related to leaking state secrets to spies, consumers were reminded of a popular saying: "alcohol can disorder one's nature" *(jiu neng luan xing)*.[113] Newspaper accounts of crimes committed by drunken and disorderly people abounded. On 12 November 1937 the *Shengjing shibao* published the court transcript of proceedings against Bai Linfu, a twenty-two-year-old man of modest means who got into a drunken altercation with Liu Zizhi, who was said to have owed him money.[114] Bai was convicted of beating and killing Liu and was sentenced to ten years in prison. After losing his appeal, Bai was imprisoned. The case illuminated the costs of drinking and crime: it destroyed lives, in this case leaving one young man dead and another incarcerated.

Immoral and criminal behaviour arising from alcohol consumption, including the case of Cai Weijian and Ms. Li above, was often blamed for ruining women's lives. But women were also criticized for drinking, and cautionary tales regarding intoxicated women were common. So many of the students at Jilin Provincial Female Teacher Training Institute reportedly drank and smoked that the virtue of its graduates was publicly questioned in the pages of the *Shengjing shibao*.[115] Women were criticized not only for drinking but also for supposedly not even understanding the intricacies of cultured alcohol consumption; citing an unnamed French source, an article in *Qilin (Unicorn)* mocked women for being unable to choose a good wine or to use a corkscrew.[116] Alcohol was also blamed for being a dangerous depressant that drove unhappy women to suicide. The final days of a thirty-eight-year-old woman surnamed Ma who lived in Harbin were recounted in the article "'Ci Liu Ling': Zui jiu shou fu chi yi nu jiu huazuo diaosigui" ('Female Liu Ling': Intoxicated and Reprimanded by Husband, Suddenly Angry and Becomes a Hung Dead Ghost).[117] The article described Ma as a female Liu Ling (the famed drunken scholar), noting that every time she had a drink, she had to get drunk. Although she was reputed to have had a happy marriage, one day her husband Liu Shunyi returned home to find that she had hung herself, with the only explanation offered being her alcohol addiction. Intoxication was increasingly blamed for ruining happy, productive lives.

Not only were problems associated with alcohol consumption described in newspaper articles and in works of fiction, the subject of Chapter 5, but they were also illustrated in cartoons. Two examples from *Qilin* highlight arguments regarding alcohol's destructive nature. The eight frames of Wu Ying's cartoon "Jiu li chunhou" (Alcohol's Strength Is Rich) (see Figure 9) begin with the first polite interaction of two men before pleasant finger games turn into a rowdy fight in which they pummel each other. Finally, they stand amid broken furniture and glassware, dazed, bruised, and with ripped clothing, trying to understand how they came to blows.[118] Another cartoon, Da Yong's "Shuang zhi yan" (A Pair of Swallows), shows in six frames the dissolution of a happy couple (see Figure 10). In the first scene, they share the "same feelings." In frame two, they flirt. Then they walk together, holding each other closely, before having a drink. After a drink, the man hits the woman, who falls to the ground. In the final frame, they run away from each other.[119] Both of these cartoons vividly depict the violence and disorder that were commonly attributed to alcohol consumption in the early 1940s.

In the final years of Manchukuo, Japanese observers regularly linked alcohol consumption with the fate of the nation. The 1941 article "Jiu wei xing Ya zhi di" (Alcohol is the enemy of the rise of Asia) in the *Shengjing shibao* summarized the opinions of several prominent Japanese.[120] Quoting Dr. Ōhira Tokuzō, a program supervisor at the Department of People's Livelihood, for the title of the article, the author notes how, in 1934, Ōhira had travelled from Nanjing to Beijing and that in Nanjing during the "so-called New Life Movement," drinking and smoking were effectively banned. Even in Beijing, where he lived, over a thousand kilometres from the Republican capital, he was surprised by the lack of drunkenness. Ōhira praised the Republic because of his perception of the regime's ability to control what he regarded as a dangerous social ill. In 1940 the influential editor Yamamoto Sanehiko published the book *Mōko (Mongolia)*, in which he wrote that despite his belief that limited drinking and smoking at night were healthful, in China he did not see pedestrians smoking, and the bars were all closed.[121] Similarly, Shimizu Yasuzo (the founder of J.F. Oberlin University in Japan), argued in the book *Shina no hitobito (People of China)* that it was extremely rare to see Chinese drunk in public; he wrote that in his more than twenty years in China, the only people he ever saw who had passed out from alcohol intoxication were Japanese and Koreans.[122] Further, he claimed never to have seen a Chinese couple lose their home or fight because of alcohol. The article then continues on, to complain about the frequency of seeing local Japanese "very

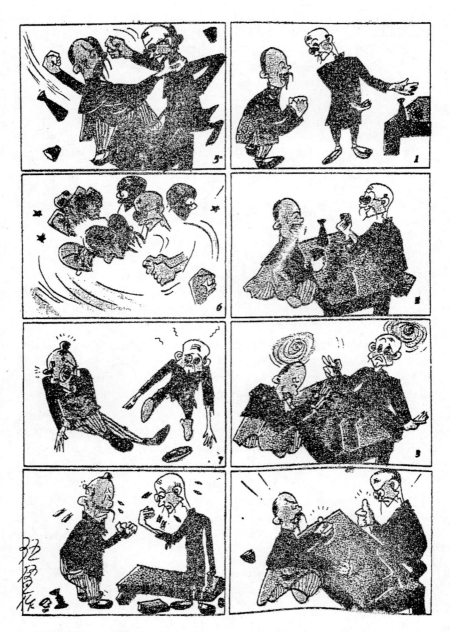

9   "Alcohol's Strength Is Rich." *Source:* Wu Ying, *Qilin* [Unicorn], September 1942, 26;
unable to contact creator.

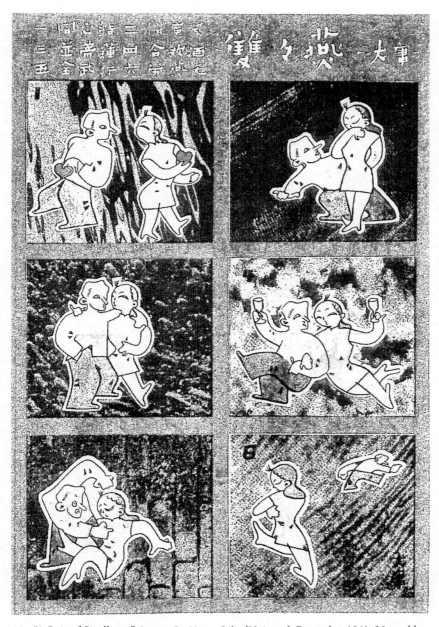

10 "A Pair of Swallows." *Source:* Da Yong, *Qilin* [Unicorn], December 1941, 26; unable to contact creator.

drunk" *(da zui)*, questioning how the Japanese, "the leading people," could guide the rest of society. The author urges the Japanese to abandon several hundred years of drunkenness and wake up to the poisons of Western imperialists, who had used alcohol to rob Native peoples in Canada and Hawai'i of their land." Alcohol is the enemy of the rise of Asia" argues that the battle against alcohol intoxication was as urgent to Asia in the 1940s as the Opium War had been to China a century before. Whether these observers of contemporary Chinese and Manchukuo society were accurate in their descriptions or not, their concern regarding alcohol consumption demonstrates the negativity that they attributed to it.

Distress over the health, stability, and fate of the empire also dominated Nakamura Kōjirō's 1945 essay "Kessenka no sake to tabako" (Sake and Tobacco in War), published in the final months of Manchukuo. Nakamura praised alcohol for its nutritious and motivational properties, yet he advocated strict control over grain allocation to the alcohol industry, drawing a direct correlation between military strength and alcohol.[123] Noting that consistent, declining rates of grain production were unable to meet the population's basic needs, he proposed that officials "should control alcohol consumption more strictly than [they] do today and prepare quickly for the final stage of the war for the soldiers."[124] Nakamura argued that since January 1943, as Tokyo was subjected to air attack and with death tolls mounting in South Asia, it was commonplace in Manchukuo's cities to see Japanese people, who he too argued were members of the leading race, "completely drunk and crawling on the street like animals in freezing weather."[125] Excessive alcohol consumption, Nakamura suggested, led Japanese to abdicate their weighty social responsibilities. He urged that sake should be available for the comfort and refreshment of soldiers on the frontlines and for workers at arsenals. But he also called for reducing the availability of alcohol for the general, especially Japanese, population to free up grain supply for food and to increase levels of sobriety, which would result in more labour available for industry and increased loyalty toward the state and, therefore, the military.[126] As the regime faced immanent collapse, Nakamura repeated narratives that had circulated to some degree since the earliest days of Manchukuo and that provided a vivid portrait of the extent to which alcohol had become demonized by the end of the empire.

The early 1930s' generally positive evaluation of alcohol, which stressed the health and social benefits of consumption, waned as socio-economic conditions declined in Manchukuo and as war spread across Asia. By the early 1940s, such an evaluation had fallen out of favour as alcohol had come to be viewed more negatively and to be used as a tool to criticize local life and governance. Instead of praising alcohol as an all-purpose medicine or as a fundamental inspiration of cultural production, critics charged that alcohol was a poison, or a deeply disruptive tool of Western imperialists, or both. Nationality-based understandings of alcohol consumption and addiction emerged, with Chinese praising their own history of alcohol while limiting discussion of Japanese practices to medical advice or to the view that these practices served as a conduit for Western ideas or values. Chinese writers did not produce paeans to sake or Japanese drinking practices; they generally ignored them. Japanese writers publicly questioned their nation's place in Asia because of what they perceived to be excessive alcohol consumption. In the early 1940s Chinese and Japanese regularly denounced alcohol as a danger to the nation, if not the empire. Despite contemporary, nationality-based assertions that the Chinese and the Japanese were susceptible to different intoxicants – opium and alcohol, respectively – both were popularly consumed and led social commentators to warn that Asian intoxication fuelled Western imperialists' sense of superiority.[127] In the short span of a decade, alcohol had shifted from a marker of modernity to a symbol of disease, disorder, and a society on the edge of collapse. The following chapter explores advertising practices that were part of the dramatic rise and fall of alcohol.

4 Selling Alcohol, Selling Modernity

In the first half of the twentieth century, the selling of "modern" lifestyles was a prominent feature in Manchuria's popular media. As Karl Gerth has documented, in Republican China "consumerism played a fundamental role in defining nationalism, and nationalism in defining consumerism."[1] Beyond the Great Wall, in Manchuria to the late 1930s, alcohol producers also promoted consumerism and, at times, invoked Manchukuo nationalism through references to the Kingly Way, the royal family, and Japan in the attempt to identify their products with healthful modes of living that reflected the best of the past and the present. Their campaigns appear to have achieved considerable success. Alcohol became so socially prominent that in 1940 Dr. Shao Guanzhi observed that it was an "essential article" *(bixu de wupin)* of contemporary life.[2] Alcohol was lauded as modern yet traditional, associated with a blend of local and foreign influences, and widely advertised as a nutritious tonic to strengthen consumers' bodies. But in the 1940s, as the Japanese Empire moved toward Holy War with England and the United States, the increasingly militarized environment and punitive economic policies took a toll on the alcohol industry and its promotion, with stress being placed on the harms of consumption and its negative effects on the nation. This chapter examines alcohol advertising in the early twentieth century, when alcohol consumption was promoted as a hallmark of good taste and modernity, before 1940s demands for strict control or prohibition to rescue East Asian peoples from Anglo-American imperialism. The chapter focuses on the most prominently advertised products: (1) the beer Asahi (sequentially, Chinese: Xu, Riguang, and Taiyang; English: Brilliance of the Rising Sun, Sunlight, Sun); (2) the red grape wine Chi yu pai putaojiu (English: Red Jade Brand Grape Wine; Japanese: Akadama; hereafter Red Ball); and (3) the health tonics Gui pai haomeng putaojiu (English: Soft-Shell Turtle Brand Grass Grape Wine; Japanese: Suppon Holmon; hereafter Essence of Turtle) and Yangming jiu (English: Life Support Wine; hereafter Life Support).

In *Jindai Dongbei shehui zhu wenti yanjiu (Research on Various Questions in Modern Northeast Society)*, Jiao Runming argues the importance that local regimes attributed to schools and newspapers for the propagation of state priorities.[3] Officials deemed education essential to state building, and considerable expenditures were made in establishing and staffing schools to create loyal subjects: technically skilled male workers to dominate the workplace as well as "good wives, wise mothers," whose skills could be selectively deployed. Less formal but equally significant means of control were attempted through a proliferation of Chinese-language newspapers and journals (many of which were owned or operated by Japanese) that were established to inform, educate, and entertain readers.[4] These publications reflected ideals of modernity by melding Chinese, European, Japanese, and North American–influenced imagery and information in their pages, at least until the start of Holy War in 1941. They attracted readers with varied editorial stances as well as with the latest advertising practices. The latter are the focus of this chapter.

The *Shengjing shibao (Shengjing Times)*, the *Datong bao (Great Unity Herald)*, *Jiankang Manzhou (Healthy Manchuria)*, and *Qilin (Unicorn)* are particularly relevant to a discussion of alcohol advertising in the first half of the twentieth century. The *Shengjing shibao* (1906-45) dated to the late Qing Dynasty and was the longest-running newspaper in the region's most important city, Fengtian. It remained one of the most popular regional publications until the end of its run, largely for its role in introducing May Fourth styles of writing to the region. *Datong bao* (1933-45) was the main newspaper of the capital city of Manchukuo, Xinjing (present-day Changchun), and was more closely affiliated with the government. For two years, *Jiankang Manzhou* (1939-40) was produced by the Manchuria Tuberculosis Prevention Association (Manzhou jiehe yufang xiehui) and published essays, editorials, and short fiction on a range of subjects, including health, sports, and the latest fashions. *Jiankang Manzhou* appeared at the high point of advertising for alcohol in the region, before a "palpable sense of the reduction in living standards"[5] hit the Chinese consumers who were a target market. *Qilin* (1941-45) was a journal produced by the Manchuria Magazine Society (Manzhou zazhi she) that aimed for an educated Chinese readership; it featured a wide range of fiction and nonfiction work. From the 1920s to the 1940s, ads in these publications for alcoholic beverages, especially grape wine, grew in number and sophistication, linking positive depictions of alcohol with traditional and modern healthy lifestyles.

Until the early 1940s, alcohol advertising generally depicted consumption in positive ways that bolstered narratives of modernity and health, while reflecting lengthy traditions of alcohol use. Alcohol consumption was often used as a marker of personal identity. One example is provided by Yang Xu, who celebrated her rebellious character (as a Muslim woman) by writing of her public intoxication and expressing her desire to do it again, which she knew did not conform to conservative ideals of submissive, obedient women but was more fully in accord with the independence to which "new women" such as she staked a claim.[6] Yi Chi, too, proudly recounted in the foreword to his 1938 volume of collected works, *Hua yue ji (The Flower Moon Collection)*, how he and other noted writers, including Gu Ding (1916-64), had founded the Arts Research Association (Yishu yanjiu hui) one night in 1937 while drinking a "moderate quality brandy."[7] The description of such behaviour was meant to appeal to cultured readers by underlining the consumer's modernity and by harking back to well-known precedents, in terms of artistic temperament, set by Chinese literary figures such as Li Bai and Tao Yuanming. This linking of notions of self-identity and quality with consumption was a consistent feature of contemporary advertising, especially in the *Shengjing shibao*.

As one of the longest-running newspapers in the region, the *Shengjing shibao* documented the growing enthusiasm for, and changing practices in, advertising. Jiao Runming notes how the first edition of the paper in 1906 had eleven ads; of these, ten were for Japanese companies (metals, construction, financial services, cloth, paper, medicines, hotels, and transportation), and one was for a Chinese medicine store.[8] Over time, ads grew in number, size, and sophistication. Many businesses that initially promoted their products with a small box of text, such as the makers of Asahi and Sapporo beers, incorporated imagery to attract readers' attention and to accentuate and reinforce their brand's presence in popular media. Jiao argues that ads in the *Shengjing shibao* illustrated not only contemporary lifestyles but also Japan's colonizing ambitions. Jiao stresses the dishonest nature of the ads, which "blot out the sky and cover up the earth" *(putian gaidi)* through "excessive praise" *(yi mei zhi ci)* of products that encouraged capitalist behaviour by promoting consumption.[9] Observing that individuals are "imperceptibly influenced by what one constantly sees and hears" *(er ru mu ran)*, Jiao argues, approvingly, that the capitalist nature of advertising weakened the Northeast's feudal society, but he cautions that its main function was not to encourage the growth of capitalism per se but to incorporate the Northeast into the Japanese Empire and thereby create a site for the exploitation of a massive labour pool, the extraction of resources, and the promotion of Japan's products.[10] Although the companies can be criticized en masse for promoting questionable Japanese and Manchukuo state priorities, the ways that they did so varied considerably, reflecting a vitality in business and advertising practices that has long since been forgotten. Additionally, it should be borne in mind that not all readers responded uncritically to advertising claims. Kawabe Taichi, for example, in his testimonial ad for Life Support Wine, noted that when he first read about its curative powers, he was leery of wasting his money but that after having unsuccessfully tried other products, he bought it out of desperation.[11] Kawabe was eventually, although not uncritically, convinced of its efficacy. Unfortunately, the extent to which his belief in the product was shaped by advertising cannot be known.

Competition between alcohol producers to convince consumers of the uniqueness of their products was intense. High-profile, relatively expensive foreign imports such as Hei'ermisi (Hermes) brandy (touted as the oldest alcohol in the world) or Hei'ermisi Scotch whiskey (which was sold in attractive round or square bottles)[12] vied with Russian vodkas. Ouzika gaoliang jiu er'shi wu hao de jiu (Vodka Gaoliang Alcohol, Brand No. 25) was advertised as being made from *gaoliang jiu* (distilled alcohol made primarily from Chinese sorghum) to appeal to local tastes.[13] These products faced further competition from domestic brands such as Xian you (Virtuous Friend) and Ju quan (Chrysanthemum Spring), both of which were produced by the Manchuria Alcohol Production Corporation (Manzhou zaojiu zhushi huishe). These latter Fengtian-produced wines were advertised as the best-quality *shaoxing jiu* (rice alcohol) wines, far superior to their southern counterparts in terms of purity, quality, and taste because of the advanced technology used in their creation.[14] Producers assertively promoted the wines as guarantors of consumers' good health and in the 1930s urged purchases of the product to honour the Manchukuo royal family; the names for these wines were even attributed to the prime minister, Zheng Xiaoxu.[15] Echoing calls for patriotic consumption directed to consumers throughout the Republican period, ads for the "national product" *(guo chan)* Bao jing (Precious Mirror) grape wine, created by Dr. Tsuboi at the Manchuria Food and Drink Research Institute (Manzhou yinshi liaopin yanjiusuo), encouraged consumers to be patriotic and to exclusively purchase domestic products.[16] Its taste, colour, and nourishing qualities were lauded, making it suitable, according to the ads, for consumption either for pleasure or for health. Ads for "medicinal wines" *(yaojiu)* frequently asserted the benefits of drinking alcohol produced with tiger bones. Brands such as Hugu huashe yaojiu (Tiger Bone, Flower Snake Medicinal Wine), Shenxiao hugu yaojiu (Magic Tiger Bone Medicinal Wine), Shen rong hugu yanshou jiu (Ginseng, Antler, Tiger Bone Prolong Life Wine), and Wanling fenghan hugu jiu (Cold Souls Tiger Bone Wine) were advertised as cure-alls effective in combating general illness as well as muscle and nerve pain.[17] The latter was prescribed especially for women having menstrual difficulties, postbirth complications, or stomach pain.[18] These ads reflect

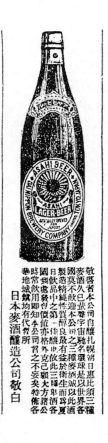

11   Asahi beer ad. *Source:*
Shengjing shibao [Shengjing
times], 11 June 1909, 1.

narratives deployed across the industry, and they all contributed to the tone
and look of the publications they appeared in.

Beer was one form of alcohol for which prominent advertisement campaigns were launched. Beer advertising dated to the end of the Qing Dynasty
and the earliest issues of the *Shengjing shibao*. Asahi and Sapporo (Chinese:
Zha huang) beers, for example, were introduced together in 1907, the year
after both the founding of the paper in Manchuria and the amalgamation,
in Japan, of the Asahi, Osaka, and Sapporo companies into Dai-Nippon
Breweries (Chinese: Da Riben maijiu zhushi huishe; hereafter Dai-Nippon).[19]
The arrival of Asahi and Sapporo was heralded through advertising that initially consisted of two brand symbols bracketing text, in Chinese, English,
and Japanese, that provided the names of both products and expressed the
hope that officials and merchants would place orders.[20] Subsequent ads featured Chinese text, addressed to consumers more generally, that surrounded
drawings of the bottles and their labels, which were in English and Japanese
(see Figure 11).[21] In 1908 Dai-Nippon strengthened its presence in the market

by establishing a distribution centre in Fengtian, and promotion of Asahi, especially, accelerated.[22] In 1910 the Chinese name of Asahi was changed from Xu (Brilliance of the Rising Sun) to Riguang (Sunlight), and by 1915 it had been altered to Taiyang (Sun) in order to avoid conflict with another product in south China produced under the same name; ads assured consumers that although the name had changed, the quality had not.[23] Asahi was one of the first Japanese alcohol brands to be introduced to the region, and its early and constant promotion was suggestive of the even more aggressive alcohol advertising that followed in the 1930s.

Ads for Asahi beer labelled it the "number-one old brand in the world," and in the early 1910s its label was emblazoned with the words "Grand Prize, Japan-British Exposition."[24] Asahi was touted as a reasonably priced, pure, hygienic drink – the number-one summer beverage.[25] It was promoted as a "specially brewed for export" beverage crafted from an age-old recipe of herbs (from south China's Fenglai Mountain) that produced a clear colour and pure taste. Ads heralded its "hygienic" nature, which worked to enhance stomach health while nourishing breath and blood. The producers invited especially Chinese and foreign merchants, scholars, and businessmen to sample the product. Most ads featured bottles with labels and a line or two of text, but an example of a drawing of a person consuming the beer can be seen in a frequently reproduced ad from the late 1910s and early 1920s. A man dressed in Western-style clothing sits beside a table on which are placed two bottles and cigarettes (see Figure 12). He lifts a glass of beer in one hand and has a cigarette in his other hand. Three beers are advertised: Asahi as well as Fu shen (Good Fortune Spirit) and Sapporo.[26] This ad was one of the earliest to incorporate human imagery in order to promote alcohol sales, although beer advertising continued to centre on pictures of the bottle. A notable exception is an ad in the magazine *Manchuria* that features a woman raising a pint of beer, demonstrating her "good judgement" (see Figure 13).[27] Other Dai-Nippon labels that were advertised, to a lesser extent, included Da yang (Big Sun)[28] and Hong xing (Red Star), for which a major factory was established in Fengtian. Consumers were encouraged to purchase Hong xing, which was described as being available everywhere and the most appropriate gift to give on festival days.[29]

Another popular Japanese-produced beer was Kirin (Chinese: Qilin; English: Unicorn), and it remains popular to the present. Promotional campaigns argued that it, too, was the best-quality and most internationally renowned beer.[30] Kirin was also proclaimed to be the oldest beer in history but produced with the newest manufacturing techniques to ensure the highest quality. Ads for Kirin, too, mostly featured bottles, whose labels were in

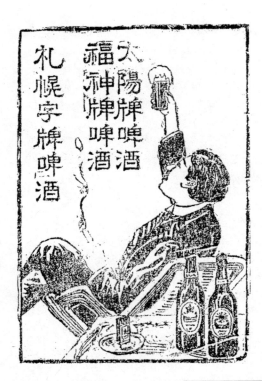

12   Asahi, Fu shen, and Sapporo beer ad. *Source: Shengjing shibao* [Shengjing times], 6 June 1920, 8.

13   Sapporo and Asahi beer ad. *Source: Manchuria,* 1 November 1937, 759.

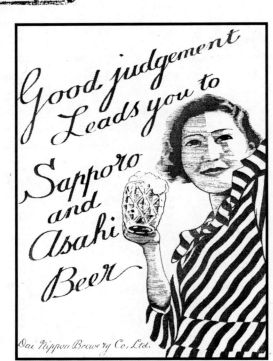

Chinese, English, and Japanese. Consumers were advised that Kirin's quality was internationally recognized and that it was the number-one beer in Japan.[31] After a distribution centre for it was opened in Fengtian, Kirin was increasingly promoted as a local, old-brand product.[32] It was also frequently described as the best beverage for relaxing and cooling down in the summer heat.[33]

The above beers competed with a considerable number of other labels for consumer loyalty. Consumers had a wide range of beers to choose from. Sakura (Chinese: Yinghua; English: Cherry) was produced from the early 1910s in Fengtian, with ads featuring Chinese, English, and Japanese text arguing that a central feature of modern society was that consumers always sought the best products, even when choosing alcohol.[34] Ads noted that people of all ages, whether Chinese or foreigners, liked to drink beer, although officials and businessmen were frequently targeted as its main market. Manshū (Chinese: Manzhou; English: Manchuria) beer was a popular Fengtian-based lager, which in the summer of 1920 held a prize giveaway, with cash prize amounts printed on the underside of bottle caps, to thank consumers for their ongoing support and to encourage more sales; Sakura held a similar giveaway in 1936, with ads featuring Mickey Mouse riding a bottle of Sakura beer.[35] Imported beers from Japan included the brands Hei (Black) and Dai-Nippon's You'ni'en (Union).[36] Ads for Hei had Chinese, English, and Japanese text, with the latter often dwarfing the Chinese name of the beer. It could be ordered from various cities in Japan, such as Fukuoka, Nagoya, and Kyoto. You'ni'en was promoted as being of the highest class and having pure German style; an ad from 1926 features the cartoon image of a man's face with Western features drinking a glass of beer as well as a picture of a bottle of the beer, which producers hailed as the mighty "conqueror of beers" *(pijiu zhong zhi bawang).*[37]

As a relatively new beverage, beer was most frequently advertised as a high-quality product in the attempt to lure consumers away from their "most favorite" wines: *gaoliang, huang,* and *shaoxing.*[38] The consistent use of the three languages, Chinese, English, and Japanese, in beer advertising accentuates the high-class local and foreign characteristics that producers were eager to attribute to the product for which they were actively seeking a market. For several decades, until advertising was sharply curtailed during Holy War, beer ads generally emphasized the brand quality that Sakura ads explicitly equated with modern consumer behaviour rather than the health narratives that drove campaigns for other forms of alcohol. And, as noted in Chapter 2, beer sales soared, as did local production.

Wines, which enjoyed a much longer presence in the region than beer, were even more prominently advertised, and one of the most heavily promoted

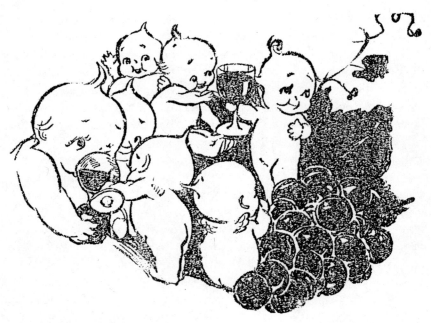

14   Red Ball cherubs. *Source: Shengjing shibao* [Shengjing times], 29 August 1920, 8.

was Red Ball. A locally produced port wine, Red Ball originated as Akadama port wine (launched in Japan in 1907) and was developed from a blend of Spanish wine, aromatic agents, and sweeteners.[39] From the 1910s to the 1940s, considerable effort was expended to publicize this wine's health and social benefits; the creator of Red Ball, Shinjiro Torii (1879-1962), founder of Suntory and "father of Japanese whiskey," was famed for pioneering advertising practices in Osaka and extended this expertise to Manchuria.[40] Jiao Runming argues that Red Ball became one of the most popular consumer products introduced by the Japanese.[41] In an early advertisement from 1920, cherubs are shown drinking and frolicking in a patch of grapes, which is situated above a detailed description of the health benefits derived from consuming the product (see Figure 14).

Significantly, by the end of the 1930s, its Japanese connections were downplayed. In ads to 1937, the Japanese name, rendered in English as "Akadama," was often prominently featured on bottle labels alongside the English words "Port Wine," "Registered Trade Mark," "natural," "sweet," "delicious," and "nourishment," with a short introduction in English. After 1937, most labels, at least as reproduced in ads, left the name illegible or replaced the Japanese name, "Akadama," with its English translation, "Red Ball." The revised labels, with Chinese and English text, thus encouraged consumer identification of the product with Chinese and English cultures, presumably for greater market appeal.

Red Ball advertising promoted the product as being the result of Chinese, Japanese, and Western influences. In 1939 a full-page ad in the *Shengjing shibao*, "Putaojiu yu putaojiu zhi shuo" (Grape Wine and Talk of Grape Wine), featured an essay outlining the history of grape wine.[42] The origins of wine-making using grapes were located in western Asia, whence, it was argued, the technology travelled to India, Greece, Egypt, and France before returning to Asia, namely China and Japan. Grape wine was positioned as a positive element of Western culture, supported by the testimony of doctors in France; it was also favourably noted that there are more than 400 references to it in the Bible, that Noah produced his own, and that Jesus promoted its consumption, especially at the Last Supper. In China the cultivation of grape vines, "the god of plants" *(zhiwu zhi shen)*, was traced to the reign of Han Wu Di (r. 141-87 BCE), thus giving grape wine a respectable Chinese lineage of over 2,000 years. A central theme of the ad was that "the life of a civilized person depends on happiness attained from grape wine." It was argued that European, North American, and Japanese families drank grape wine to increase familial "warmth" *(wenqing)*, thus encouraging consumers to learn from Japanese and Western experiences in order to improve local life. The extent to which Red Ball actually reflected Western tastes was questioned by Shi Zhizi, who argued that French travellers (to whom he attributed a wine expertise) derided Red Ball and another popular Japanese red wine, Hachijirushi Kozan Budoshu (Fragrant Wine), as excessively sweet beverages; in his opinion, "cultured people" *(wenhua ren)* would be wise to do the same.[43]

In accordance with longstanding Chinese and Japanese beliefs, the most acclaimed attribute of Red Ball was its application in health regimes for adults and children.[44] Ads cited seven (nameless) university doctors, from Asia and the West, who praised the product and testified to its efficacy.[45] As a medicinal wine argued to have been recommended for decades by doctors, it was "number one in the medicine world for everyone" *(yi jie zhi zhu quan wei)*.[46] It was touted for alleviating problems associated with "old age and weakness, working hard, hard labour, insomnia, lost appetite, insufficient yin-yang nourishment, giving birth, disabilities, foot problems, stomach ailments, postillness anemia, cholesterol problems, nervousness, stomach ulcers, indigestion, daydreams, and inconsistencies in the brain and blood."[47] Red Ball promised quick recovery for all of the above conditions, with fastest results guaranteed for those engaged in physical labour. Red Ball was also praised for preserving youth and improving facial colour; it had the "power to turn the aged into youth" *(nianlao fan tong zhi li)*. Red Ball was so nutritious that it could help consumers to gain weight. In an ad titled "Pang!" (Fat!), readers were invited to sample the wine and benefit from its special grape and fruit sugars, iron, and calcium.[48] The sugars were argued to improve the absorption of vitamins and minerals that would help consumers to gain weight, while improving blood circulation and bone strength. The wine's health benefits were said to be wide-ranging, but consumers were also warned that physical damage could result for "those who are too greedy" *(tu tan duo liang)*. Red Ball wine, readers were informed, was to be consumed for "nourishment" *(yingyang)*, "comfort" *(wei'an)*, and the "improvement of society" *(shehui gailiang)*, not to satisfy an "addiction" *(shihao)* – a reference to emerging linkages between the habitual consumption of alcohol and disease.

Red Ball ads appeared with greater frequency and flair than promotions for other alcoholic beverages, reflecting the promotion of Akadama wine in Japan, which engaged in the most up-to-date practices, blending text with imagery of the product, other objects, and individuals. A regularly reproduced 1939 ad features a mature gentleman in Chinese-style robe, vest, shoes, and cap surrounded by Chinese and Western accoutrements of culture (see Figure 15).[49] Holding a glass of wine, he sits on a plush Western-style chair in front of Chinese furnishings and beside a table with two bottles of Red Ball. Behind the man is a couplet referencing elements that link nature and cultivated life, setting Red Ball alongside other, more firmly established cultural symbols. The wine's name is placed to the left of the scene, and above is a commendation: "Gentlemen, if anaemic and weak, drink for recovery. This wine will immediately develop your strength." The wine's long-term health benefits are made even more explicit by a slogan at the bottom left of the ad: "A thousand cups for strength, Ten thousand years of health." The ad effectively connects male strength, obtained through the consumption of Red Ball, with Chinese and Western imagery suggestive of the blending of cultures that Manchukuo supporters insisted was the state's raison d'être.

Several ads are notable for their depiction of women and provide what Sherman Cochran has identified as distinctly modern representations of parts of the human body.[50] A 1921 ad, with Chinese and Japanese writing, features a drawing of a Japanese woman from the chest up holding a tray with two bottles of Red Ball and four glasses. The ad encourages housewives to use the product to best serve their guests.[51] An even more forthright promotion of the wine is found in a 1939 ad that features a woman's hand holding a glass of red wine in front of a picture of grapes on the vine (see Figure 16).[52]

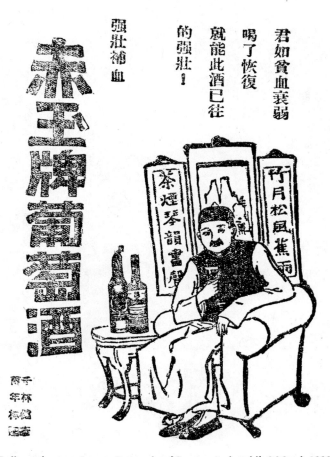

強壯補血

赤玉牌葡萄酒

君如貧血衰弱
喝了恢復
就能此酒已往
的強壯！

15 Red Ball gentleman. *Source: Datong bao* [Great unity herald], 3 March 1939, 7.

In addition to the name of the product, there is also a small image of a Red Ball bottle. In the bottom left-hand corner is a variation of Red Ball's slogan, "One hundred cups for health, One thousand cups to prolong life." This ad underlines a wife's care for, and knowledge of, her husband's health. She prescribes drinking a few glasses of wine to start every morning: "Husband! You must take good care of your health. Please, every morning drink a few glasses!" The husband dutifully agrees, "Yes, when the opportunity arises, I will drink grape wine." The wife's expressed concern for her husband reflects idealized roles of the "good wife" and demonstrates her knowledge of health, an important element of the domestic sciences in Manchukuo education for women. If Red Ball is consumed every morning, it is promised to enhance

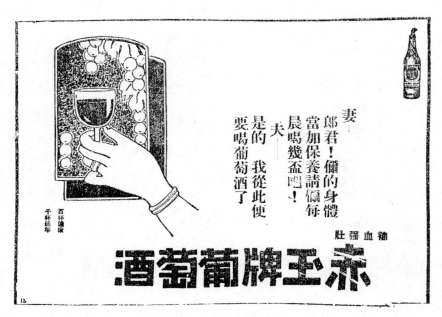

16   Red Ball ad. *Source: Datong bao* [Great unity herald], 26 March 1939, 4.

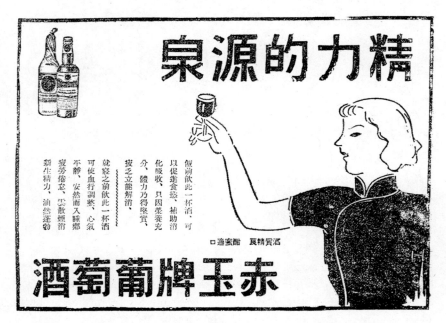

17   "Source of Energy." *Source: Datong bao* [Great unity herald], 3 November 1941, 4.

work, and if consumed every evening, it will ensure a sound sleep: "One cup in the morning and evening surpasses one hundred medicines" *(chao xi yi bei you yu bai yao).*[53] In the 1941 ad "Jingli de yuanquan" (Source of Energy), an illustration of the upper body of a woman with a short modern hairstyle raises a glass of wine toward a pair of Red Ball bottles (see Figure 17).[54] The benefits of consuming a glass of wine are suggested: before dinner, to raise an appetite and to aid digestion; and before going to bed, to ensure good circulation and sleep. This 1941 ad explicitly links the consumption of grape wine with contemporary notions of healthful living and modern imagery but does so with noticeably less force than similar ads of 1939. Consumers were no longer encouraged to start their mornings with wine but rather to consume wine in the evening. The wine was advertised to middle- and upper-class consumers as an essential component of modern healthful living.

Even more stress on alcohol's health benefits can be seen in ads for Essence of Turtle, which were featured regularly in *Jiankang Manzhou.* Its promotion shared many similarities with that of Red Ball, especially in the depiction of the product as a nutritious, all-round restorative (see Figure 18).[55] The wine afforded benefits similar to those of Red Ball, including the promotion of health and happiness, healthy pregnancy, physical vigour, and relief from sleeplessness and constipation. The product's most acclaimed ingredient was turtle essence, a long-valued medicinal element believed to enhance blood and strengthen the gallbladder; turtle was marketed as a special product of Manchukuo. Essence of Turtle blended hormones harvested from the blood of local soft-shell turtles with grasses grown on the banks of the Nen River, grape juice, and alcohol. This quintessential regional drink was deemed suitable for everyone and was said to impart youthful energy, maintain physical strength, and enable long-term labour. Essence of Turtle was labelled an "incomparable high-class beverage" *(wubi gaoji yinliao),* an assertion underlined by the impressive colour enhancement of its ads. Unlike ads for Red Ball, explicit connection with Japan was maintained through the prominent placement of the brand name in Japanese text alongside Chinese and English. Further, ads often stressed that Essence of Turtle was produced and distributed by the Japanese-operated Manchuria Wine Producers Alliance and was available for sale in Manchukuo's best department stores and restaurants, Manchukuo military hospitals, various departments of the Guandong Army, and Manchukuo troop stations. Promotion for Essence of Turtle stressed the wine's high class and medicinal value, linking local specialities with leading Manchukuo institutions and Japan.

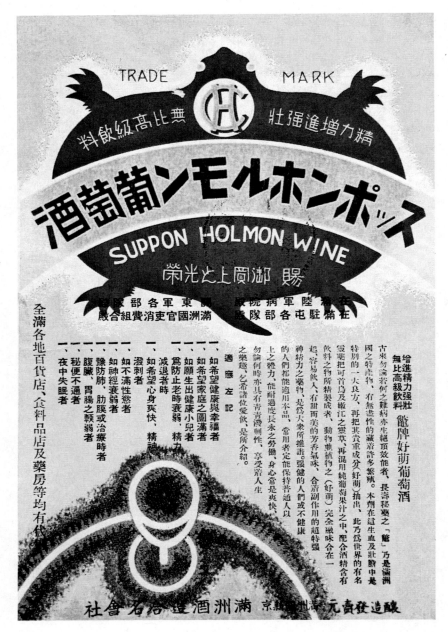

18   Essence of Turtle ad. *Source: Jiankang Manzhou* [Healthy Manchuria] 1, 4 (1939): back outside cover.

19   *(facing page)* "Strong Prosperous Asia." *Source: Jiankang Manzhou* [Healthy Manchuria] 2, 2 (1940): back outside cover.

The physical benefits of consuming Essence of Turtle are vividly depicted in the 1940 ad "Fasheng xing Ya zhi zhuangli" (Strong Prosperous Asia) (see Figure 19).[56] A young, shirtless cartoon strongman flexes his right arm to demonstrate his virility, which is further reflected in his facial expression, hairstyle, upright posture, and fist – above the product's name in Japanese text. He flexes under a backdrop of grapes and beside a bottle of Essence of

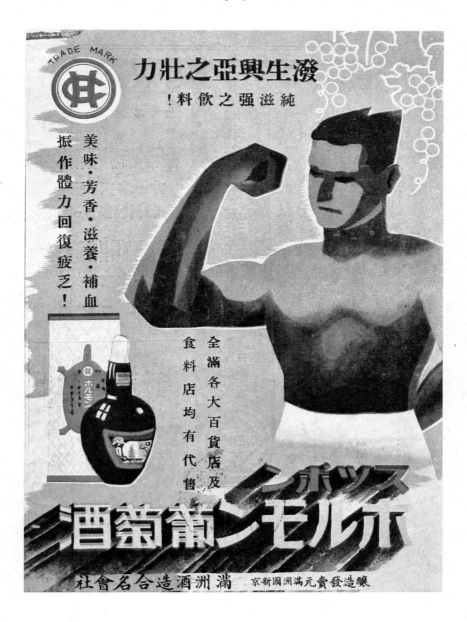

Turtle, which is acclaimed for its strength-enhancing and nourishing qualities: "The drink of pure, strong nourishment ... delicious, fragrant, nourishing,
and enriching to the blood – enables vigorous physical strength and recovery
from exhaustion!" This ad assertively links enjoyment of the wine with the
health of the consumer, Asian strength, and by implication, the Japanese
Empire. To drink Essence of Turtle, the consumer is told, is to attain a potency
befitting the resurgence of Asia and its peoples. Essence of Turtle advertising
featured explicitly political messages that seemingly failed to win it as prominent a place in the hearts of Manchukuo consumers as Red Ball.

Another brand of medicinal wine that was aggressively advertised to the
mid-1940s was Life Support. In comparisons with Western alcohol and
gaoliang wine, consumers were advised that its taste was more delicate than
either.[57] The light Japanese-style taste was argued by its producers to be an
improvement on other beverages made in Fengtian. As a special product of
renowned Japanese companies of long standing, including Shinano Kyōkoku
and Shiozawa ke, its promotion focused on its status as a health tonic produced by a family business through eighteen generations and for over 300
years. The health-inducing ingredients, including medicinal herbs and grasses,
were argued to have been harvested from a natural mountain environment
1,000 metres above sea level.[58] Ads described the wine as an incomparable
medicine, supported by practical results for consumers, approval from medical doctors, and as claimed in a 1937 ad, the United States government.[59]
Ads informed consumers that the product was available at all pharmacies
and grocery stores but warned that they had to beware of fake products.
Consumers who had not tried the product were encouraged to mail the
company's head office in Tokyo for a free sample.

As with other wines, promotion for Life Support argued that a wide variety
of ailments could be treated with it. Consumers were cautioned that over-
working, insomnia, and weather extremes depleted strength and increased
vulnerability to colds, stomach or intestine problems, and depression.[60] As
with early ads for Red Ball, malnourished people were encouraged to drink
Life Support in the morning and at night for best results.[61] Consistent consumption of the wine could fatten and strengthen weak bodies, for men and
women, and thereby restore an impressive vigour.[62] Spiritual, mental, and
physical strength would improve as youth was restored. Anaemic, weak individuals, and those with prematurely aging faces and bodies, could regain
their *joie de vivre* through use of the product. Women, especially, would
benefit from consuming the wine if they worked in extradomestic employment without adequate exercise.

In the early 1940s, a special feature of Life Support advertising was consumer testimonials, with photographs and text attributed to (mostly Japanese) consumers. Often, ads in *Qilin* were favourably placed facing the first page of the table of contents. The photographs were generally formal shots of the face and upper body of the letter writer beside a table with a bottle of Life Support, the box it was sold in, and a glass. Some identifying information about the writer was provided, either place of residence or membership in a group as well as the name of the person. In a testimonial in the *Shengjing shibao* in 1941, Ye Fengsheng argued that consuming Life Support increased his physical strength. He quoted a folk adage, "laughter in the family brings good fortune" *(xiao men fu lai)*, and asserted that Life Support could provide consumers with both laughter and good fortune. He claimed that the medicinal ingredients had the power to restore life to the nearly dead. He recommended drinking one or two glasses in the morning and at night to nourish the body, intestines, and inner organs. Ye particularly noted that the wine was effective for women, as it improved their circulation after giving birth and guaranteed healthful breast milk for stronger babies.[63] Also in 1941, in *Qilin*, Kin Mitsunari testified that the wine was useful in treating gastroenteritis, insomnia, and neurasthenia. Kin recounted how he was attracted by the claims in Life Support advertising. He argued that since he had begun drinking the wine, no matter how hard he worked, he did not feel tired.[64] Both of these testimonials highlight the restorative claims that dominated Life Support advertising.

A key component of Life Support promotion was advocating the product as a salve for weakness and exhaustion. Fujī Kyūta wrote that because he generally lacked adequate exercise, he suffered from nerve and waist pain, constipation, and no appetite. Gradually, through his consumption of Life Support, his body temperature was restored, his appetite and bowel movements returned to normal, and his pain subsided. He recounted how before using the wine he had been very thin and embarrassed to have his photograph taken, but in the picture accompanying the testimonial, he looks confident and self-assured in a Western-style suit.[65] Imamura Masu, photographed in formal Japanese attire, wrote that she had begun to drink Life Support because her body had been weak and skinny: she had suffered from a cold waist and feet, insomnia, and a lack of appetite. Since she had begun drinking the wine, her body temperature had returned to normal, as had her appetite. Happily noting that she had gained weight, she affirmed the benefits of drinking the wine day and night.[66] Miura Keiko, the mother of three children, wrote that her husband had started drinking the wine and had persuaded her to use it.[67]

She found it to be an effective and tasty remedy for her exhaustion from excessive household and society responsibilities, which caused her neurasthenia, insomnia, indigestion, and difficulty walking.[68] Higashimoto Hide, chair of a branch of the Japanese Patriotic Women's Association, concurred that contemporary women had to work day and night to fulfil their family and society obligations. Overworked, too, her body was weak, and she was exhausted. She testified that since starting to regularly consume the wine, her health had been restored and that she felt more capable of performing her duties.[69] The consistent appearance of such testimonials placed Life Support at the forefront of advertising for medicinal wines.

In the final years of Manchukuo, such prominent promotion of alcoholic beverages began to wane, although Life Support was less impacted than other brands. In *Jiankang Manzhou*, for example, Essence of Turtle ads lessened in number before the journal ceased publication in late 1940. By 1942 the confluence of expanded war operations and rationing, the start of the Second Five Year Plan, and more negative reflection on alcohol consumption across Manchukuo popular culture had signalled the decline of such high-profile alcohol advertising campaigns. Although positive alcohol narratives still circulated in advertising and popular literature, the latter tended to focus not on the nutritional values so loudly hailed by advertisers but rather on alcohol's use to relieve bad moods, as a social lubricant, or as an inducement to writing – as expressed by the writers Yang Xu and Yi Chi. For the most part, even potentially positive characteristics of alcohol consumption tended to cast negative light on Manchukuo society. After all, Red Ball, Essence of Turtle, and Life Support advertising stressed the ill health and widespread exhaustion of the population, and Yang Xu praised drinking as a mechanism to cope with miseries in her life and to publicly challenge ideals of submissive, obedient women. Alcohol was increasingly criticized for destroying lives and tearing families apart and for being a gateway drug to narcotics, with certain calamity for individuals, their families, and by extension, the state.

As the promotion of alcohol diminished, ads for products that sought to alleviate the harm of alcohol came to the fore. The Fengtian-produced supplement Ruosu (Basic Element), a compound developed by Japanese scientists, was one of the most prominent; it is discussed in more depth in Chapter 7 as a cure for opiate addiction. Ruosu was marketed as an ideal remedy for ills pertaining to alcohol poisoning. Ruosu's prominence has been noted by Jiao Runming, who observes that it was one of the only nutritional supplements available to Chinese consumers in the late-Manchukuo period.[70] The 1940 ad "Pohuai jiankang de si da dusu: Bianbidu, jiehedu, jiudu, yandu" (The Four Big Poisons that Destroy Health: Constipation, Tuberculosis, Alcohol, and

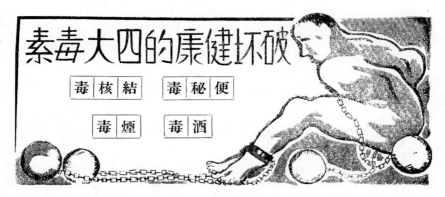

20 "The Four Big Poisons that Destroy Health." *Source: Jiankang Manzhou* [Healthy Manchuria] 2, 5 (1940): 36.

Smoking), in *Jiankang Manzhou,* is indicative of the sea change in alcohol narratives (see Figure 20).[71] Instead of depicting a relaxed or robust person, the ad features the image of a naked, shackled man who is bent over beside the names of the four poisons. Below him is an essay condemning alcohol as a poison plaguing Manchukuo, Europe, and North America.[72] The essay argues that people may know how to combat constipation and tuberculosis but that problems associated with drinking alcohol and smoking tobacco are even more difficult to guard against and require scientific solutions. Alcohol is described as causing great harm to the body for "alcohol drinkers" *(yin jiu jia),* making them susceptible to life-threatening "addiction" *(shihao).* The ad urges readers to buy Ruosu, the most modern medicine for curing "evil intoxication" *(e zui)* and "longstanding intoxication" *(su zui).*[73] Alcohol is criticized as a poison deployed by European imperialists to decimate Native communities in North America and Hawai'i; consumers are warned not to let their tragic fates befall them.[74] Doubtless, readers were aware that it was in fact Japanese, not Europeans, who were dominant in Manchukuo's alcohol trade, but prohibitionists and other critics of alcohol consumption surely agreed that imperialism was a factor in rising levels of consumption.

The alcohol consumption that health professionals such as Shao Guanzhi described as an "essential element" of Manchukuo life was decried in Ruosu ads as "bad hygiene" that caused heart attacks and premature death.[75] Ads outlined in detail how ethyl alcohol was absorbed into the stomach and spread through the body to harm the brain, heart, and nervous system. The dangers of excessive levels of alcohol in the blood were stressed, and it was argued that people with a quantity of alcohol in the bloodstream of 0.5-1.0 percent would die.[76] An ad from 1940 contained the following chart linking levels of alcohol in the bloodstream with certain responses:

  .2 = especially happy
  .2-.3 = talk nonsense
  .3-.4 = dizzy
  .5 = drunk as mud
  .5-1.0 = immediately drop dead[77]

According to the chart, only people with a reading of 0.2 percent experienced positive effects from alcohol, beyond which they would suffer or die. The ad warned that "ordinary people think that the more they drink the happier they are, and that they must drink till drunk." Such incorrect habits, the ad argued, necessitated that alcohol be placed under a critical spotlight.

With the start of Holy War in 1941, alcohol advertising began to be curtailed, campaigns for the promotion of alcohol consumption waned, and products such as Ruosu stressed alcohol's dangerous nature even more. For nearly four decades, alcohol consumption had been linked in popular media with modernity, health, and at times in the 1930s with the Manchukuo state, its royal family, the Kingly Way, or Japan in ads that contributed greatly to the look and tone of the publications they appeared in. Consumers were consistently advised on how to attain the best-quality products and on how, when, and where to consume them for greatest effect. Beer was promoted as a fashionable beverage of the highest quality. Grape and medicinal wines were argued to be products of the best traditional wisdom and the most up-to-date technical processes that ensured good health for all. But war, rations, and the collapse of the region's nascent consumer culture changed the ways that alcohol was viewed and the ways that it was represented. What had once been equated with good fortune and health was labelled a "big poison" or an Anglo-American imperialist weapon.

The alcohol promotion discussed in this chapter does not significantly differ from current campaigns for products such as China's most famous beer, Qingdao, which is promoted as "the beer which is loved among beer drinkers from all over the world."[78] The producers of Ha'erbin (Harbin) beer regularly boast of brewing the oldest beer in China, made of top-quality, pure, and natural waters. What is perhaps China's most famous brand of alcohol, Kweichow Maotai, has been linked with political personages of the highest rank: Premier Zhou Enlai (1898-1976) reputedly believed that the liquor had almost "magical qualities," and it was allegedly drunk by Henry Aisin-Gioro Puyi's relative the Empress Dowager Cixi (1835-1908) to help her "maintain her youthful and beautiful look" – a claim that would have been unthinkable in the Maoist era.[79] Kweichow Maotai has been used for toasts on important state occasions, such as at the founding of the People's Republic of China and at China's entry into the World Trade Organization.[80] The repeated, insistent claims of Kweichow Maotai's fame, quality, and consumption by such prominent people on such lofty occassions are meant to convey to consumers the belief that they, too, might benefit from alcohol. Such promotion displays tendencies similar to those of advertising in the first half of the century that is criticized by Jiao Runming and that Karl Gerth has argued firmly linked consumerism with nationalism and vice versa. The alcohol promotion described in this chapter encouraged consumers to pursue a modernity based on what advertisers posited as the best of Chinese tradition and foreign influences. During the Manchukuo era, what exactly constituted "the best" shifted: whereas in the early 1930s positive elements of Manchukuo or Japan were often invoked, by the 1940s most advertising campaigns had begun to downplay such associations in favour of promoting healthful abstention and warning against the evil of the empire's enemies. Changing with the times, advertisers actively linked their products to what they believed consumers might want to associate themselves with or to what they believed consumers could be inspired to buy. Whereas the nation of China proved an effective totem for consumers south of the Great Wall, in Manchukuo it was the culture of China that endured since the state could not.

An additional, striking similarity between the industries of today and a half-century ago is that of ownership. Today, some businesses – the producer of Kweichow Maotai, for example – are state-owned enterprises, echoing earlier state-backed monopolies. Others blend local and foreign control; the second highest shareholder in Qingdao is now none other than Japan's Asahi Breweries, the forerunner of which held a large market share in Manchukuo.[81] This combination of state and foreign ownership has not to date inspired the negativity attributed to the industry during the late-Manchukuo era, when critics condemned alcohol as a poison to the people or an imperialist weapon to destroy Asia. Advertising now, as then, is done in earnest by competing producers who invest considerable time, effort, and money in attempting to attract consumers and to convince them to believe in whatever qualities the product might provide. Doubtless, many producers today believe their own advertising. In Manchukuo such advertising was once reflective more of capitalist or Chinese cultural promotion than of Japanization – regardless and because of Japanese ownership, which advertisers knew could not register well with a majority of consumers who had since the late-Qing era been urged to buy Chinese goods in the face of foreign imperialism. In the 1940s alcohol advertising declined as consumer markets diminished, as war ravaged Asia, and as any sheen that Manchukuo may once have had was wiped away. The heavy-handed Japanese military and prejudicial social policies encouraged advertisers who sought to popularize their products to think ever more strategically about just how notions about the Chinese, Japanese, and Manchukuo were understood by consumers. Ironically, the latter years of the "narco-state" Manchukuo were marked by state prohibitionist tendencies aimed at intoxicants whose social roles came under closer scrutiny by all, including the Chinese writers whose work is the subject of the following chapter.

5 Writing Intoxicant Consumption

> The near and distant lights are uncountable, and although the levels
> of their brightness differ in strength and weakness, all of them are
> exerting themselves to wage a war of resistance *(kangzhan)* against
> the black night, like some fine young little swords piercing my eyes.
>
> SAN LANG, "ZHUXIN" (CANDLEWICK) (1933)

In one of Xiao Jun's (1907-88) earliest works, the author (writing under the
name San Lang) describes stars shining in the night sky above Harbin. The
"war of resistance" that he attributes to them might also be the product of
writers working within the increasingly burdensome regime of surveillance
and censorship that came to define Manchukuo's literary world as social
realism became the dominant literary form in local newspapers and journals.
With the establishment of Manchukuo in 1932, cultural functionaries attempted to dictate local cultural production through regulations designed to
curb dissent and foster support for the state. Under their watchful eyes, writers
increasingly criticized the recreational use of intoxicants, reflecting anti-
opium and, eventually, anti-alcohol public campaigns as well as the state's
shortcomings.[1] At the time, Zhou Zuoren, the pre-eminent writer living in
Japanese-occupied China (in Beiping, present-day Beijing), argued that "the
backdrop of society is reflected in literature. Because of the influence of
literature, at the same time the backdrop can gradually change. This is the
reason we must respect literature."[2] Zhou's belief in the ability of literature to
effect social change was shared by young writers in Manchukuo, such as Xiao
Jun, who criticized intoxicant consumption in their work. This chapter outlines Chinese-language fictional work that was published in Manchukuo and
describes the consumption of alcohol and opium, mapping the writers' efforts
to raise mass consciousness of the dangers of intoxicants.

Following the establishment of Manchukuo, officials quickly promulgated
cultural and literary guidelines to muffle criticism of the state and its relation

to Japan and foster "independent" cultural development. This early Man-chukuo literary world has been described by Prasenjit Duara, who argues that during the early 1930s "writers such as the feminist Xiao Hong and her partner Xiao Jun, nourished on [Maxim] Gorky, [Nikolai] Gogol, and other European writers, produced a radical literary culture that survived even after their departure from the region in 1934."[3] The radical literary culture that they created sheds important light on contemporary social issues, includ-ing recreational alcohol and opium consumption. The state's highly publicized anti-opium platform encouraged writers to critique its consumption, even at risk of violating Manchukuo's publication laws, which prohibited criticism of the state.[4] By the end of the 1930s, as war spread across Asia, alcohol had joined opium as a target for criticism.

Xiao Jun left Manchukuo in 1934. Before he departed, he published the short story "Zhuxin," in which opium smoking is cited as one of the charac-teristic sounds of the then one-year-old state:

> From various corners, different noises are emitted – is it the plaintive cry of girls selling their bodies for the first time? Is it the secret words of young lovers embracing under peach-coloured lights? Is it the rustling sounds of opium being smoked? Is it the whispering of daughters-in-law? Is it the silent tears of the wrongly imprisoned? Is it the howling sound of the prison guards' leather-thonged whips? Is it the gasping for breath of the sick? Is it the ravings of the dying? Is it the sighs of poets? Is it the shouting of soldiers, at war because humanity is not at peace? Isn't it a pity that these shocking sound waves are so weak? How is it that they can't reach my ears?[5]

Emulating China's foremost social critic of the early twentieth century – Zhou Zuoren's elder brother Lu Xun (1881-1936) – Xiao aspired to heighten public consciousness, through his writing, of the "shocking sound waves" of Manchukuo society. He depicts Harbin as "a hell of this world" echoing with horrifying sounds, including those of opium smoking, torture, and widespread suffering. His depiction of a society "not at peace" clearly outlines his percep-tion of the regime and suggests the reasoning behind his departure to Shanghai.

In 1933 a contemporary of Xiao Jun's, Bai Lang (1912-94), published the short story "Panni de erzi" (Rebellious Son), in which she describes the miser-able life of the poor, who fight with dogs for food, and men who use women as the stuff of barter.[6] The rebellious son, Bai Nian, is a young man from a wealthy family who sympathizes with the poor, whereas his father, mother, and their cook disparage them. When Nian asks for food to feed the poor, the cook retorts, "Sympathy for the poor has what benefit? When you aren't looking, he'll just steal your things. Burn and kill, plunder, kidnap ... aren't these all things poor people do?"[7] The poor are rejected as men engaged only in destructive acts. Nian views such contempt as a poison of the "enemy."[8] Ultimately, Nian is estranged from his father, whom he regards as a member of the enemy class, because of Yin Na, a young woman from the countryside. At seventeen, Na was married to a man who spent his days playing mah-jong, smoking opium, and visiting prostitutes; Na was powerless to make him change or to leave. After three years, their money was gone, and in order to buy opium, Na's husband sold her to a brothel for 1,000 yuan and then disappeared. Na tried refusing clients and twice attempted suicide before Nian's father bought her contract and took her home. As a poor woman, she was powerless to overcome her subjugation, but with the help of Nian she becomes conscious of the class-based nature of her oppression. The two announce their intention to leave and become "perfect people," thereby challenging social contradictions through their rejection of selfishness and prison-like families.[9]

In "Panni de erzi," Bai Lang paints a portrait of a money-obsessed society that denigrates and dehumanizes the poor and women. Recreational opium consumption is depicted as a major influence on contemporary life that devastated Na's life, resulting first in her sale to a brothel and later to Nian's father. Na describes herself as a "weak woman" *(nuoruo nüzi)* who lacks the personal and financial resources needed to save herself but finds them through her relationship with Nian – her male saviour. The author emphasizes the class nature of Na's oppression while demonstrating how her particular oppression is also gendered. Like Xiao Jun's short story "Zhuxin," Bai Lang's Manchukuo-produced publications do not explicitly criticize the Japanese but rather local society, which is blamed for a lack of justice that compels youth to rebel against their elders, who are blinded by their class backgrounds and consumption of opium.

The complications of life in Manchukuo, which included living under expanding Japanese rule, the implementation of a racist socio-economic system, and natural disasters, led the region's most prominent Chinese writers, including Bai Lang and Xiao Jun, to leave in the mid-1930s. A few years after their departure, a new generation of young writers emerged to embrace the social realism that had characterized their predecessors' work. Japanese intellectuals living in Manchukuo, such as Kobayashi Hideo, Abe Tomoji, and Kishida Kunio, encouraged writers' depiction of economic hardship, social disorder, and the low status of women in their work as realistic portraits of life in the new state. Left-wing Japanese writer Shinichi Yamaguchi approvingly noted that "realism seem[ed] to predominate among the main literary trends" in Manchukuo.[10] By the late 1930s, the literary world was enlivened by literature that promoted official anti-opium and, eventually, anti-alcohol campaigns.

State attempts to control the opium industry are mocked in literature that depicts the Opium Monopoly as ineffectual. Mei Niang's (b. 1920) short story "Zuihou de qiuzhenzhe" (The Last Patient) (1939) depicts a young family's visit to a health clinic.[11] The woman ostensibly seeks treatment for anaemia, but it is really the couple's opium addiction for which they seek relief. The doctor suspects from the woman's "pale grey" face that she is addicted to opium.[12] Dishevelled, dirty, and constantly yawning, they appear incapable of caring for themselves or their baby, who is filthy from neglect. Devoid of social and parental skills, the couple bickers over who really abuses opium and what type of "medicine" they are seeking; they both refuse the doctor's proffered needle as too costly, but the implication is that they are seeking a drug to share later.[13] The man convinces the doctor to prescribe laudanum, an opium-based liquid.[14] As the pathetic couple shuffles out of the clinic, having achieved their goal, a light glints across a badge bearing the national flag on the man's cap, thus linking their condition with the colonial state.

In one of her most prominent novellas, "Bang" (Clam) (1939), Mei Niang describes a wealthy family's heir, Elder Brother, who aspires to be rich like his father only so that he, too, can purchase opium in large quantities. He complains that the Monopoly is manipulated by the wealthy who flout restrictions on the sale of opium, leaving a system that is unable to satisfy him since the limited amounts of officially sanctioned opium to which he has access are more expensive than, and inferior to, drugs that he bought before the Monopoly was established and that he continued to buy privately.[15] With little effort, he bypasses the Monopoly to purchase illegal opium. Filling his younger sister Meili's room with the "peculiar smell" of opium, Elder Brother pleads to borrow money from her wages until he receives his allowance.[16] He insists that since few adequate employment opportunities exist for men, he is better off staying at home, smoking opium, and being "comfortable" (*shufu*); Meili retorts that what he believes to be a comfortable life has left him "not far from death" *(li si bu yuan)*.[17] Meili's work ethic contrasts with Elder Brother's drug-centred existence: she works as a secretary for a pittance, which often ends up in his pipe. By the end of "Bang," despite her hard work, Meili's life is devastated by rumours of a love affair, and she loses her job, her fiancé, and her dignity. Meili is destroyed by her ambition to forge an independent life outside of her home while her brother stays in his room fuelling a ruinous addiction. Both siblings are denied their potential, but Meili pays an even higher price than her brother, who actively pursues opium consumption and compounds her subjugation.

That same year, Wu Ying (1915-61) published her story "Gui" (Deceit), a fictional work that portrays a female opium addict. A maid and her husband (the cook) treat their employers – a wealthy man, his wife, and his opium-addicted concubine – as objects of ridicule.[18] The servants steal opium from them to support their own habits while openly mocking the concubine's attempts to overcome her addiction: "If she can quit opium, the sun can rise from the west."[19] To raise the funds necessary for smoking opium all day, the concubine ingratiates herself with the master of the house by deceiving him that she is pregnant, which leads him to lavish money on her. Eventually, her barren state and her compulsion for opium expose her deceit. The concubine's erratic behaviour compels the master back into the arms of his wife as her deception leaves her powerless, a theme common to fictional accounts of the upper classes who while away the potentials of their lives. "Gui" was published in Wu's volume of collected works, *Liang ji (Two Extremes)*, which was awarded the Number One People's Award for its realistic depictions of contemporary society.[20]

The following year, the opium industry was the focus of a play written by Li Qiao (1919-91), *Xue ren tu (Bloody Sword Scheme)*. Li links the opium industry with individual treachery and the state of the nation.[21] The play opens with the female protagonist, Qian Hong, anxiously awaiting the late-night return of her husband, Lin Lang. He is a "courageous and upright" manager who loses his job after co-workers discover that "trafficking in opium is the easiest way to make lots of money!"[22] They conspire to get him fired so that they can deal opium under the cover of a legitimate business. Their immoral activities are contrasted with a positive depiction of the police investigation, which is conducted in a professional and courteous manner. As gunfire rings out, the neighbours are unsympathetic to the "bastard" conspirators and cheer on the colonial authorities.[23] Hong and Lang conceal their former colleagues from the police, and lie about it, at their peril. The chief conspirator, Xiao Peng, eventually betrays his colleagues, who are taken into custody, where Peng argues they will be comfortable in a safe environment with adequate food and clothing. Ironically, they are saved by their imprisonment.

In *Xue ren tu*, turmoil in the family is cast as a precursor to national decline: "when families hasten to difficulties, the nation is cast into difficulties" *(you jia nan ben, you guo nan tou).*[24] The two women in the play, Qian Hong and the boss's concubine, tear their families apart by having affairs with Lang's duplicitous co-worker, Xiao Peng, the man with a "monster's heart."[25] Hong confesses to having committed the "biggest, biggest crime" of adultery with Peng; she is also revealed to have unwittingly inspired Peng's drug conspiracy.[26] Lang denounces Hong as a "traitor to China" *(Hanjian),* linking her conspiratorial behaviour with the fate of the nation and tarring her with a harsh epithet that was applied to writers like Li Qiao, who continued to work in Manchukuo.[27] The other member of the love triangle, the "bewitching" concubine of the company owner, aspires to elope with Peng.[28] She is dumbfounded to discover that Peng is actually in love with Hong, who rejects his final advances. Hong rebukes Peng, swearing that "to destroy other people is to destroy yourself."[29] At the end of *Xue ren tu,* Hong's self-fulfilling prophecy is realized as Peng kills Hong and her husband before committing suicide. In this morality tale, all of the main characters are tainted by opium and betrayal, and they die. The fate that attends them augured ill for the state, which was similarly riven by the disparate desires of opiate dealers and those whose lives were shattered by the industry.

Li Qiao, Mei Niang, and Wu Ying condemned the recreational use of opiates, using such behaviour to engage in sweeping criticisms of local society and culture, as Bai Lang and Xiao Jun had done before them. The writers supported official Manchukuo anti-drug policies while contravening literary guidelines through their denigration of contemporary society. In January 1941 Wu Ying's husband, writer and editor Wu Lang (1912-57), published an analysis of Manchukuo's literary world, "Women de wenxue de shiti yu fangxiang" (The Substance and Direction of Our Literature). Wu lauded the writers' critical stances, arguing that since the late 1930s writers had exhibited commendable vigour in developing local literature, "completely expressing their staunchest, indomitable courage, fully determined to pursue the arts."[30] The writers, he argued, were "all speaking the language of the masses" *(dou jiangzhe dazhong de yuyan)* and shared a "worldview" *(shijie guan)* aimed at destroying harmful traditions.

The following month, officials who had wearied of such worldviews promulgated the Eight Abstentions (Ba bu), which provided sanctions ranging from censorship to imprisonment for dark, pessimistic writing that cultural functionaries argued denigrated Manchukuo and Japan.[31] The Eight Abstentions reflected the critical nature of popular literature being produced almost a decade after the founding of the state. Officials soon supplemented them with the Summary of Guidelines to Art and Literature, or Artistic Guidelines (Gangyao yiwen zhidao), which dictated the adoption of Japanese literary traditions and professional organizations as models for Manchukuo.[32] Manchukuo's writers responded suitably. Gu Ding (1914-64) pronounced the Artistic Guidelines the "most significant matter" of the year.[33] Wang Qiuying (1914-97) mourned the "need to sweep away descriptions of the dark side."[34] Over the following months, media chief Muto Tomio published even more missives condemning "the very troublesome matter" of dark literature – which did not diminish regardless of the regulatory framework.[35]

This dark literature is epitomized by Wang Qiuying's 1941 novel, *He liu de diceng (The Bottom of the River),* in which opium is denounced as a causal factor of the Japanese invasion.[36] The novel is set in 1930s Fengtian and criticizes the elite for a "dissipated bourgeois lifestyle" at a time of national crisis.[37] Their profligate lives are contrasted with those of the poverty-stricken, virtuous country folk who pine for the long-lost Qing Dynasty; rural life is a world apart, yet it is also vulnerable to devastation by the occupying forces. Wang extols rural society yet is critical of the brutality of the occupation and the privileged Chinese who did not prevent it. The novel recounts the male protagonist Lin Mengji's move from the countryside to attend university in Fengtian. Mengji ignores his parents' warning to avoid their urban relatives and is "contaminated" by them.[38] Ultimately, he fails in his studies. Further, his involvement in the Common Sense Society (Changshi hui), a group of youths dedicated to consciousness raising among the masses, is ended by the invasion.

Wang blames Japanese occupation on a Chinese dereliction of duty that has its genesis in the elite's opium addiction. The wealthy shirk their responsibilities and are negative examples for their children, who become wastrels. The "yellow and skinny" matriarch is most ravaged by opium addiction.[39] During the invasion, on "a night of terror in history" *(lishi shang de yi ge kongbu zhi ye),* she toys with her pipe, and the servants hurry about flustered, without a trace of the patriarch.[40] The invasion encounters no resistance and exacerbates youth's "intoxication" *(mizui)* with petty affairs.[41] Mengji's cousins don't smoke opium but spend their lives gambling, eating in expensive restaurants, and pursuing love affairs. Mengji, unable to focus on his studies, returns home defeated. At the conclusion of *He liu de diceng,* Mengji revisits Fengtian to find his uncle dead and his lonely aunt cradling her opium pipe. With the servants discharged, the family scattered, and the region under foreign occupation, the full price of their intoxication is realized.

In the early 1940s, such social decline also came to be linked with alcohol consumption. Li Zhengzhong's (b. 1920) 1941 novel *Xiang huai (Homesickness)* depicts a young man named Jin Xiang who lives in a big city yet yearns for the purity of his home village. At the start of the novel, Xiang enjoys reading and self-reflection, not the mah-jong and coffee houses that attract his peers.[42] His life is turned upside down when his girlfriend, Bai Xueru, unexpectedly marries a rich man for security.[43] Xiang then returns to his home village to discover that the local life he idealized during his seven-year absence is gone. He dreamed of a peaceful life in the village but discovers that society there now consists of "staggering drunkards making wild and absurd drunken talk" *(liangqiang zuihan zuo zhao kuang dan de zui yu)* and ghostly people kneeling alongside the houses, quietly throwing coppers on the ground.[44] His friend Li Shuang explains to him that "before, life was very proper, now it is this evil; before, villagers were so diligent, now they waste money like this. The people here are as though they don't know if they have a future."[45] Propriety and diligence have been replaced by general social malaise, drinking, and gambling. Xiang learns that his childhood girlfriend, Hui Gu, has been engaged to another man, and despite her pleas, Xiang has neither the courage nor the money to ask her to cancel her pending marriage. Gu decries women's pitiful status, which forces them to rely on men of means for support "without a speck of freedom!"[46] Breaking Gu's heart, Xiang returns to the big city and works at a gruelling office job; he also begins a clandestine relationship with his former girlfriend, Bai Xueru, who funds their affair with money she takes from her husband.

Alcohol is central to the plot of *Xiang huai*. To Jin Xiang, drunken Fifth Uncle Zhu represents all that has been corrupted in his hometown, for he is an honourable man who has been felled by addiction to alcohol. Further, Xiang is repulsed when he learns that after his girlfriend Bai Xueru married, she began "smoking, getting drunk, wearing expensive clothes, and enjoying sex."[47] Despite this criticism, Xiang soon begins to act like Xueru. On his return to the city, Xiang accompanies two friends to a bar, where they discuss their lives.[48] Xiang's initial inability to drink is readily apparent to him: his face turns red, and he immediately feels dizzy. Too embarrassed to admit his intoxication, he continues drinking to impress his friends with his "manly" behaviour. Xiang later criticizes Xueru's drinking ability and urges her not to get drunk, but she counters that "only alcohol can tell me what kind of lonely corpse life is" *(zhi jiu neng gaosu gei wo shengming shi zenyang jimo de shiti).*[49] In response to Xiang's further protestations, Xueru retorts, "to not understand an intoxicated person is to not understand life" *(bu liaojie zui de ren shi bu liaojie rensheng de a).*[50] Xiang begins to lead two lives: he works to exhaustion during the day and then smokes and drinks all night long. After a year, he has a nervous breakdown and is hospitalized for two months. When he recovers, Xueru suggests that they break up. Xiang convinces her to leave with him and start a new life, but her husband sends her away on the eve of their planned departure. Alone again, Xiang returns to his hometown to find Gu and his grandmother dead, and he begins to comprehend that "one must do what is proper or suffer loss and loneliness."[51] Throughout *Xiang huai*, the characters are beaten by "the whip of life."[52] As in Wang Qiuying's *He liu de diceng*, Li Zhengzhong's novel is replete with references to society's "pain and destruction" – in this instance, stemming from drinking alcohol, poverty, and long working hours.[53] In the city, Xiang discovers that "reality is so dark, so cold. His days are without dreams; he is like an animal that has lost its idealism, doing things without any consciousness."[54] *Xiang huai* ascribes catastrophic loss to excessive alcohol consumption and urban life, linking them with a decline in morality.

The social decline and addiction that wracked Chinese in Manchukuo also afflicted local Russian expatriates.[55] In Fan Ying's 1941 story "Beidi lian'ge" (Northern Love Song), a Chinese man, Li Xia (who the author notes is a fan of the Russian social-realist writers Alexander Pushkin and Maxim Gorky), has an extramarital affair with a Russian girl, Shaling, and it is through their relationship that Russian love of alcohol is argued.[56] Shaling convinces Xia that her mother, who disapproves of their relationship, will allow them to date if he buys her whiskey. He purchases a half-dozen bottles of whiskey, saying to himself, "Russian people all love to drink!" *(Eguo ren quan shi shihao yin jiu de!).*[57] The mother's "greedy for whiskey inferior nature" *(tanlan wei-shijijiu lie xing)* is denigrated by Shaling, who seeks to turn her mother's desire for alcohol to her own benefit.[58] Xia attributes Russians' love of alcohol to their "sadness of not having a fatherland," which has forced them to eke out miserable existences in other countries.[59] As Shaling predicts, once her mother is given the whiskey, she approves of her daughter's relationship with the older, married Chinese man.[60] But their relationship is ill fated: Xia's son falls ill, and he hurries back to his marital home to find his son dead. By the time he returns to Shaling, she has also died. Whereas her mother tried to find solace in alcohol, Shaling was unable to deal with the depression caused by what she believed was the end of her relationship with Xia. Their "Northern Love Song" was made possible because of the social dislocations that compelled Russians into Manchukuo, but the tragic ending tells of their failed efforts to cope with their trauma.

Russian misery and alcohol also feature in Zhi Yuan's 1943 short story "Bai tenghua" (White Vine Flower).[61] A Chinese man is befriended by a Russian woman whose husband, a former general office superintendent of a Russian railway, is out of town.[62] They live in poverty in a city that is described as filthy; the Russians live in homes with a "distinctive mildew smell."[63] The woman comes from a wealthy background but has fallen on bad times and lives in an area populated by heroin addicts, or "silver-needle guests" *(yinzhen ke)*.[64] The woman is thin and delicate (characteristics that the author notes distinguish her from other Russian women), and she often cooks meals for the Chinese man in her home.[65] As their friendship grows, he begins to wonder how she earns her money, noting that she often leaves home early and returns late (sometimes even the next morning) and that Russians generally sell heroin or work as drivers, coolies, or beggars to survive.[66]

Alcohol plays a central role in the development of the story. One night, the Chinese man takes a bottle of whiskey to the Russian woman's home to drown his sorrows. They drink, and the woman shows him pictures of her younger days and, sadly looking at rain outside the window, paraphrases a line from a Charles Baudelaire poem: "Our grief redeems our happiness."[67] She continues, citing from memory lines from Leo Tolstoy's *Anna Karenina:*

> To now, forty years of life, this life has made me see that life is an illusion. Only when I am drunk do I feel alive. But when I sober up, I see that life is such a swindle, it is so phony. In the future, I'm just going to leave behind a set of rotting bones and countless maggots. Besides that, there is nothing.[68]

The woman drinks alcohol to cope with her lost prestige, poverty, and absent husband. One day, the woman's husband returns, looking like a "perennially ill convict."[69] The three start drinking whiskey. Her husband drinks quickly, one shot after another, until he puts his head on the table, saying that it is best not to think about life because it causes only misery: "Alcohol can make you not have the pain of life, alcohol can also make you not have the shame of life" *(Jiu keyi shi ni meiyou shenghuo de tongku, jiu ye keyi shi ni meiyou shenghuo de chiru)*.[70] He drinks alcohol to forget the pain and shame that dominate his life. In a "morbid state of drinking alcohol" *(yin jiu de bingtai),* he swears, "I use alcohol to exist. Without alcohol, I have no life" *(Wo shi yi jiu shengcun de, meiyou jiu, jiu meiyou wo de shengming)*.[71] The Russian argues that even the cleverest people can survive only by doing degenerate, vulgar, and despicable acts.[72] Disturbed by such excessive drinking and despondency, the Chinese man leaves them and goes out of town. When he returns a few days later, he is told by a neighbour that the couple was arrested by the authorities on the night that he left.

In "Beidi lian'ge" and "Bai tenghua," Russians' misery is rooted in their loss of national, economic, and social status. Russians consume alcohol to cope with their loss, which is compounded by the negativity with which their Chinese peers and the authorities view them. In both stories, the Chinese protagonists look down on Russian drinking capacity, which they cannot match and do not admire. Instead of providing users with the strength to overcome their pain and shame, alcohol exacerbates their losses and sadness. The Russian husband in "Bai tenghua" swears that he drinks alcohol to live, blinded to the self-destruction that is made readily evident to the reader and that eventually causes the couple's incarceration. Alcohol consumption destroys their lives, and both stories implicitly suggest parallels between Russian and Chinese losses in Manchukuo.

Alcohol's destructive capacity is also detailed in Zhu Ti's (b. 1923) 1943 story "Yuantian de liuxing" (A Shooting Star in a Faraway Sky), which depicts a chorus girl named Madan, whose failed relationships drive her to suicide after a night of drinking. At the start of the story, Madan's boyfriend ends their relationship, and she boards a boat to travel on the Heilongjiang River.[73] Searching in vain for love that she believes will make her life complete, she collapses from melancholy and slips into unconsciousness. After the ship's doctor revives her, she believes that she is in love with him. To celebrate what she believes is their new romance, Madan goes to the boat's nightclub, where she "drinks a great quantity of whiskey" *(yin le daliang de weishiji)* and mistakenly believes that she rules over her "kingdom" of men, which comprises the doctor and the captain.[74] Her fantasy is shattered when she is raped by the captain. Madan convinced herself that she loved him, but she is shocked and detests his "excessive brutality" *(guo fen de canbao),* which she blames for destroying her youthful innocence.[75] The story concludes with her death, underlining the futility of using alcohol to cope with life's challenges, the cost of Madan's drinking, and the source of her predicament, namely women's reliance on their relations with men.

The "women's tragedy" *(nüren de beiju)* that Zhu Ti linked with alcohol in "Yuantian de liuxing" was also regularly associated with opiate addiction.[76] In Zuo Di's (1920-76) novella *Meiyou guang de xing (A Lustreless Star)* (1943), an actress, Luoli, recounts her life story to a neighbour. She reveals how her "ruthless" father, a senior official with "three wives," brought her mother into his house as a concubine and then drove her out after she gave birth to her second daughter, Luoli.[77] When he discovers that Luoli has received a letter from a boy at school, he demands that his daughter kill herself for "rebelling" against decency.[78] Luoli refuses, runs away, and is rescued by an uncle, who then conspires to sell her into prostitution. Luoli escapes again, finds true love, and begins to live with the man, and they have a baby. Her uncle re-emerges, threatening to reveal that her long-lost mother leads an "extremely tragic" life of drug addiction.[79] He takes Luoli to the opium den where her mother lives with other "ghostly" *(youlingban)* men and women; their casual intermingling on an opium bed shocks Luoli into acknowledging the depth of her mother's addiction.[80] Her mother's "shameless and addicted hell" *(wuchi er beini de diyu)* is attributed to the loss of her home and her children.[81] After Luoli visits her mother, she is forsaken by her lover, who is convinced by her uncle that she went to the opium den to satisfy her own addiction. Luoli is thus left penniless to raise their daughter. In *Meiyou guang de xing,* three generations of women are victimized by the misogynistic expulsion of Luoli's mother from her home, instigating a descent into addiction that awaits women who are denied the right to family life and independent employment.

Lan Ling's (1919-2003) "Guxiang de jia" (Native Place Home) (1943) also describes the impact of the opium business on women: a widow is abused by relatives who deal in opium.[82] Ming returns home to discover that his mother is overwhelmed by opium addiction, reduced to a mere pawn of his scheming aunt and her brother, who obtains illicit opium through his work at the Opium Monopoly. He learns how their drug dealing has darkened the family name and has cost his sister, Yu, her fiancé because he refused to marry a woman with drug-dealing relatives. Ming's mother is aware of the family's predicament but contends that she is powerless; she would "rather go without food than give up opium."[83] Instead of confronting the drug dealers who have devastated his family, Ming resolves to convince Yu to embark on a new life with him and to send for their mother later. Although Ming questions whether his sister has "a man's bravery and courage" to forge a new life elsewhere, Yu proves ready, willing, and able to go; before Ming approaches her, Yu has already quit her job and packed.[84] In song, Yu expresses her yearning to escape:

> Why can't I be like that white bird above the river,
> To spread my healthy wings,
> And dash out of this dense fog atmosphere?
> Ah! I'm chasing hopes,
> I am looking for brightness,
> Fly, fly, fly, ah, fly![85]

Despite her brother's apprehensions, Yu is buoyed by idealism to escape the "dense fog" emitted by her mother's addiction. Yu rejects the passivity that is ascribed to ideal women and personified by her mother. The two siblings' disavowal of opium reaffirms their bond and, as exemplified by Luoli in *Meiyou guang de xing,* underlines the potential of young women to escape the passivity and addiction that plagues their mothers – on their own volition and without the use of intoxicants.

In the final two years of Manchukuo, cultural functionaries, harried by war demands and continuous, negative Chinese cultural production, adopted a martial tone in their public pronouncements on cultural production. On 4 January 1944 the Manchuria Arts Alliance initiated use of the slogan "wielding pens as swords" *(yi bi dai jian)* in order to incite writers to assertively support the state and in order to steel the hearts and minds of Manchukuo subjects for an intensified war effort.[86] In September 1944, in *Qilin (Unicorn)*, Gu Ding published the poem "Ji mie" (Attack, Extinguish), vowing,

> We will kill you world-destroying Americans and English,
> We want to establish a thousand-year dynasty, in peace
> The gods' lights will shine in all four corners
> Greater East Asia will sparkle with light.[87]

Gu Ding clearly articulated the empire's Holy War ambitions and urged the creation of a unique Manchukuo culture to reflect the positive contributions of Manchukuo culture to Greater East Asia. In November 1944, also in *Qilin*, Xiao Song (b. 1912) urged, "Literati – hurry up and get martial! The Greater East Asia war is becoming very fierce now."[88] These calls to duty came as increasingly aggressive anti-alcohol, anti-opium campaigns encouraged even more in-depth depiction of the Chinese suffering of addiction, economic deprivation, and adversity through the end of Manchukuo, in 1945.[89]

The perils of alcohol dominate Shu Shi's 1944 short story "Zui" (Intoxication), which describes the narrator's intoxication with a few friends.[90] Playing drinking games, they "pour" alcohol into their stomachs and talk loudly, "as if they own the whole world."[91] Gradually, they quieten to play in earnest. The narrator's appearance and demeanour change, as his eyes turn red, his tongue stiffens, and he mumbles, yells, and argues for no reason. The narrator starts wondering why people are looking at him, teasing him. Why aren't others drinking like him? Don't they realize that "one intoxication solves 1,000 worries?" *(yi zui jie qian chou).*[92] He doesn't care and downs even more. He wonders why his friend, Xu Hai, is not drinking but is starting to sway back and forth, along with the cups on the table and the entire room. He puts his head on the table. Hai lectures the narrator, "To drink alcohol to lessen worries, only makes the worries more worrisome" *(yi jiu shao chou chou geng chou).*[93] The narrator rejects Hai's words of warning, believing that Hai doesn't know how to live. How could he know the pleasures of this type of "floating like celestials high?" *(piaopiao yu xian).*[94] He glares at Hai, who replies,

No matter what sorrow you have, whatever unhappiness, the past is past, what has to come will come. This is not a thing that you can use alcohol to get rid of ... Alcohol cannot kill and bury the past or protect against the future. It is merely moments of intoxication. After you regain consciousness, bitterness and hardship are still carved into your brain and standing in front of you. Whatever you have to do, you still have to use your own hands to finish it. Alcohol only wastes your precious time. That is no solution![95]

The narrator is repulsed by Hai's nagging and raises his head but cannot reply; he starts to vomit as Hai continues to lecture him. Hai gradually fades into the distance, and the narrator's head rests on the table again as he loses consciousness. Drunkenness is described as a time-wasting, vomit-inducing form of intoxication that does nothing to improve one's life.

The inability to recognize the dangers of addiction is clearly described in Yang Xu's "Laomazi riji" (Nanny's Diary) (1944), a fictional nanny's diary that recounts how a "good lady" married a rich man, began to play with opium as a "toy" *(wanyir)*, and then wasted her life to "seek death" *(zuosi)*.[96] Eight years of "half-death" have followed the marriage, punctuated by three or four daily hour-long sessions of smoking opium.[97] Much to the hardworking nanny's chagrin, the life of her privileged mistress consists of little more than lying on a bed smoking "life-killing opium" *(songming de yan)*.[98] With a blend of righteous indignation and jealousy, the nanny curses the fact that whereas she is forced to scrimp, save, and toil all day, her "opium ghost" *(dayan gui)* mistress wears expensive clothing and accessories but doesn't lift a finger to do housework or care for her son.[99] The abuse fostered by her mistress's addiction eventually forces the nanny to resign. The opium use that started as a leisurely diversion has become the lady's "half-death" and costs the poor nanny her livelihood.

The impact of opium on women's lives is also the focus of Jin Yin's (b. 1916) short story "Muchang shang de xueyuan" (Blood Ties on the Pasture) (1944), in which teacher Ma lectures his girl students on how to maintain their "purity" and pressures Wen Jiamin to explain to him her falling grades.[100] Jiamin reveals the tremendous toll opium has taken on her life. Jiamin's mother, who grew up in the countryside, gave birth to her out of wedlock and, unable to bear the scorn of neighbours, abandoned her and fled to Harbin, where she was forced into prostitution. Within a few years, she was addicted to opium and had a son and skyrocketing debts. After the Japanese invasion in 1931, she used stolen money to open an opium den with a lover in Fengtian, where dens sprang up like "bamboo shoots after a spring rain."[101] Jiamin recounts how the 1937 Opium Law forbade private sales but enabled dealers to reap a fortune through the sale of contraband heroin. After an accident, Jiamin's mother returned to Harbin, where she was reunited with her daughter, whom she then tormented to support her habit; Jiamin's schoolwork suffered as she stole from her father, and her brother was eventually expelled from school for stealing. After her mother dies from her addiction, teacher Ma encourages Jiamin to resume her studies. Jiamin is thus rescued by a male authority figure who "restored [her life] to its proper place," returning the young girl to a "proper" pursuit of ideal womanhood.[102] In "Muchang shang de xueyuan," a young woman is victimized by opiate addiction, which devastated the life of her mother, but is rescued by a man who aspires to restore her "purity." The young woman is emancipated from opium addiction by the reinscription of patriarchal ideals in her life.

The terrible toll of the opium industry on a larger community is the topic of Wang Qiuying's short story "Lou xiang" (Vulgar Alley) (1944). Wang describes an opium business in a suburb that the narrator characterizes as a "festering finger."[103] The poverty-stricken community revolves around a den owned by the "greedy ruffian" Gao, who uses his profits to make loans to neighbours at usurious interest rates.[104] Even though none of the residents appear addicted to opium, they are all "trampled on in the evil environment" fostered by Gao's business.[105] Their misgivings regarding the Opium Monopoly are expressed through debate regarding whether Gao's lucrative business is licensed. Negativity toward the state is accentuated by the neighbours' apprehension over Gao's business and the eviction to labour camps of all residents without "regular" employment, a threat to almost all of the Chinese. Their misery is relieved only by the occasional drinking binge, which in one instance provides the backdrop for the ironic deployment of a Manchukuo wartime slogan: "Dedicated Service to the National Economy, Exterminate Dark Behaviour" *(jingji baoguo, pumie anxing)*.[106] The dedicated service to the national economy that lies at the centre of the "festering finger" is the operation of an opium den, which fuels the dark behaviour that "suffocates to death" *(dusi)* its Chinese inhabitants.[107]

In "Lou xiang," Wang links the opium industry with degeneracy. Opium dealer Gao is greedy and lascivious, his son is an inveterate gambler, and his daughter is "loose."[108] Gao forces an aging entertainer to become his mistress in order to pay off her debts; she resigns herself to being "played with" by men.[109] Gao's son exposes himself, urinates in public, and screams obscenities at young women. The only positive act attributed to the family is performed by the daughter, who gives a student some money to save his sick friend. But she steals the money from her father and gives it to the student only in order to pressure him to have sex with her. "Lou xiang" climaxes as Gao is stabbed to death by a poor worker who mourns the love of his life, the aging entertainer. In a final insult, Gao's fatal stab wounds are compared to his daughter's "big gaping mouth."[110] At the end of "Lou xiang," the aggrieved worker stands stoically beside the dead Gao. Neighbours gather around but are reluctant to summon the authorities because to them justice has seemingly, and unexpectedly, been served. Gao dies with a violence that befits his life and for the betterment of a community ravaged by a lack of morality, an indictment of the opium industry and those who profited from it.

Perhaps the harshest condemnation of intoxicants can be found in a 1944 special, fifth printing of Zhang Chunyuan's (1920-88) 1938 novel *Hen zhong hua (Flowers among the Hate)*, which links alcohol and opium in the destruction of the protagonist, Wang Ruichang. Ruichang is an innocent rural man searching for his mother, who has been forced by poverty into the city to look for work. After Ruichang arrives in the urban environment, his life is destroyed by addiction. From his first drink of wine with a meal to prove his sophistication to his hosts, he is incapable of controlling his compulsion for alcohol and, soon afterward, other drugs. Ruichang begins binge drinking: "every time drinks, must get intoxicated" *(mei yin bi zui)*.[111] Ruichang wonders why his compulsion for alcohol and opium is so strong after only three months when his new friend, Yu Shide, has been drinking alcohol and smoking opium for years and is apparently able to stop whenever he wants.[112] Ruichang is depicted as incapable of coping with the difficulties ensuing from the loss of his parents and with the complexity of social interactions in the city, which suggests that the roots of his addiction lie between himself and his environment. Ruichang's addiction becomes so debilitating that a taxi driver wonders why someone "with an illness" *(you bing de)* would request to be taken to a bar instead of to a hospital.[113] Ultimately, Ruichang loses all of his friends and possessions. His attempts to abstain from alcohol and other drugs fail, despite his move to another city to make a fresh start, and when he takes another drink of wine, it leads him directly back to opium.[114] The novel climaxes as Ruichang dies alone, freezing and nearly naked, on a deserted street. Shortly thereafter, his cold, emaciated, lifeless body is found by his mother. *Hen zhong hua* is a cautionary tale that links alcohol with other drugs, addiction, and the dangers of the urban environment.

The literature described in this chapter demonstrates the ways that authors linked alcohol and opium consumption with social decline and moral decay. The writers depict characters who indulge in intoxicants for leisure or to escape from reality or who sell them for profit, to their ruin; more altruistic, proper behaviour is needed to save individual lives and the state. The lower classes are shown to be trebly oppressed – by addiction, local Chinese elites, and an immoral society. These stories bolstered official condemnation of intoxicants, yet whereas Manchukuo officials tended to emphasize the economic ramifications of addiction, these writers cautioned of moral decline and its toll. Alcohol and opium are depicted as incapable of comforting or strengthening users. Although both may once have been considered elements of polite society, occupation and war spawned a culture that spurned their consumption. Chinese writers used social realism to shape anti-intoxicant narratives. Critiquing intoxicants proved an ideal vehicle for critical reflection on individual, family, and social life. The narratives outlined in this chapter bolstered Manchukuo policies, as they heightened awareness of the dangers of drugs – to the detriment of those who sought to profit from the industries. These criticisms were not perceived by officials to be directed at the Japanese per se but rather at Chinese weakness and wilful disobedience of the law, discourses officialdom also promoted.

The above writers shared a proclivity to condemn addicts, to scorn efforts at rehabilitation, and to deride the Opium Monopoly, without explicit criticism of Japanese rule. In their narratives, a critical disjuncture attests to contemporary gender constructs. Male writers tended to interrogate the relationship between a world that "is not at peace" and drugs, in work rife with stereotypes that their female counterparts seek to dispel. Stereotypes of lusty, devious women parallel those of abusive men who destroy their families. Male and female characters condemn intoxication for its destructive nature, but men tend to more explicitly link this destruction with society or the state, whereas women associate it with the family and, especially, its patriarchal foundations. Women are depicted as reliant on, or undermining, the men who are their supposed saviours: women distract men from their duties, seduce them, or inspire them to deal drugs even though they rely on men to help them break the cycle of addiction. These narratives not only underline Confucian maxims that consigned women to the domestic sphere but also reflect deep-seated anxieties over the health, status, and self-identities of the Chinese in Manchukuo – not the economic or industrial obsessions that came to dominate official rhetoric. In narratives crafted by women writers, female characters are more often depicted as victims of male abuse; addiction compounded the subjugation of women in Manchukuo society. Writers such as Lan Ling, Mei Niang, and Zhu Ti depicted intoxicants, poverty, and patriarchy as constituent elements of "women's difficulty" *(funü de kunnan)*.[115] The narratives that emerge from their writings are consistently negative, and although they support anti-intoxicant campaigns, they are also more critical of the state than might be expected of a colonial literature.

The Chinese writers discussed in this chapter echoed the Manchukuo regime's anti-alcohol and anti-opium platform because it appealed to them, as it did to many officials, who treated intoxicants and popular culture with a similar disdain: they acknowledged that both required supervision, and laws were drafted to control them, but Manchukuo officialdom never mustered the willpower, resources, or legitimacy necessary to bring either fully to heel. In Manchukuo, writers' support for official anti-intoxicant campaigns enabled the production of a Japanese-sponsored Chinese-language literature that did not simply parrot official policy but also added fuel to the fire of anti-Manchukuo narratives and forged a legacy that consistently reinforced negative memories of the regime. Although the Japanese escaped explicit criticism, dark portraits of addiction and subjugation were implicitly critical of their rule. Despite its military might, the Manchukuo regime proved unable to fully silence its critics or to fully implement its own policies; in fact, certain forms of criticism were encouraged. But the condemnation of intoxicants and, by extension, imperialist subjugation proved as damaging to the Japanese and Chinese who lived in Manchukuo as such narratives had to the English, who to this day bear the burden of the Opium War legacy. In mainland China, for decades after the collapse of Manchukuo, those who had attained high-profile careers during the colonial era, such as Li Zhengzhong, Mei Niang, Wang Qiuying, and Yang Xu, had their personal lives and careers devastated, as they were hounded as traitors for their career achievements under Japanese occupation, regardless of the critical nature of their work. With regime change and the shifting of historical narratives, those whose work battled intoxicants were consumed by the condemning memories that they had played no small part in creating. The next chapter examines fictional and nonfictional accounts of the women who were most prominently engaged in work in the opium industry – hostesses.

6 The Hostess Scare

In the spring of 2009, Hubei waitress Deng Yujiao made international head-lines for killing one official and injuring another at her workplace, in what she argued was self-defence from rape. Deng's case and the judicial, media, and Internet users' responses to it cast a spotlight on the status of women in China's service industries. That same year, Zheng Tiantian published her study of women engaged in sex work in the Northeast, *Red Lights: The Lives of Sex Workers in Post-Socialist China*. Zheng examines women working in a setting different from that in which Deng was employed, but the women share many similarities. Zheng argues that women in China have had "to use their looks and sexuality – the only accepted talents of women – to get ahead."[1] Zheng traces women's status to longstanding collaboration between the state and patriarchy: "The Chinese state has always served the interests of masculine power."[2] *Red Lights* details how women's lives in Dalian have been structured by gender constructs and socio-economic conditions that have led to women being in positions as precarious as that described by Deng Yujiao in her court case. This chapter focuses on hostesses in the opium "retail outlets" *(ling-maisuo)*[3] of Manchukuo in the 1930s, when debate ignited over what consti-tuted the "accepted talents" of women and how they should be deployed in the workforce. Contemporary *Shengjing shibao (Shengjing Times)* reportage, which provides insight into perceptions of hostesses, influenced the creation of fictional accounts of them and other women service workers, such as Mei Niang's 1940 short story "Zhui" (The Chase). Locating their work within debates over early-twentieth-century "new women" reveals the conflicted nature of women's roles in the service and intoxicant industries.

Women have been employed in service industries in China for centuries. By the Tang Dynasty at least, women were regularly hired by wine shops and restaurants to tempt customers to consume the products and atmosphere on offer. In the Tang capital, Chang'an (present-day Xian), young women of "exotic origin" were sought for service; those with light-coloured hair and blue eyes were called "western courtesans."[4] In the late imperial period, women also worked in wine shops, restaurants, and other service industries, as vividly depicted in contemporary novels, including *Shui hu zhuan (The Water Margin)*. The millennia-long practice of employing women in such professions did not diminish the controversies that attended it: these working women were deemed by their critics to be of questionable virtue.[5] Waitresses and hostesses were often accused of wearing "pretty and coquettish" *(yaoyan)*[6] clothing and cosmetics with the aim of selling their products, as well as their bodies, to customers. One commentator, You You, argued that customers could not resist being "intoxicated" *(taozui, mizui)* by the women.[7] In the late-imperial period, as recreational opium consumption spread throughout society as alcohol, tobacco, and other consumables had before it, women came to have a major presence in establishments dedicated to opium sales.

In the Northeast, during the Zhang Zuolin era, "new women" rose to prominence especially in the urban centres, further complicating gender ideals in the multicultural "frontier" region. Local Manchu women were long famed for leading more independent lives than their Han Chinese counterparts. Manchu women did not bind their feet and often practised martial arts and horseback riding. Han migrants to the region found themselves surrounded by more varied gender ideals and distanced from stricter adherence to relatively conservative cultural ideals that predominated in "China proper."[8] The rigours of pioneer life also mitigated sexual segregation and women's seclusion. In addition, "overwhelmingly male"[9] migration heated debate over ideals of womanhood as larger numbers of men sought exclusive relationships with women. By the 1920s young urban women were demanding control over their bodies and rights to pursue educational and professional opportunities.[10] Following similar May Fourth–inspired activism in other parts of China, the women staked out what they envisioned to be "modern" forms of bodily and economic independence. "New women" became symbols of modernity that mirrored their counterparts elsewhere in China, Japan, and the West. However, Shen Kechang, for one, pondered why in the West female professions elevated the status of women whereas in China the reverse appeared to be the case.[11]

During the 1930s, in Manchukuo, Chinese-language newspapers, journals, and other media regularly featured discussion of the "Woman Question" and responses to it. Prasenjit Duara, in his study *Sovereignty and Authenticity: Manchukuo and the East Asian Modern,* argues that during the Japanese occupation an ideal of "tradition within modernity" developed, encouraging women to engage in extradomestic activities while subordinating their interests to men and the state.[12] But such tradition within modernity was not without contention. From the late 1930s, prominent women, and some men, writers penned anti-patriarchal, anti-state critiques that testify to the contested nature of shifting gender mores, the Sino-Japanese colonial environment, and the frontier conditions for which Manchukuo was famed.[13]

Gender was central to the "Manchukuo modernity" that emerged in the 1930s. As in most twentieth-century societies, schools in Manchukuo aimed to shape individual and social identities – and to create loyal subjects. Basic education focused on literacy and "proper" socio-political cultivation. Education for girls was modelled on the conservative Confucian ideal of the "good wife, wise mother" *(xianqi liangmu),* which appealed to officialdom, conservative-oriented parents, and likely not a few of the students. In primary and secondary school, girls' courses were at times augmented with "modern" sciences such as physics or mathematics so that the students could incorporate the latest learning into their domestic duties. Advanced educational opportunities existed but were limited in number, and most were conducted in Japanese; there was further competition, too, for the rare chance of study in Japan.[14] Graduates of the system pursued careers in a range of occupations that included clerking, secretarial work, teaching, writing, and editing. Such work did not provide lucrative salaries but rather degrees of personal fulfillment, economic support, and status. These women worked outside of the home, filling social and economic roles that fitted within accepted notions of propriety.

Hostesses in opium retail outlets, as well as workers in restaurants, coffee houses, and bars, were not generally considered within this same framework of model behaviour. These women were often criticized for work in industries that were perceived to be morally suspect and sexually charged.[15] One photograph from the 1934 book *Manchoukuo: A Pictorial Record* is accompanied by the following text: "The service-maid in an ultra-modern bar using her wiles on the guest in co-operation with the two hostesses. A great number of Russian girls are engaged in such bars in Manchoukuo" (see Figure 21).[16] Laughing, smoking, or drinking, the women workers are described as deploying their "wiles" on the male guest, whose face is hidden from the camera. The women are depicted as an essential part of the business, which depends on their social interactions with, and attraction of, customers. The dangers of working in such an environment were regularly recounted in newspaper articles that described opium retail outlets as sites of sexual violence. An 18 August 1935 report in the *Shengjing shibao,* for example, recounts the rape of a fifteen-year-old village girl who ventured into an urban opium retail outlet in search of relief from stomach pains.[17] Her innocence is contrasted with the evil of the business and those who work there – the bosses, customers, and

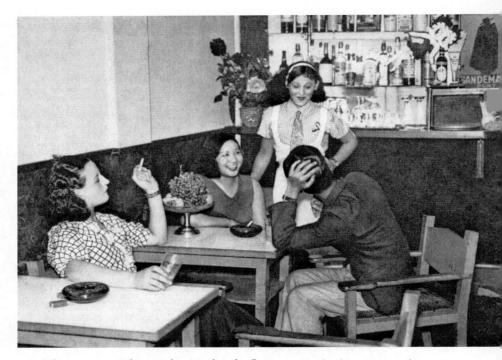

21   "The service-maid in an ultra-modern bar." *Source: Manchoukuo: A Pictorial Record* (Tokyo and Osaka: Asahi Shimbun, 1934), 74. Copyright of the Asahi Shimbun and used with permission.

serving women, the latter of whom are called "hostesses" *(nü zhaodai)*, a compound word composed of three characters. Tani Barlow has detailed the entrance of the first character, *nü* (female), into contemporary parlance and how it symbolized a shift in understandings of gender and women's roles in familial and extradomestic contexts.[18] Meanings of the second character, *zhao,* include to beckon, enrol, attract, provoke, tease, trick, and infect.[19] The third character, *dai,* means to deal with or to entertain.[20] A *nü zhaodai* was thus a female who attracted, tricked, or infected others by dealing with or entertaining them. Each of these characteristics was, for better or worse, attributed to hostesses in Manchukuo's opium retail outlets, which in local slang were often called "flower opium dens" *(hua yan guan).*[21]

Hostess activities varied widely. So, too, did the work environment, which differed from outlet to outlet and from other service-oriented businesses, such as restaurants, bars, or brothels. Minimally, hostesses in opium retail outlets prepared opium for smoking and assisted customers with operation of the pipe. This required specific skills that were either taught at the work-place or learned at home. Often, hostesses engaged in conversation with customers and served drinks or food. Sexual services might have been pro-vided, too, either on the premises or at a nearby hotel, to which the hostess might go from the workplace accompanied by the customer. Hostesses were expected to mingle with men, who (according to contemporary accounts) were the majority of the customers. Not all women engaged in sexual activ-ities. The nature and extent of interactions with customers varied according to the establishment and the individuals involved. Although some proprietors no doubt demanded that the women have sex with their clients, hostesses could grow so popular that they attained degrees of individual autonomy; Su Qiu, for example, deigned to deal only with certain customers and refused to speak with others, an attitude that appears to have increased the appeal of the most renowned hostesses.[22] The majority, however, were not so priv-ileged. Their livelihoods, if not their lives, relied on keeping both customers and management happy. After 1932, when most hostesses had their daily wages replaced with a "tip-only" system of payment, the women found them-selves even more at the mercy of customers for their earnings, which no doubt influenced what kind of activities they would do. The wide range of roles that hostesses filled challenged notions of what "accepted talents" of women were suitable for the workplace. The women's proximity to unfamiliar men, amid erratic application of the Opium Law, made many question what actually transpired in opium retail outlets.

In the early to mid-1930s, discussion of hostesses became a regular feature in newspapers and even inspired the 1933 publication in Tianjin of Yu Zhizhu's *Nü zhaodai quan ji (Hostess Complete Collection)*. The tone of critical re-ports on hostesses is vividly illustrated in the following extended excerpt from the *Shengjing shibao* article "Yan guan nü zhaodai shangfeng baisu: Wushun dangju yinhe bu qudi?" (Opium Den Hostesses Corrupt Public Morals: Wushun Authorities – Why Can't They Ban Them?):

When Manchukuo was established, it was based on the Kingly Way, money-making enterprises, and the discouragement of corruption. The country was to be rich, the people strong. From the start, the private production and im-portation of opium were forbidden. Then opium retail outlets were established and people could openly smoke opium. When this first began, there were only a few smokers. The product could not be sold, and expenses could not be covered. Shop managers wanted to make money, and they did not care about anything else. Step by step, they expanded their shops and hired hostesses who made the business sound. They attracted smokers, did not care about morals and manners, and just satisfied their own desires. These types of hostesses, because of their personal backgrounds or because of their addiction to opium, are all different, but they do the same job and nothing but. A lot of them are shameless. From dawn to dusk, they wear thick cosmetics in order to please the smokers. During the day, they call their jobs burning smoke; in the night, they have skin and flesh careers. Well-organized opium retail outlets have become dens of prostitutes, and leisurely players have stopped going to brothels. Instead, they go to opium retail outlets and choose a hostess to smoke with and flirt with. The customers are very happy with what they get. But if this kind of business continues, what kind of world will this be? I cannot imagine the future. Our Manchukuo, which has the Kingly Way as its basis, should respect the gods and Buddha and honour Confucianism's three cardinal guides and five constant virtues, as well as the country's natural rhythm. If we do not clean up this mess, how can we stand up in the world? Each city has already seriously banned hostesses to emphasize morals and manners. But some proclaim their wealth and become curious [to play]. Because of this, ordinary young people are tempted by the hostesses. The whole day long, "once they lie down and play with the flute" [*yi ta heng cheng duan die cui*], they will gradually become addicts and then a blacklist person.[23]

This excerpt outlines major criticisms of hostess work and the opium industry in Manchukuo. Hostesses are described as greedy, self-centred, narcotic-selling, unlicensed sex workers manipulated by unscrupulous business owners out to undermine the moral foundations of a state grounded in religion and devoted to economic development. Hostesses are blamed for tarnishing the new state's reputation on the world stage. They are blamed, too, for bankrupting brothels. The women are not criticized for sex work per se but rather for displacing licensed sex workers and for their harm to this industry; reporters noted that brothel owners began applying for licences to turn their facilities into opium retail outlets.[24] Further, hostesses are condemned for creating addicts through a fatal combination of narcotics, sex services, and degenerate behaviour. This depiction underscores contemporary debate regarding what constituted suitable work for women and the state of local society, which, it should be noted, is here described as having had "only a few smokers" before Manchukuo's opium retail outlets were established. The description of a hostess-fuelled, expanding industry challenged both the claims of Manchukuo's critics, who argued that solely Japanese domination of the opium trade in a bid to "poison the whole world"[25] was responsible for increasing recreational opium consumption, and the claims of Manchukuo's supporters, who depicted widespread opium use and addiction as one justi-fication for the occupation. Hostesses may have been viewed favourably by management and their clients, but social reformers and those whose busi-nesses were negatively impacted by their work vociferously denounced their roles in the opiate industry. The Opium Law mandated reduction in the consumption of opiates and, eventually, an end to the employment of host-esses, but for years women played central roles as servers, customers, and symbols.

In 1936, four years after enactment of the Opium Law and two years after the explicit banning of hostess work, hostesses still worked in many outlets and loomed large in social commentary. Police records from Fengtian in 1936 recount physical examinations performed on hostesses, explicitly rec-ognizing their continued employment while implicitly comparing them to prostitutes, who underwent similar examination; these records note that many hostesses simply did not report to the police as requested, so the numbers of hostesses examined, forty-nine, does not represent how many women were actually still working as hostesses in Fengtian.[26] Many retained their illegal positions since operators continued to employ hostesses to boost sales and increase profits. According to Hua Jiangrong, author of a 1936 series of eleven articles outlining the state of hostess work, "Yan lou suohua: Ge lingmaisuo nü zhaodai sumiao" (Trivial Talk about Opium Dens: Sketches of Opium Retail Outlet Hostesses), the number of hostesses in Harbin alone was 1,400, with seventy establishments each employing an average of 20 hostesses.[27] Since hostesses were employed across Manchukuo, thousands of women must have been engaged in this work to the mid-1930s despite the ban. The 6 March 1935 article "Lingmaisuo nü zhaodai: Ji qin, ji zong – shi wei quidi!" (Opium Retail Outlet Hostesses: Several Times Captured, Several Times Set Free – The So-Called Ban!) explains that hostesses were retained as "bait" *(er)* for customers, arguing that, just as fish could not be caught without good-quality bait, customers would not be "hooked" *(shang-gou)* without the women.[28] The article contends that men who wanted to consume the opium or alcohol served by the hostesses were actually few in number. Rather, they were enticed into consumption by their attraction to the women. In communities characterized by high rates of seasonal migration and disparities in the numbers of men and women, the social draw of host-esses must have been considerable. The presence of fewer women also con-tributed to anxieties regarding their independence, as women faced greater numbers of men seeking their company on an exclusive basis. Thus women working in jobs that necessitated social interaction with multiple men could become very popular and targets of criticism.

Hostesses began work from a variety of backgrounds and for diverse reasons. Whereas some accounts suggest that close to one-half of their number came from "good" (i.e., bourgeois) families, Hua Jiangrong estimated that the number was closer to one-third.[29] Hostesses who came from such families were typically argued to have been "defeated" by life, suggesting that only low-class and unfortunate women would choose such a career path, if indeed they had any agency at all.[30] In her work on hostesses in Dalian, Zheng Tiantian argues that "social change," in the form of Japanese imperialism, war, and economic depression – all of which contributed to the expulsion of farming families from their land – was the driving force determining women's participation in hostess work.[31] Financial and family pressures could compel women into the profession. So, too, could addiction. Contemporary commentators reflected that if one or both parents were opium smokers, daughters likely learned at an early age how to prepare the opium and operate the pipe and could thus be sent out to work with a skill set they had acquired at home. If the hostess still lived with her family members, which was not uncommon, they likely encouraged her into the business. Some took the job to contribute to the household income, to gain an independent livelihood, or to avoid family or husband control. Others were forced into the job by a relative, partner, or their own addiction. The varied ways that women entered the profession added to its contentious nature: women could be coerced or might otherwise not willingly be there, or they could be in pursuit of freedom, money, men, or narcotics. Thus hostess work could be subjugating or empowering – and it was consistently linked to questions regarding the woman's individual moral character as well as the status of women more generally.

Throughout the 1930s, the issue of "suitable professions" for women was greatly contested. With no consensus regarding women working outside of the domestic sphere, let alone women engaging in hostess work, women's professions were a constant topic of discussion in newspaper articles and editorials. Ruo Xue, for example, argued that hostess work should be perceived as a first step in promoting women's professions.[32] In the 1936 essay "Nü zhaodai de shouce" (A Hostess Handbook), Zheng Zhi recounted how she had once believed hostessing to be an ideal profession for her, lauding the independence and status that such work could bring. Whether Zheng was in fact a hostess (or even a woman) cannot be known for sure, but the handbook expresses a positive view of hostessing and its potential for women in Manchukuo. It is with considerable pride that Zheng wrote of embarking on her career: "Starting tomorrow, I will begin to be an independent *(duli)* person. That is to say, from tomorrow on, I will be a professional *(zhiye)* woman ... From now on, my finances will be independent. I can make some money to help the family. This is really a memorable event in my life."[33]

Unaware or unconcerned that the "memorable event" of which she wrote entailed work in a highly contentious position, Zheng anticipated the financial independence that she might earn from work as a professional woman, framing this independence in terms of her ability to contribute to the family income. She cited two main benefits of working as a hostess: strengthening her family's finances and acquiring longed-for status as an actively contributing member of the household. Unbeknownst to her, becoming a professional woman had serious drawbacks, which forced re-evaluation of her choice:

> When I am hostessing, there are many guests who in a thousand and one ways joke with me and tease me; some even put their hands on me. Heavens! Is this a woman's profession? Does a woman's profession require this kind of being played with by men? Despite much thought, I cannot understand it, and it makes me suffer. I dare not tell my boss the truth, and I do not dare tell mother. I would not even dare to tell the boss that I am not willing to do this job.[34]

Zheng wrote of the lack of respect accorded her in her newly acquired woman's profession. Before she became a hostess, she understood professional work to be respected, extradomestic paid employment, not physical and mental harassment that she had no recourse to resist. Her perception of what professional women's work was, and what she believed the expectations of her mother and boss to be, restrained her from expressing her dissatisfaction, lest it should reflect badly on her or cause her to lose the job that she no longer really wanted but still depended on. Zheng went on to denounce the economic dependence that structured her life as a woman and that forced working women like her to tolerate physical and mental abuse from men. Zheng's expectations of a woman's profession were not met; they were undermined by abusive treatment with which she did not know how to deal effectively.

Zheng's transition from a dependent daughter to a professional woman required not only her employment in an alien, extradomestic environment but also tolerance of harassment and a change in her appearance. Both factors encouraged in her a growing sense of solidarity with other women engaged in similar occupations. Zheng wrote of how she had once been critical of "rouged, powder-smeared women, with permed hair, wearing red and green clothes, sitting in cars with big-bellied men whose hands were around their waists. I despised them."[35] Initially critical of women whom she perceived to have decadent makeup, hairstyles, and clothes and inappropriate relationships with men, Zheng's opinion of them changed after she embarked on her own career and dealt with the challenges facing her. To explain and justify her changing attitude, Zheng recalled her mother's assertion that it was an insignificant matter to change one's appearance in order to raise money for the household. One's moral behaviour, however, was another matter entirely, and she argued that it was not necessarily linked to one's appearance, as she had once believed. Hostessing led Zheng to re-evaluate her perceptions of other women and their lifestyles and to publicly question what she identified as her former prejudices.

According to Zheng, and most other observers, money was a prime motivating factor for women to become hostesses. Accounts from Harbin in 1936 suggest that hostesses in opium retail outlets there could expect to earn between 3 and 5 yuan a day; popular hostesses could make as much as 7 or 8 yuan.[36] These figures were substantial, providing some with monthly incomes comparable to bank tellers, teachers, and lower-level government workers – perhaps even more than the reporters who wrote about them. The sums earned by the women no doubt contributed to criticism of them. Hostesses were chastised in the press for spending money recklessly, especially on clothing and accessories. Hostesses in Manchukuo were denounced for wasting their wages on opium, gambling, and relationships with men that often involved hotel rooms. It is remarkable how closely these critiques mirror those of their "modern woman" counterparts in Republican China.[37] The *Shengjing shibao* regularly published articles critiquing hostesses for profligate spending or, even worse judging from their critical tone, for using their earnings to support their own addictions or those of their lovers or relatives. It was also noted that, in addition to the casual visits of hostesses or their male clients to hotels and restaurants, at least half of the hostesses in Harbin lived in hotels, a sizable contribution to the local economy.[38] However, Hua Jiangrong warned that despite hostesses' considerable incomes, missing a single day of work would leave them unable to meet basic living expenses given that most could not save money and that many were not in control of their wages.[39] Hostesses were constantly criticized for making money in an industry that many viewed as illegitimate, if not immoral, and for not "properly" employing their earnings, or ill-gotten gains. These criticisms underline the considerable economic impact of hostesses in Manchukuo even if they did not personally prosper.

The economic benefits that accrued to opium retail outlets through the hiring of hostesses meant that in the early 1930s, when hostessing was still legal, businesses aggressively advertised their most popular hostesses.

Contemporary observers noted how large banners were often hung on the exteriors of outlets to advertise the merits of the venue as well as the women working within. Customers could be greeted, for example, with banners that proclaimed, "this opium retail outlet sincerely thanks customers and especially hires hostesses to serve them. All those who want the best leisure should come in."[40] Hostesses were advertised for their inducement to the "best leisure" in the outlets, supporting critics' condemnation of their promotion of opium consumption. On North Second Street in Harbin, for example, outlets hung banners listing hostesses by name, distinguishing between them and lauding their attributes: "eighteen years old," "soft and warm posture" *(titai qing wen)*, "attentive social intercourse" *(ying chou zhoudao)*, and "beautiful and pleasant" *(xiuli ke ren)*.[41] Youth, physical beauty, and interpersonal communication skills were cited with the ambition of attracting customers. Some hostesses, especially those with a perceived abundance of these "talents," were able to change employment when they wanted, as in the case of Lian Zhi, who is discussed later in this chapter.[42] This advertising of women in support of an addictive product to be consumed in a seductive environment worked. Newspapers and other media consistently decried men who were attracted to outlets because a particular hostess had launched them on their path to destruction.

The public, aggressive promotion of hostesses and the establishments that hired them enraged critics, who pointed to the Opium Law as a measure to curb recreational opium consumption, not to increase opium use for those who "want the best leisure." In a barrage of anti-hostess reportage in the early 1930s, critics demanded that the industry minimize and eradicate, not glamorize, recreational opiate consumption. Further, they argued that such unbecoming publicity encouraged hostesses to behave with impunity and engage in dissolute behaviour. They criticized hostesses for openly flaunting their wealth and popularity; in a 1933 *Shengjing shibao* article, "Lingmaisuo quxiao nü zhaodai" (Opium Retail Outlets Abolish Hostesses), hostesses were decried for behaving like "Kings of Fengtian" *(Fengtian wang)*.[43] They were also attacked for a lack of professionalism. Student Jun Jun wrote in *Qilin (Unicorn)* that in 1938, when she returned from Japan to Manchukuo, she was shocked to discover that local hostesses were far less professional than women working in service industries in Tokyo.[44] She argued that the ban on hostesses should not lead anyone to regret the loss of a women's profession but rather that it should be cause for celebration given the need to "wipe out the shame of vases" – that is, to end women's use as objects to beautify workplaces. Jun urged that the banning of hostess work increased the validity of "proper" extradomestic employment for women in more dignified positions. Hostesses faced continual denigration in popular media for creating social problems even as critics recognized the personal challenges the women faced, which ranged from opium addiction and dealing with corrupt police and officials to associating with "sex maniac hooligans" *(sekuang liumang),* all of which was said to lead only to "dissolute, resentful matters" *(fengliu yuan shi).*[45]

Hostesses were repeatedly cautioned about the risks to their good family backgrounds of using opium and mixing with men. Even the most "progressive" *(jinzhe)* hostess, critics argued, might first only serve opium to her customers, but within six months she would become "curious and do it just for fun" *(haoqi wanpiao),* which would inevitably lead to her own addiction and destruction.[46] Estimates of hostesses who were addicted to opiates ranged from one-third to virtually all of them. Hua Jiangrong suggested the varied understandings of addiction by arguing that one-third of the women were addicts, another one-third were half-addicts, and the rest were addicts in waiting.[47] Elsewhere, Hua guessed that 85 percent were addicted.[48] Although no precise description was provided of what constituted addiction (full, half, or in waiting), this sliding scale indicates that distinctions were made but that opium use of any kind was believed to lead straight to addiction, destruction, and death. Negative examples of women on the road to such ruin are plentiful. Hua related the story of Cui Yu, a young woman from Tangshan who migrated to Manchukuo for work and was said to be so addicted to opium that it had marred her once beautiful features.[49] Cui was renowned for her "dissolute" *(fangdang)* character, which Hua reasoned may have been inherited from her mother, who was also an addict. Cui was noted for fabricating stories to increase client sympathy for her, urging them to buy her out of her contract. As her addiction grew stronger, and her need for money increased, she allowed clients increasing liberties, including paying to watch her bathe, an activity that particularly repulsed Hua. Hua described another hostess, Yi Ting, who had once been "first class," a status she lost due to an inherited addiction from her mother, an argument that appears with some regularity.[50] As Yi aged, her addiction grew all-consuming, the drug became unaffordable, and her cravings overpowered her, destroying her life.

One of the most serious and persistent accusations levelled against hostesses was that they lured law-abiding young men (students were characterized as especially vulnerable) to opium retail outlets, where they were turned into addicts.[51] Narratives such as this one lasted well into the 1940s, as illustrated by Figure 22, which depicts modern-looking seductresses and a sickly male victim in a 1948 book, *Jiankang zhi dao (The Path of Health),* published by the Yao Shi yiyuan (Yao Shi hospital), which operated in Fengtian from at least the mid-1930s.

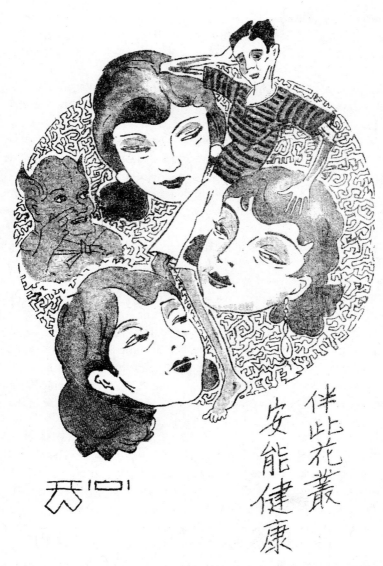

22   "With this flower cluster, can your health be safe[?]" *Source:* Yao Jibin. *Jiankang zhi dao* [The path of health]. Shenyang: Yao Shi yiyuan, 1948, 189.

Reports consistently argued that the outlets lured young men who accident-ally wandered down "the wrong road," lost forever to the women and addic-tion. Men who were not addicts but rather womanizers, or who were attracted by a particular woman's character and/or physical attributes, were at risk of succumbing to opium primarily because of their interest in the women.[52]

Hostesses were criticized for glamorizing opium, selling sexual services, and attracting innocent men and criminal elements alike.[53] Fu Chen argued that hostesses' wilful and aggressive behaviour "cause people to be disgusted by the sight" *(ling ren jian er sheng yan)* of them.[54]

The anxieties generated by hostesses, public interest in them, and the media's depictions of them are demonstrated by the article "Nü zhaodai jian ying fu ye, yin chu cha jin" (Hostesses Holding Jobs as a Side Business, Should Be Quickly Investigated and Forbidden) in the *Shengjing shibao*.[55] The brief article is placed in the centre of the page. The title is composed of characters three times the size of the regular font on the page, having been designed to attract readers' attention. The article denounces hostesses who "trick and bewitch by cajolery" *(humei shouduan)*, entrapping vulnerable young men who are not interested in drugs but are attracted by their beauty and personalities. Hostesses are accused of undermining stable family life by using opium retail outlets as secret meeting places for sexual liaisons. These activities, the author stresses, threaten national social stability.

Perhaps most of all, hostesses were criticized for being "fashionable" *(shimao)*, a term that was applied to women who were considered especially outgoing. Hua Jiangrong provided several illustrative examples. Lian Zhi, eighteen or nineteen years old in 1936, was a young woman from Shandong who worked sequentially at several Harbin establishments, including Ju ying lou (Gathered Flowers Building) and Tong chun lou (Same as Spring Building), where her reputation grew until she was hailed as the Red Flower of the Zui xian ge (Drunken Fairy Pavilion).[56] Hua described Lian as a modern, low-class woman with a "trendy" *(fengtou)* style and "a skin and flesh career" *(pirou shengya)*. The considerable popularity that Lian attained derived from the very characteristics that Hua disapprovingly cited. Similarly, the hostess Su Qiu (original name, He Yujie) was described as a young pretty woman with a mysterious past.[57] A "Temptress Moon" *(fengyue)*, she was deemed dangerous for her looks, with skin like polished jade, and had an admiration for all things "*modeng.*" After she failed to marry an opera actor whom she had pursued, in desperation she wed a man named Wang Chaobin, who was reputed to have been a short, unattractive stutterer. When their marriage ended in a divorce that Su initiated, she returned to her mother's home and worked as an "opium prostitute" *(yan ji)* to support herself, her mother, and a brother. Su's most renowned attribute was her ability to drive young men crazy with desire; they flocked around her wherever she went. Hua also noted that describing her character was easy: she beat her mother, behaviour that Hua believed was sufficiently revealing as to require no further comment. Like Lian Zhi and Su Qiu, the opium prostitute Bin Tou was described as unfailingly attractive to men, gathering groups of them whenever she went to the market. Bin was criticized for her "skill in bewitching by cajolery" *(humei shu)* and for her "indulgent" *(fangren)* and "romantic" *(langman)* nature.[58] Hua attributed to her an arrogance that enhanced her allure. Each of these three women was characterized as a popular, prominent member of her social circle, which consisted mainly of men. All appeared to engage in sexual relations with, or sold sex to, various men, with varying degrees of independence. These portraits of beautiful outspoken women contrast with the depictions of "women in the sewers" or "pitiful maggots in a rouge hell" that characterized most other critical depictions of women in Manchukuo's service industries.[59]

Hua Jiangrong criticized opium retail outlets for treating hostesses like commodities in "a human meat market" *(renrou shichang)*.[60] He argued that the industry was not focused on the restriction of opium consumption but rather on the business of selling women's bodies. Like other critics, Hua noted that even the toughest, repeated warnings from police and government officials fell on deaf ears. Businesses were denounced for their "designs on luring" *(sheji you)* young male smokers through the sale of women's bodies, thereby increasing calls for a total ban on hostessing to maintain "morals and manners" *(fenghua)*.[61] Although most newspaper articles lauded attempts to ban hostesses, Hua also cautioned that bans forced poor, powerless hostesses into sex work, pointing to distinctions between sex work and hostessing, intimating that the latter had greater status to him. Most critics, however, accused the women of being no more than "wild prostitutes" *(ye ji)*, condemning the lack of morality with which they moved from more respectable restaurants, bars, or teahouses to the opium industry.[62] Once employed in the outlets, hostesses were accused of indecent behaviour and indiscriminate sex with their customers, which lured them away from licensed brothels to an opium industry that was supposed to be diminishing. Thus, to retain their livelihoods, legitimate, licensed sex workers were then forced to seek employment in opium retail outlets, where they continued their profession within an illegal drug-fuelled environment, further pressuring other hostesses to also engage in sex work and risk opium addiction.

Demands to ban hostesses and maintain "morals and manners" date from the inauguration of the 1932 Opium Law to the mid-1930s, demonstrating the difficulty of, and resistance to, law enforcement. In Fengtian, bans were demanded by critics who condemned hostesses' outgoing behaviour and blamed them for spreading venereal diseases.[63] In Harbin, in 1934, several bans on hostesses were promulgated.[64] All outlets were forbidden to hire hostesses or to allow customers to linger on the property; authorities even recommended altering provisions of the Opium Law to ban all women under the age of forty from entering an outlet. In 1936 Harbin police again attempted strict implementation of the law, purportedly to maintain morals and manners.[65] Also in 1936 police in Xiaogangzi, in violation of the statutes of the Opium Law, proposed eliminating hostesses by banning all women and men under the age of twenty-one from entering outlets, regardless of whether the person was an addict or not.[66] Authorities argued that if this principle were followed, sex in the outlets would certainly cease.[67] The increasingly serious application of the law caused some social commentators to reflect that a full ban would negatively impact hostesses' families, who had become dependent on their incomes; life would be made even more difficult for the poor women and their families. Hua Jiangrong, for example, suggested that some of the women might be able to apply to the police for a licence to work in the sex industry or to work in a restaurant, but he warned that those who were "old and ugly" *(nianlao maochou)* could have no option beyond working the streets at night as the opium retail outlets emptied, causing even graver problems for the women and public security.[68] Hua's concern for the so-called "old and ugly" hostesses underlines the extent to which youth and beauty constituted these women's "accepted talents" and the latent misogyny that informed many critiques.

The nature of hostess work ensured that the women had varied relations with law enforcement. In Fengtian the police extended the deadline for banning hostesses so that the women could find alternate employment and – as noted in the 1934 police hygiene yearbook – thereby reduce financial strain on their families.[69] In contrast, in Harbin the vice-chair of the municipal police, Yoshimura, ordered full implementation of the ban and earned a reputation for seriously dealing with transgressors.[70] Under his purview, outlet operators who defied the ban faced prosecution or fines. Such fines, however, were openly mocked in newspaper articles, for hostesses were famed for immediately paying fines, buying their freedom with what often constituted only a fraction of their daily wages. In fact, Hua Jiangrong wrote that the women should not be treated as criminals, arguing that the term "ban" was merely a synonym for donations to the authorities; through payment of their fines, the hostesses were performing the valuable social service of supporting law enforcement.[71] But whereas Yoshimura was reputed to have been steadfast in his duties, other officials and police ignored orders or abused their positions. A particularly difficult aspect of hostess work included dealing with officials and police who went to opium retail outlets demanding services without pay and threatening the women; at times, this could occupy the entire night.[72] Hostesses were rarely in a position to oppose such demands, yet as

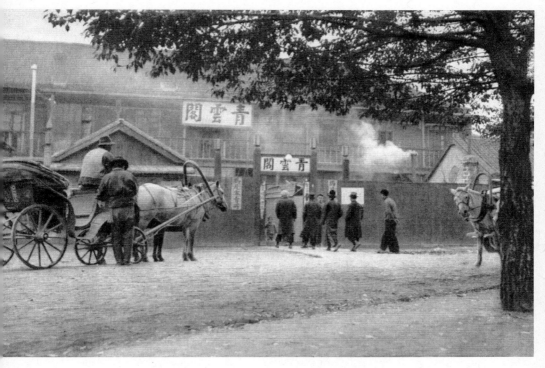

23 Young addicts about to enter an opium den. The signboard reads, Qing yun ge (Blue Cloud Pavilion). *Source: Manchoukuo: A Pictorial Record* (Tokyo and Osaka: Asahi Shimbun, 1934), 280. Copyright of the Asahi Shimbun and used with permission.

contemporary observers noted, hostesses were not entirely victimized by this behaviour. The women may not have received income, but they could potentially parlay such relationships into later favours, including, for example, being warned in advance of raids or being set free on arrest.

Outlet operators, too, responded to bans in a variety of ways. The outward appearances of outlets were transformed as banners lauding the hostesses and the leisurely environment of the institutions were banned and removed. Figure 23 illustrates the bland outward appearance of the Blue Cloud Pavilion.[73] Inside, management forced hostesses into even less tenable positions. Hostesses did not disappear. Many outlets retained the women; they were too lucrative to lose without a fight. Operators might bribe officials or police to disregard their activities or even to work with them. Enforcement officers were frequently accused of being bribed and giving secret notification if a raid was forthcoming. Coded messages alerting outlet employees to an imminent raid included flicking lights on and off or pressing an electric bell.[74]

Hostesses could then hide in a secret room or under the beds, although the latter were noted for being extremely unhygienic – and dangerous when zealous inspectors suspected what they were doing and shoved clubs and other objects under the bed to force them out.

In response to bans and a claimed reduction in business in 1932-33, operators reduced costs and gave the appearance of compliance by transferring responsibility for the hostesses' wages from the outlets to the customer. Some outlets registered the women as customers on their entry of the premises, and they were then paid for services by the actual customers. Hostess fees for preparing opium and pipe lighting or for serving food and alcohol were no longer included on bills, so hostesses had to increasingly rely on self-promotion and approval from customers. For the businesses, this shift had two clear advantages: money could be saved by not paying wages, and the operators appeared to support the law by not having hostesses registered on the payroll. In terms of the hostesses, one advantage for popular women was that they might earn more income directly from the customers, although monies were often clawed back by the business. For most hostesses, the major disadvantages included increased reliance on customers for their income and even further dimunition of their professional status. Hostesses reported declining incomes. With tips generally ranging from 0.5 to 1 yuan, most hostesses had to service many customers to equal former salaries.

Hostesses did not quietly accept the calls to ban their profession. In 1933, when opium retail outlets in Harbin began implementing the ban and firing the women, they responded by creating petitions. They argued that the ban should be reconsidered, postponed, or cancelled so that they could retain their jobs, seek other employment, or not starve to death.[75] On the ninth day after the ban took effect, Dong Guxuan presented an application on behalf of fifty-seven business representatives of the inner-city outlets for the ban to be revoked.[76] In Fengtian hostesses continued their work and began a movement to reverse the decision. They wrote proposals that hostessing be continued as a women's profession and presented their request to the Ministry of Civil Affairs; the women were told that there were no grounds for an appeal but that their application would be forwarded to the Fengtian provincial office for an official denial.[77] Not just in Manchukuo but also elsewhere in north China similar protests took place. Hostesses in Tangshan, for example, established a city-wide hostess association under leaders Jin Xiaoru and Sun Yushan to protest excessive taxation there.[78] Protests continued for several years, pointing to an important feature of the early Japanese occupation. Hostesses complained publicly in the media and to officialdom in order to save their jobs. Their actions suggest that they believed that if they spoke out, the authorities would favourably, if not fairly, adjudicate their cases – because of connections between the management, officials, and law enforcement; because of their own connections; or due to faith in the new Kingly Way system that was being promised. That they did not receive the response they anticipated does not lessen the significance of their assertive actions.

Overall, hostesses were ascribed a negativity that cast long shadows, extending to their fictional representation. The hostess profession is poignantly described in the 1940 short story "Zhui" (The Chase), by Mei Niang,[79] which links addiction and patriarchy in the life of an "opium prostitute."[80] A young girl, Guihua, starts working at an opium retail outlet after her father dies in order to support her drug-addicted mother and brother, who also drinks heavily. As the only member of the family who is not incapacitated by addiction, she earns money by employing the one skill that her mother taught her: how to prepare an opium pipe. Through her work, Guihua becomes addicted to opium at the cost of her youthful beauty, her ability to earn a living, and her dignity.[81] On New Year's Eve, as she joyfully anticipates telling her mother about a new rich client, her brother returns home demanding her wages. When Guihua refuses, he berates her and storms out. Traumatized, Guihua turns to the mirror and sees "a monkey-shaped face in the mirror, with two cheeks dead-red and lips painted blood-purple."[82] Transfixed with horror at her unrecognizable appearance, Guihua's eyes fill with tears, which summon memories of her father's funeral. In a swell of self-consciousness, she comprehends the family burden that has cost her her "virgin's body and heart."[83] Her brother's outburst, which has destroyed her celebratory mood, has finally made her cognizant of the "life-killing addiction" *(yaoming de yan yin)* that has taken such a toll on her.[84]

Guihua's life is devastated by addiction and subjugation in a business regularly condemned by Manchukuo officialdom. But Guihua comes to see the full impact of her misfortune only when she looks in a mirror and mourns her perceived loss of beauty. Both Guihua and her mother in "Zhui" are victimized by men, and Guihua is further oppressed by her mother's addiction. Guihua's free-spending father left the family with inadequate savings and no means of support. Her brother's character is reflected by his appearance: he has a skinny green-white face, dishevelled hair, rotting teeth, and the odour of a dog. Neither man has a positive influence on Guihua's life, and "Zhui" climaxes as Guihua returns to the brothel, where she is fired. Her male boss verbally abuses her in front of co-workers, cheats her out of her wages, and pummels her, tossing her like garbage into the alley. When she lifts her bloodied face from the curb, her wretched fate is played out in front of her as a dog feasts on the flesh of a cat before tossing its skeleton aside.

Beaten, starving, penniless, and craving a fix, Guihua peers out from the alley to see her brother "walking past accompanied by a young simple girl. Her elder brother's face looked as if he'd just caught a fish."[85] With Guihua's use expended, both her brother and her boss turn to new, "young simple" girls to prey on. In "Zhui" the female characters are utterly consumed by men and life-killing addiction.

Opium also impacted the lives of women working in other service professions, such as sex work and waitressing. In 1944 Ye Li's "San ren" (Three People) was published in a volume of his collected works titled *Hua zhong (Flower Tomb)*. In "San ren" sex worker Ye Fen narrates her tragic life to a man who she eventually discovers was her primary school teacher, Liu Linggen.[86] Following a night of drinking, Linggen passes out in an unlicensed brothel in the company of his former student. When he regains consciousness, Fen recounts to him how her mother, who resented being married to a poor teacher, began entertaining men and smoking opium. In short order, her mother spent her days with "opium addicts" *(yan ke)* and "morphine ghosts" *(mafei gui)*.[87] Fen reveals how her father divorced her mother after she burgled the family home for money to buy morphine. Fen and her mother then lived with a woman who sold Fen to the brothel in order to support their morphine habits. Fen is depicted as a victim of "patriarchal society" *(zongfa shehui)* who suffered from subjugation as a young woman.[88] Unable to comprehend the addiction that tore her family apart, Fen asks teacher Linggen, "in the past, wasn't Lin Zexu's refusal of narcotics ... entirely for the nation, for the people, for our later generations? But the people don't know their sad history."[89] Fen links the fate of the nation and its people with the forgotten "sad history" of China's engagement with narcotics, the famous anti-opium Qing official Lin, and the Opium War. Moved by his former student's predicament and her reminder of China's sad history, Linggen resolves to save himself and rescue Fen from her "evil environment."[90]

In Wei Cheng's 1942 story "Kuilan de du shi" (The Festering, Poisoned Tongue), waitress Yu Zhen transforms from a Manchukuo-based Taiwanese professional woman into a waitress and finally a sex worker with a disease that rots her tongue.[91] The male protagonist, twenty-five-year-old Wang Jun, goes with friends to Rose-Mary's Bar to drink and "toy with the women."[92] Zhen flirts with Jun, her boss's guest; he reciprocates on account of her charm and good looks. Two years later, on another drunken spree, Jun encounters Zhen in a brothel, where he recognizes her, is curious about her disfigured beauty, and convinces her to tell him her life story. She reveals that she was educated and once held a government job before turning to bar work. She blames her father for spoiling her, which created her "dissolute nature" *(fang-dang de xingge)*[93] and encouraged expensive, bad habits she paid for with wages she was able to spend as she wanted. Zhen recounts how she was a social butterfly from the age of seventeen, pursuing males, using their money, and taking advantage of them. Her female co-workers started behaving like her, envying her relations with men. Zhen complains about the bother of toying with men and the time that she has to set aside to deal with them; the narrator interjects that she has forgotten her own responsibility in the creation of her problem.[94] After three years of affairs, she lost her job, started smoking opium, and drifted into bar work. When Jun warns her that smoking opium will be the end of her, she agrees but continues to smoke in front of him. Jun believes she is unsalvageable and blames himself for being a low-class man who is always playing with honest women like her, driving them to their destruction. Terrified of Zhen's disease and worried about his descendants if he has sex with her, Jun stays awake all night. At the break of dawn, he hastily abandons Zhen to her fate.

The pitiful lives of the women in these works by Mei Niang, Ye Li, and Wei Cheng no doubt reflect the realities of many employed in Manchukuo's service and intoxicant industries. They certainly reflect the critiques of the women that dominated popular media in the early to mid-1930s. In these fictional works, the women's lives are devastated by addiction, their relations with men, and their generally subjugated positions as women. Each of these stories seeks to foster sympathy for the young women, whose lives are clearly devastated by their experiences, and to evoke disgust for the socio-economic conditions and addictions that lead to their ruin. The stories also relate how the women at times employ, or believe that they do, a certain degree of agency or independent thought, although rarely to positive effect, as their reliance on their looks and sexuality – and personalities – is shown to be futile. Significantly, in each of the stories, the male protagonists drink to excess, although only in Mei Niang's "Zhui" is the man depicted in a wholly unflattering manner. In "San ren" and "Kuilan de du shi" the men are drunkards who redeem themselves by awakening women to societal or familial responsibilities. In only one story, "San ren," is the woman saved, and her saviour is a man, not herself. For the others, a bleak and pitiful fate awaits, as depicted in media that detailed the pitfalls of this women's profession.

The sources in this chapter attribute central roles to women in the opium industry. They also demonstrate the conflicted nature of the positions they occupied; the women could be outspoken and independent even while being profoundly disempowered and subjugated, thus provoking their critics to demand that officialdom maintain "morals and manners" by banning hostess work. Social commentators were outraged that some women were forced into hostess servitude and that others used their bodies and personalities to choose their own employers in a contentious industry that spread across Manchukuo. Some, including the editor of *Nü zhaodai quan ji*, Yu Zhizhu, argued that hostesses faced common, widespread problems: "the life of a hostess, one could say, is the life of the masses" *(nü zhaodai de shenghuo, yi keyi shuo shi dazhong de shenghuo).*[95] In a similar vein, You You argued that hostesses, like other women in Tianjin, were destroyed by the "gradual corrupting influence of evil society" *(e shehui de xunran).*[96]

In 1923 Lu Xun famously queried what would happen to the playwright Henrik Ibsen's character Nora if she left home in China. He answered that women's forced economic dependence on men left women few options other than returning home or becoming a sex worker. In Manchukuo in the early 1930s, she could also have been a hostess in the opium industry. Although the profession was banned, through inconsistent application and observance of the law, hostesses remained in their jobs into the mid-1930s. The women were engaged in an illegal activity, which encouraged critics to attack them as complicit in, if not the actual perpetuators of, the opium industry and addiction. Although many were victimized by the opium industry and their own addictions, they were also victimizers of those who sought their services. Their livelihoods depended on the effective promotion of an addictive substance and of themselves, which inspired criticism in media that now underlines the significance they attained. Perceptions of hostesses and their work were structured by an industry that was riven within by competing forces, namely other businesses and individuals impacted by the opium industry's expansion, the law, enforcement practices, and the women themselves. These perceptions were also influenced by shifting gender ideals. Critics attacked the industry for putting women in positions far too precarious for their own good and the hostesses for not conforming to certain ideals of propriety. Ultimately, critics rejected the women as dangerous sex workers who were unlicensed yet armed with narcotics and coddled by officials and law enforcement.

Zheng Tiantian has argued that a "dynamic interaction" existed between sex workers and the state in late-twentieth-century China.[97] In Manchukuo similar relations developed among hostesses, business owners and operators, officials, and law enforcement. All were engaged with a legal industry that proved impossible to dislocate from the illicit drug trade with which it was paired throughout the occupation and by which it was irreparably tarnished. Officials and police were unable to implement the Opium Law to full effect even if they were willing because the opium industry was so lucrative and impacted so many levels of society. In the opium retail outlets, management, hostesses, and customers negotiated interactions amid a deeply flawed regulatory framework that ultimately served no one properly. Contemporary newspaper reportage and fictional works demonstrate that hostess work was one of the most contentious of the "new women's" professions because of the controversies that surrounded the industry and their perceived influences on women's characters. Widespread recreational opium consumption and the general economic subjugation of women were powerful stimulants to criticism of hostesses in opium retail outlets. So, too, were the women's personalities and their relations with men. Anxieties over hostessing put the profession at the centre of debate over the state of Manchukuo society and the place of women in it. The following chapter engages in a closer examination of what constituted addiction and the attempts to deal with it.

7 Reasoning Addiction, Taking the Cures

> There are many kinds of hobbies *(shihao)* that harm people; the most poisonous is opium, which can degrade heroes and often teaches the rich to be poor. It harms human life even more than alcohol and lust. It destroys people's property worse than gambling. If you are not careful, you will become an opium addict *(yan yin)*, and your whole life will be pain without borders.
>
> "JIE YAN GEYAO" (QUIT SMOKING BALLAD)

In the "Jie yan geyao" opium is listed as the most poisonous of four "hobbies" – opium, alcohol, sex, and gambling – that are commonly associated with addictive behaviour. In *The Chinese and Opium under the Republic*, Alan Baumler highlights the introduction to China of Western narratives of addiction, including debate over whether addiction should be considered a question of sin or will.[1] Baumler demonstrates how, through the late Qing Dynasty and early twentieth century, various words denoting cravings and illness were applied to what many considered hobbies, with one of the words, *yin,* entering into English usage as "yen." In China the term "scientific" (*kexue* or *xueshu*) was often used to legitimize new understandings of addiction, which were, by nature of the foreign influences, believed to be inherently scientific and modern. In Manchukuo, anti-opiate legislation was hailed for being "mighty scientific" *(ji kexue)* and for being created with a "pure medical spirit" *(chun yixue de jingshen).*[2] Received scholarship has demonstrated that Western missionaries and doctors were major vehicles for the transfer of such scientific knowledge to China. So, too, were Chinese, Japanese, and Manchu health professionals, bureaucrats, and anti-opium activists, whose work in China's Northeast has been forgotten or dismissed as inconsequential because of the region's early-twentieth-century warlord and Japanese colonial regimes. Dr. Wang Luo (chief of a medical administrative unit in Fengtian and later procurator of the Department of People's Livelihood), for one, argued that beyond government policy implementation, those engaged in research in the physical and social sciences had to work even harder than they were doing if they hoped to combat opium consumption.[3] This chapter interrogates how people such as Wang Luo understood opium addiction and the means by which they believed that it could most effectively be treated. Of the many products and institutions that were created to deal with addiction, this chapter focuses on the Japanese-produced gastrointestinal supplement Ruosu (Japanese: Wakamoto), a popular dietary supplement that was frequently marketed as an explicitly political "Kingly Way medicine" *(Wangdao yao)*, and on state-sponsored Healthy Life Institutes (Kangsheng yuan).

As demonstrated in Chapter 2, opium loomed large in local life. Opium was so widely used that some argued it was impossible to ban, whereas others argued that its eradication was vital to the future of the human race.[4] The medical doctor Xiang Naixi (director of the Fengtian Quit Smoking Office), for example, argued that narcotics caused more damage than bombs, which constituted only a short-term problem.[5] Similarly, Wang Shigong, a medical doctor and professor at Manchuria Medical University, argued that opium was more dangerous than the bubonic plague because the latter inflicted and scared people for a short time, whereas opium had a long history and was seen by many to be no more than a recreational or medicinal product.[6] Wang also noted that addiction seemed to strike down people in the prime of life, from the ages of twenty to forty.[7] Bai Chun concurred, writing that historically opium was the most difficult substance to control and that addiction stuck to one's bones like a wound that could not be cut out.[8] Bai urged users to become conscious of the need to quit opium lest all harm reduction and prohibition measures the government introduced be in vain.[9] Despite his appeal, Bai was pessimistic that the Manchukuo government would achieve eradication because "there are none who do not indulge" *(wu you bu guan)*.[10] In June 1941, at the New Citizens' Movement to Get Rid of Opium Forum (henceforth New Citizens' Forum), Kudō Fumio, director of the Xinjing Healthy Life Institute, argued that the economic and social losses caused by addiction impacted the middle class and youth most heavily, noting that according to records from his institution, from 1934 to 1940, of 4,286 patients treated, 2,974 had been employed and nearly 80 percent had been around the age of thirty or under.[11] Kudō's assertion countered dominant Japanese representations of addicts as coolies.[12] At the same forum, the director of Xinjing's Opium Prohibition Office, Han Kunjin, argued that it was not the use of opium that was problematic but rather the creation of addicts. Citing a popular saying, "opium addiction is worse than sex addiction" *(yan yin shen yu seyin)*, Han argued for careful control over opium and questioned what it was that made addiction to opium so difficult to treat and the trade so impossible to stop.[13]

Opium's critics roundly condemned it as a "chronic poison" *(manxing zhong du)*, which lured users into addictions that destroyed them in their entirety.[14] In 1930 Ru Gai, a former addict, distinguished addiction from other illnesses on the basis of its ability to afflict both the body and "spirit" *(jingshen).*[15] Whereas physical impacts manifested in various, readily identifiable ways, spiritual damage, Ru argued, was more abstract and difficult to treat. In "Yapian yu renti" (Opium and the Human Body), Yong Boping argued that opium's poison gradually elicited habit-forming physical responses that developed into addictions that then killed users' bodies and spirits.[16] Opium's destructive powers were argued to be unparalleled. Bai Chun characterized opium as "a poison stronger than that of snakes or scorpions, with strength greater than a tiger. The strong man thinks to conquer it and the Monkey King to outsmart it, but their cleverness is actually stupidity."[17] In 1939 T. Nagashima argued that addiction was a stage of "drug poisoning" that dulls one's mental capacity and moral character, making users fall "into a retroceding stimulation, feeling semi-consciousness and phantasm interchangeably."[18] In 1941 Liu Guojun distinguished between alcohol and opium, warning that both were poisons: "the poison of [being] drunk and numb, especially must be known" *(zui yu bi zhizhong du, you buke buzhi).*[19] Users were warned in no uncertain terms that opium was a dangerous poison and that what once may have been considered a hobby or medicine could cause life-threatening addictions.

In October 1941, in "Yinshi" (Addicts), Su Jianxun questioned why people became addicts when it was so widely recognized that addicts' lives were pitiful. Su contrasted their tragic circumstances with an idealized portrait of contemporary society:

> Alas, addicts why do you do it? The Kingly Way is clean and cultured. Politics are honest and enlightened. We do not have the desolation of armies and revolution, we do not have hungry peasants all over the place, and the sun is shining beautifully. Everyone is singing, the autumn moon is clear in the sky, and the whole world is enjoying happiness. The empire is full of kindness and love, the generals are protecting the country and our neighbours. Culture and education emphasize loyalty and filial piety. The kingdom and the people are united in one body. Everyone is loyal and filial.[20]

Su argued that addiction was incomprehensible in Manchukuo with its moral society, good economy, and peaceful unity. Su posited a correlation between social stability and low levels of addiction that may have been accurate, but the society that he described was far removed from the realities of the majority of the population, which faced impoverishment in a racist and militarized regime on the brink of Holy War. Su went on to underline differences between two words that have the same pronunciation, *yin*, yet have different meanings: "hidden from view" and "addict." Su argued that "hidden from view" had positive connotations in the tradition of remaining "aloof from politics and material pursuits" *(qinggao)*, while condemning addiction as immoral and debased. The irony of Su simultaneously lauding Manchukuo and a form of exemplary behaviour historically employed by Chinese subjects who found themselves living in a regime to which they did not believe they owed allegiance would not have been lost on readers and suggests that Su's description of the Kingly Way was more ironic than accurate. But no matter how Su's article was read, addiction was laid bare as the antithesis of health and happiness.

In "Yapian huo zai Manzhou de jinhou" (Opium Calamity in Manchuria from Now On), Qiu Shan argued that opium addiction derived from four dominant factors, the first two of which were linked with alcohol.[21] First, elderly, weak, or depressed people sought "stimulation" *(ciji)*, which he argued made opium equivalent to alcohol and tobacco; he noted that relatively few of these users became addicts.[22] The second factor was socializing in homes, in brothels, or at banquets, especially after drinking alcohol. The third was sexual stimulation, in the belief that smoking opium would increase pleasure during sex. The fourth was medicine, for its use as an "anaesthetic pharmaceutical" *(mazui ji)*. Qiu argued that the path to addiction could be broken down thus:

1   Recreational use: 30 percent of addictions.
2   Medical use: 30 percent of addictions.
3   Stimulation: 20 percent of addictions.
4   Family worries and social instability: 20 percent of addictions.

Each of these factors, Qiu argued, led to addictive behaviour if opium were consumed on a regular basis. Together, they demonstrate that Qiu viewed nonmedicinal consumption as the primary genesis of addiction. Significantly, Qiu did not provide any commentary on the fourth group – family worries and social instability – whereas commentary accompanied the other three listed factors, suggesting a reluctance to offer in-depth discussion of instability and its contribution to levels of addiction.

Qiu Shan detailed varied reasons for opium consumption, whereas others focused on medical use. Jin Long, director of the Dongbei jieyan (Northeast Quit Smoking) Hospital and subsequently director of Liaoning's Xinmin

(New People) Hospital, argued that users were drawn to opium for its ability to intoxicate as a "scientific anaesthetic" *(xueshu mazui).*[23] Parents, health professionals, or other concerned persons might introduce opium to a sick person because of the effective therapeutic and medicinal relief it provided for many ailments. After taking it, the sufferer may feel better, but with continual use for several days, it became increasingly difficult to stop. Personal testimonies of users who became addicts from first using opium for medical reasons were frequently published as warnings to others. Ni Fuzhi, for example, recounted that addiction first struck him as a result of his use of opium to treat an illness at the age of fifteen or sixteen.[24] Ni argued that young people like him were not careful regarding clothing, nourishment, and accommodation, and so in the cold winter they could get serious illnesses or joint pain, which they treated with opium. Local housing conditions were also blamed for causing addiction. Chikamori Kansuke (a medical officer in the Department of People's Livelihood) argued that unhygienic housing in China and Manchukuo, especially the lack of adequate lighting, caused psychological problems that left occupants vulnerable to the influence of opium.[25]

At the 1940 Exultant Forum on Resolving Addiction (henceforth Exultant Forum), a Russian woman, Dariasha (Dalasuo), noted that although over 70 percent of addicts were commonly believed to have started using opium because of illness, she had observed that among the forum's seven participants who had overcome addiction to opiates, three had started because of illness, two out of curiosity, and two due to depression.[26] Another Russian woman, Liubin'ka (Liubinaijia), added that peer pressure and boredom were also contributing factors. Liubin'ka recounted how, as a waitress, she had befriended a Japanese co-worker and begun smoking heroin with her. Dariasha, who worked as a waitress at a dance hall, had begun injecting heroin to relieve illness and pain when her employer would not allow her to rest.[27] A Chinese woman, Yao Xia, blamed her own addiction on depression. She had been raised in a wealthy household and had married a man with whom she fell in love, not realizing that he already had a wife and a child. Having received a modern education, and having what was noted to be "a pretty face," her depression from becoming a concubine had compelled her to use opium, which was readily available in the house. Yao related how she had eventually quit on the advice of a neighbour, the wife of the Japanese police chief, who had urged her, as an educated woman, to set an example and stop for the sake of the nation.[28] As forum participants recounted their use of opium, the chairperson interjected to ask whether the Russian women had started using heroin to lose weight. The women responded that they had not but observed that this was an important factor for other Russian women over the age of twenty-five, when they tended to gain weight.[29]

Men – wealthy, married, and young – were often described as being especially vulnerable to addiction. Dr. Zhang Guochen linked addiction to wealthy families, observing that addiction was not due to the power of the father or grandfather but rather a result of financial status because opium smoking was treated by the wealthy as a form of entertainment that poorer families could not afford on a regular basis.[30] At the New Citizens' Forum, Mr. A. (who was in recovery at the Xinjing Healthy Life Institute) described addiction as a contagious disease spread by wealthy men who were expected to smoke opium and have concubines. He queried, if wealthy men did not use opium – and if not them, then who? – how were they expected to enjoy themselves?[31] In a similar vein, Qiu Shan described opium as a "mystical maiden" *(moxing nülang)* that lured men into its consumption.[32] In "Xiang guomin zhuwei ji ju hua" (A Few Words to Citizens), addicts were told that if they had "a kind of husband's will and a man's bones" *(yi zhong zhangfu zhi, yi fu nan'er gu),* then opium addiction could be eradicated and with it the East Asian "sick man" image, as opium was linked with the weakness of Chinese men and the weakness of the state of China.[33] Based on findings from a 1934 investigation, Wang Shigong argued that 96 percent of Fengtian's male opium addicts were married, 87 percent had children, and 35 percent were businesspeople.[34] If wealthy men were believed vulnerable to addiction, so, too, were young men (especially students), as shown in Chapter 6, as popular media in the early 1930s exploded with anti-hostess rhetoric that depicted the women as dangerous sirens who lured unsuspecting young men to their ruin.

Commentators were perhaps most disturbed, if not outright horrified, by women addicts. At the New Citizens' Forum, Yong Shanqi (director of the Opium Administration in the Opium Prohibition Department) argued that both young and women users should not be overlooked by popular preoccupation with older wealthy men.[35] Women, Yong also asserted in his writings, constituted 30 percent of addicts and were especially vulnerable to opium because of their exhaustion from professional work and their interactions with customers and others who might introduce them to drugs.[36] As with men, women were argued to have begun to smoke in order to treat pain, including menstrual and birthing pains.[37] Others argued that women became addicts because they were mentally weak or tempted by family.[38] Women were told that if they could stop the habit of binding their feet, they could also stop smoking opium and thereby transform themselves from "too weak to stand a gust of wind bound-feet girls" *(ruo bu jin feng de guozu guniang)* into "healthy-feet modern females" *(jian jiao de jindai de nüxing).*[39] In "Funü xiyan zhi hai" (The Harm of Women's Smoking), women, especially, were advised to respect "scientific progress" *(kexue de jinbu)* in the pursuit of healthful living. Good health, Yu Li reasoned, was the foundation of the physical beauty that, he mused, everyone desired.[40] Yu argued that women's achievement of health and beauty was reliant on proper "hygiene" *(weisheng),* which opium destroyed. Yu denounced women users for shaming their families, neglecting household responsibilities, rebelling against the family system, and bankrupting families. Yu wrote:

> Women's responsibilities in the home are huge. To strengthen the country's races, we must pay attention to women's bodies. This responsibility is not easy to deny because a person's basic education and physical strength rely on the mother. For example, America has attained its strong position in the world due to the moral politician Mr. Washington. Washington became so great because behind him he had a good and kind-hearted mother. It is by this [example] that we can know what a mother's duty is.[41]

Yu believed that women's use of opium destroyed their maternal instincts, weakened their bodies, and cost them their beauty. Women users also endangered children who relied on them and potentially turned their babies into addicts before they were born. Yu stressed the importance of their maternal duties by praising the first American president and his mother. He strongly criticized women users for their inability, or refusal, to realize the contemporary conservative ideal of the "good wife, wise mother," thereby threatening the structures that held society together. Yu rejected women addicts as "a rubbish heap of bones of the dead" *(lajidui de baigu).*[42]

What exactly caused addictive behaviour in women and men is the focus of Jin Long's 1930 series of articles, "Yapian yin zhi yanjiu" (Opium Addiction Research). Jin argues that four characteristics can be analyzed to determine the nature of opium consumption, whether such use constitutes an addiction, and the severity of the addiction:

1 Analysis of morphine. Based on the composition of the opium, as it enters the body, percentages of morphine increase and one becomes an addict. Depending on the strength of the drug, the quantity of smoking increases.
2 Physical resistance to the poison develops. In response to the composition of the opium, a form of poison-resistance system develops and results in addiction.

3 Acidification. As morphine enters the body, this kind of resistance develops and results in addiction.
4 Feelings are reduced. The body blocks the effects of opium, the character is weakened, and this results in addiction.[43]

Jin describes opium addiction as an impermanent condition that is dependent on congenital factors, absorption or "affinity" *(qinheli)* rates, and the strength of the drug being consumed; human responses to opium are as divergent as the drug itself. Individuals have varied physical responses to the drug, as levels of opiate in the bloodstream fluctuate in response to absorption ability.[44] In the first stages of addiction, Jin argues, physical reactions to opium gradually decrease as the blood's ability to absorb the drug increases. Addiction develops as changes in absorption patterns and percentages needed for intoxication occur.[45] These shifts are accompanied by physical and spiritual changes with poisonous consequences.

Both the physical and spiritual effects of opium addiction were subjects of analysis. In 1941 Dr. Kudō Fumio argued that addicts were physically weakened by gradual but consistent increases in their intake of opium, which sapped their energy while increasing opiate capacity, leaving them weak and unable to work.[46] Addicts were described as "early-stage development foetuses" *(chun zhi yu tai)*, with little energy or ability.[47] Opium addicts were popularly called "smoke ghosts" *(yan gui)*, reinforcing observers' estimations of their pitiful combination of poor health and weakness.[48] Bao Kun detailed changes that he believed were wrought to addicts' bodies and personalities, as numbness and fear became dominant physical and spiritual states.[49] Prolonged opium consumption was argued to reduce the production of saliva, increase perspiration, decrease pupil size, and make the body skinny and weak.[50] Constipation, indigestion, insomnia, pain, and sexual dysfunction plagued the body as the user came to fear that withdrawal would bring uncontrollable pain, vomiting, diarrhea, and, ultimately, death. Su Jianxun warned addicts that their belief in opium's efficacy as a stimulant was misguided and that habitual use fated them to become quiet and melancholic, with sadness, fear, and nervousness overtaking all other emotions.[51] Qu Kezhong dramatically spelled out the problems of opium use in 1941 in "Jin yan bai zi ci" (Banning Smoking One Hundred Word Poem).[52] In the first diamond-shaped entry, Qu recounted the physical and social ramifications of opium use, detailing the catastrophic consequencers for users, their families, and the larger society. In the second entry, pleading with users to abandon their bad practices, Qu outlined the benefits that accrued to quitting smoking and that would help to make Manchukuo a "paradise land":

Ah
Opium
Lets people fall
Into incalculable damage
With yellow face and dull eyes
The body weak and the nerves in disorder
Clothes are a total mess, the material is very common
Falling to the extent that relatives and friends only look down on you
Your brothers and wife, all of your flesh and blood, leave and scatter away
Father's and mother's eyes watch you, expecting you to put a stop to the smoke
What a pity that all the ancestors' money in the thousands is spent and gone
In the daytime you knock on every door begging for food
At night you sleep in the temple courtyard
A brick for a pillow, torn blanket
Soon, the north wind comes
Big big snowflakes
Instantly you die
Really deep
Sigh

Wish
You addicts
Much happiness
Early to stop the smoke
March onto the bright path
Your body will be strong as a tiger
Jump out of the bitter sea and into paradise land
From then on, save your money to put toward the country
The nation will be strong, the people will be rich, such happiness
Turn back to become a human, if not you can't toss away the bitterness
For you to stop smoking today, it would be as great as could be
Do not remonstrate from now on, the future can be mended
Observe kindness, be good to neighbours, be sincere
Instruct children in the civil and military
Live in Manchuria paradise land
Poultry feast, beat a drum
Early to quit
Blessing
Wish

Critics charged that the physical and social dysfunction that ruined addicts' lives impacted the people around them: once addicted, users were interested only in smoking, talking, eating, gambling, and sex.[53] Although most recognized that prolonged usage resulted in declining interest in the latter, a popular folk saying in north China asserted that "when men become addicted to opium, they destroy their families and become lascivious; when women become addicted to opium, the belt holding up their trousers slackens."[54] Critics of recreational opium use charged that addicts stopped caring about family, responsibilities, and reputation as their lives were consumed by compulsions for opium. They worked less. Creative abilities disappeared. Kudō Fumio argued that all addicts lied and lost any sense of shame even, he noted, to the extent of selling their wives – although he did recognize that women became addicts as well.[55] Addiction was said to bankrupt families and to force wives and children to be pawned without remorse, driving women into illicit relationships or sex work.[56] When drug supplies ran out, addicts would do illegal and immoral things for more. Finally, they became beggars and died, usually on the street. These are the narratives that dominated critics' descriptions of addicts' lives in the 1930s and 1940s. Although there can be no denying that many experienced this devastation in their lives, opium was also used by people who did not become "addicts." Others became what might be considered "addicted" and lived productive and meaningful lives. Discrepancies in responses to opium problematized efforts to determine the most appropriate interventions for ending addiction or for reducing harm to those whose lives were most at risk.

Even more dangerous than opium in terms of the potential to create addiction was opium's derivatives, such as heroin and morphine, which Jin Long named a "wonderful, supernatural powder medicine in this world" *(renjian shen dan miaoyao)*.[57] First isolated in the early 1800s in Europe, morphine had become widely demonized in Manchuria by the 1920s. Either consumed orally or injected, it was used to treat pain, exhaustion, and hunger. Like opium, morphine was used recreationally. Morphine was also prescribed to wean addicts off opium, frequently leading to morphine addiction; in 1935 this withdrawal method was condemned as a conspiracy of greedy European businessmen.[58] Although medical professionals assured addicts that morphine treatment could end opium addiction without pain, the increasing consumption of the drug over a prolonged period tended to numb the nervous system, damage the body, and result in addiction as well.[59] At the Exultant Forum, recovered addicts Dariasha, Jin Chengrong, and Xing Canlü recounted their experiences with morphine. Dariasha argued that when deprived of morphine, she thought only of how to get more and would do anything for it. Jin agreed, adding that morphine users gained a sense of calm when using but lost their conscience. Jin also described overwhelming anxieties and feeling as though someone were watching him all the time, especially when he was hiding his drugs and paraphernalia. Xing reported similar feelings of anxiousness. The chairperson mused that these anxieties were likely a psychological response to engaging in illegal activities. Xing responded with outrage: he had started using morphine to quit opium under a doctor's orders but soon found himself addicted to morphine and hating his doctor. Xing was not alone. In October 1939 anger over another doctor, Zhao Yinglin, and his constant prescription of morphine led to public protests in Harbin.[60] Prominent dissatisfied customers, claiming to have been cheated out of hundreds or thousands of yuan, gathered outside of the Huaying yishi in the afternoon of 13 October. Facing the angry crowd of business managers and representatives of local organizations – many of the men and women, and their positions, were mentioned by name in the *Shengjing shibao (Shengjing Times)* – Zhao attempted to convince them of the efficacy of his treatments and his well-meaning intentions. Coverage of the event noted that Zhao was ultimately unsuccessful in calming the crowd. Such a public protest suggests that the outraged believed that their demonstration could be effective. It certainly proved newsworthy.

Morphine was denounced not only for its addictive potential but also for the forms of consumption in which users engaged. Taking a pill or using a needle were activities far removed from the culture, accoutrements, and sociability that gave smoking opium or drinking alcohol their airs. Additionally, the unsanitary use of hypodermic needles left scars and wounds that were pictured in newspaper photographs to terrify readers. Reports of morphine-induced deaths became regular features in media from the late 1910s to the 1940s; representative titles included "Mafei wei lu" (The Dead End of Morphine) and "Su yu mafei" (Dead from Morphine).[61] The devastation associated with morphine resulted in even less sympathy for these addicts than for opium addicts. Zhao Kuiru argued that under no circumstances, even on the coldest days of winter, should anyone give money to morphine addicts – despite their inadequate clothing, food, and accommodation.[62] Zhao argued that if they were given money, they would spend it only on morphine, which would further encourage them to steal and lie later. Condemning addicts as thieves and miscreants, Zhao suggested that they only needed to become conscious of their self-inflicted damage and they would stop poisoning themselves and end their predicament. Zhao was convinced that it took only conscious awareness to overcome addiction.

Despite Zhao Kuiru's certainty, no consensus existed regarding effective methods to quit using opiates. Zhao Min, a recovered addict, argued from personal experience that there were two main approaches: to naturally reduce intake or to medicate.[63] Natural reduction could be accomplished on a day-to-day basis, without causing pain, over a period determined by the user. During withdrawal, the consumption of mild salt water was recommended in order to dilute the blood and assist in ejecting the poison; temptations such as tasty food, overeating, and areas where people smoked were to be avoided. If medication was used, withdrawal could be achieved more quickly, in ten days, with the first few days being crucial. During the first three to five days, medicine, exercise, and relaxing would ease the transition and reduce pain, while reading and other hobbies could provide useful diversions; sleeping on one's side rather than flat on the back was suggested. Drinking alcohol was forbidden, as it would directly lead to smoking opium again. Zhao noted that hospitalization was preferable, with supervision to ensure optimal outcomes. Dr. Itō Ryōichi (a researcher of pharmacology under the supervision of professor Kubota Seikō at Manchuria Medical University) agreed with Zhao that the first three to five days of withdrawal were most important.[64] After a week the pain would subside, and in about ten days the appetite would return, along with one's complexion and body weight. Itō argued that although to quit using was simple – one could just stop – there was no avoiding the danger and pain that accompanied withdrawal, no matter how it was achieved. Hospital administrator Jin Long cautioned that addiction took slightly longer to dissipate, five to six days, and that to suddenly stop without medication could have drastic consequences for one's health.[65]

In "Manzhouguo yapian wenti" (The Manchukuo Opium Question), Dr. Wang Shigong outlined the three methods that he believed were most effective in assisting users in overcoming addiction's physical and spiritual effects.[66] The first was to replace opium with another drug, such as cocaine or morphine, as prescribed to such disapproval by the Huaying Clinic's Zhao Yinglin. Wang noted that this popular method was dangerous but effective if professionally supervised. Zhang Jiyou, director of the People's Livelihood Department, also warned of morphine's addictive nature and that if it were not properly dispensed, it could be worse than opium: users would "drive a wolf into a tiger's mouth" *(qu lang ru hu)*.[67] Other alternate replacement treatments included aminopyrine, hydrocotarnine hydrochloride, insulin, sedatives, and spamidol. The second method suggested by Wang Shigong was hypnosis, which could accomplish withdrawal as quickly as in one week but was dangerous because of disruptions to metabolism. Wang noted that the first-week recovery rate by this method was 50 percent and that full treatment often took two weeks to a month. The third method was, as Zhao Min suggested above, for the user to gradually reduce the consumption of opium. This, Wang argued, was the easiest, least painful, and lengthiest of the procedures.

Zhang Jiyou urged users to put aside fears that their bodies would not survive withdrawal and to begin treatment without hesitation. Despite admitting that economic oppression in Manchukuo created an unfavourable environment for most people to quit successfully, Zhang argued the efficacy of three main methods of treatment for domestic or institutional withdrawal: "ban and stop method" *(jinduan fa)*, "gradual reduction method" *(jian jian fa)*, and "rapid reduction method" *(ji jian fa)*.[68] Each method had positive and negative features and different proponents. Zhang cited Western researchers' support for various methods: the ban and stop method was praised by German researcher Wolff; gradual reduction was preferred by Bonhoeffer and Meyer, which they argued enabled the addict to better regain body strength; and the gradual method was also recommended by Erlenmeyer (eight to ten days), Lambert (fourteen days), and Dupouy (twenty-one days) if patients were thin, weak, or had swollen glands. Zhang noted that the rapid reduction method was often used in state facilities, where the user's physical, not psychological, needs were prioritized. The rapid reduction method met with what many officials viewed as the obligation to "fulfil the medical treatment capability" *(yi jin yiliao zhi nengshi)*, ending addiction without the "formalities" *(shouxu)* and expense of treating the totality of addiction as described by the specialists and recovered addicts in this chapter.[69] Wang Luo and Xiang Naixi, too, argued for a "stop and ban symptom" *(duanjin zhengzhuang)* approach, or as they phrased it, with explicit reference to German research, "abstinenz-erscheinung" (abstinence-appearance).[70] Zhang, Wang, and Xiang studied international developments in addiction treatment, evaluated rehabilitation in Manchukuo, and with a critical tone shared their findings with readers.

Most recovered addicts, health professionals, and commentators argued that "will" *(yizhi)* was an essential factor in treating addiction.[71] Zhang Jiyou cited European research in support of his assertion that psychological conditions determined addictive behaviour.[72] Xiang Naixi argued that "the weak-willed easily acquired addiction" *(yizhi boruo yiran gai shihao)*, as they were susceptible to what he perceived to be the psychological aspects of addiction.[73] Bai Chun and Liu Lang argued that even the best medication and strictest government regulations were in vain if one lacked the resolution to quit.[74]

These opinions were not new, but by the late 1930s they had become ascend-ant. As early as 1906, in "Jie yan baihua" (Plain Talk about Quitting Smoking), Takeo Akiyoshi had argued that users must admit their addiction and daily recognize its ramifications for their lives.[75] Takeo defined addiction thus: "Addiction is attraction. Addiction is waywardness. Addiction is habit" *(Yin shi yin. Yin shi ren. Yin shi guanyin).*[76] Takeo linked firm and patient commit-ment to abstinence with the effectiveness of any treatment; "in the end it is up to your determination" *(zhong zai hu ni lizhi).*[77] Takeo stressed that such resolve could be generated by fostering patriotism and community spirit.[78] Personal development was often linked with success in overcoming addic-tion. Ru Gai, a Manchu and former addict, argued that it was also important to train the body with exercise, including *gongfu* and traditional Manchu sports such as riding and shooting: "The customs of the Manchus are very important to virtue."[79]

For those who sought medical help to quit opium, a wide range of products was promoted by commentators such as Yong Boping, who argued the neces-sity of combating the poisons of opium with "antitoxins" *(kangdusu).*[80] Several of these stand out for their prominent advertising.[81] Ebosi (Aibiaosi), for example, was a nutritional supplement and brewers' yeast composed mainly of vitamin B. It was produced by the Japanese Asahi beer company (Dai-Nippon Breweries) and was targeted at the excessive acidification that profes-sionals such as Jin Long linked with addiction.[82] Ads for Ebosi were regularly featured in the *Shengjing shibao* and *Qilin (Unicorn).* Other lesser-known medications were credited to individual doctors or clinics, especially via testimonial ads and articles. Liu Lang, a recovered addict, stressed that ad-dictions varied among the afflicted and that the efficacy of medications, too, should necessarily vary; he recommended treatment from the Harbin-based doctor Zhang Xinglou as well as a Tianjin product made from egg yolks.[83]

Injectable anti-opium medicines were very popular, preferred by some because they did not have to be swallowed, so they would not be smelled, vomited, or excreted. Figure 24 depicts a patient in a clinic being injected to treat opium addiction.[84] Brands included Anqimaoqin, a Japanese medicine invented in Osaka, which was promoted for being able to cure "light addic-tions" in as little as four injections; "heavy addictions" could require up to twenty.[85] Nie'ou'moxi'en (Neo-Mohyn) was advertised as a product used in Germany and tested in Japan by chemists Takase and Kikuchi. It was touted as a nonaddictive medicine that was three to five times as effective as mor-phine in getting users off opium or heroin.[86] The locally produced Puluojiabing was advertised as a painless product to wean users from opium, morphine,

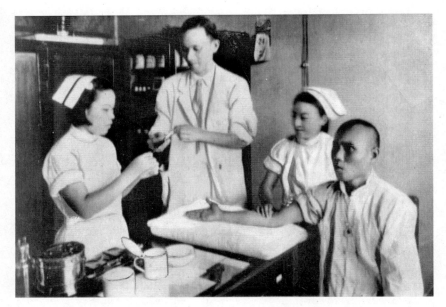

24   "Treating an addict." *Source: Daily Times,* photograph dated 26 February 1937, company name unclear.

red pills *(hongwan)*, and heroin.[87] Puluojiabing was produced in Xinjing with state sanction and sold in pharmacies at relatively inexpensive prices; each box cost 2 yuan and contained ten vials. Ads promoted Puluojiabing as a safe product with no side effects of pain, vomiting, or diarrhea; government workers and businesspeople were assured that they would not need to miss a single day of work during withdrawal. Ads attributed to it an "above average" success rate and explicitly assured consumers that it was not one of those medicines in the markets that were ineffective or dangerous. A late addition to the roster of cures was the amphetamine Dongguang ji (Eastern Light Agent), which Qiao Enrun, director of the Fengtian Ban Smoking Office, argued provided the fastest, absolute cure for opium addiction.[88]

The lofty advertising promises for anti-opium products generated considerable controversy. Itō Ryōichi argued that although there appeared to be many ways to treat opium addiction, none were very effective and that all addicts had to be wary of products or institutions that offered pain-free withdrawal since the process necessarily involved pain.[89] Xiang Naixi, too, warned against ads for commercial products that boasted one could quit without pain because it was not true and wrote that relapses occurred in about 80 percent of cases; in the academic journal *Dongfang yixue zazhi (Far Eastern Medical Journal)*, Xiang detailed seventy-nine distinct Chinese medicines and methods of treating addiction.[90] Wang Shaoxian, director of the Anti-Opium Department in Rehe, railed against commercial products, charging that most were ineffective and that products containing morphine were especially unsuited for quitting smoking opium since morphine was even more dangerous.[91] Consumers were also warned against purchasing fake replications of the ineffective or dangerous goods. Warnings about medicines and treatments were conveyed to consumers in articles by bureaucrats such as Wang as well as in news stories that recounted tragic deaths. One official in Yingkou, Shi Ziheng, aged twenty-seven, was reportedly killed by a powdered formula called Lingyiji (Supernatural Pharmaceutical).[92] He purchased a bottle for 12 yuan, and within hours of consuming it, he began vomiting and died. Addicts like Shi faced the perils not only of withdrawal but also of products that could be ineffective, fake, or fatal. Prominent advertisers consistently reassured consumers that their products were effective and safe.

The most heavily publicized anti-opium product was Ruosu, a dietary supplement created in 1929 in Tokyo by the joint-stock company Society for Nutrition and Raising Children.[93] Ruosu was developed by the Japanese scientist Sawamura Makoto, who built on Nobel laureate Ilya Mechnikov's theory of longevity, which advocated the use of lactobacilli to counter the loss of friendly bacteria in the intestines and thereby protect health and prolong life. Ruosu consisted of vitamins (especially B1, B2, and D), spermin, lecithin, cholesterin, and other substances, which together were credited with producing three healthful enzymes (protein, fat, and starch) that could enrich and extend human life, reduce the harm of alcohol and opium consumption, and assist users in withdrawal.[94] Ruosu ads promised to make consumers' bodies "as strong as steel and brass," as reflected in the product's symbol, a shot-put thrower.[95] The supplement was kept affordable through the 1930s and 1940s for at least middle-class, urban consumers at 1.6 yuan for either a twenty-five-day supply of pills or a thirty-day supply of powder. Ruosu was advertised as less expensive yet more effective than other supplements that promised to treat addiction while improving digestion, circulation, and intestinal fortitude.[96]

Ruosu was launched with great fanfare in the Northeast and became a leading consumer product, with a prominence noted by historian Jiao Runming, who observes that by the late-Manchukuo period it had become one of the only nutritional supplements available.[97] Ruosu ads were standard features in journals and newspapers, ranging in size from a few columns to the whole page. In *Qilin*, ads most often showcased images of strong, healthy, and happy adults or children, hardy pine trees, or pastoral landscapes. Ads in the *Shengjing shibao* often appeared as essays under headings such as

"Common Medical Knowledge," providing readers with reports on the latest medical breakthroughs and linking them with the consumption of Ruosu. Such essays were frequently located on pages featuring news reports and editorials on achievements in the battle against opium or alcohol addiction. The placement, prominence, and great variety of Ruosu ads underline the ambition of its producers to win over, and improve the health of, local consumers.

Ruosu ads in the *Shengjing shibao,* especially, often featured expressly political messages. The producers of Ruosu extended their congratulations to the regime with an impressive full-page advertisement titled "Qingzhu chengren Manzhouguo" (Celebrate the Recognition of Manchukuo). The following praise for the state was published on 16 September 1932, two days before the first anniversary of the military action that had led to its founding:

> Manchukuo's creation still has yet to reach one year, yet it has already attained healthy development. What is the reason? You must know that the primary element is the Kingly Way ideology. It is by agreement of the 30 million people so that they can fully develop. Already closely interdependent, the progressive Japanese government was the first to extend recognition. This is such a lucky, such a glorious affair. We can expect that from now on, Manchukuo's own capacity and survivability will be stronger, such that various kinds of minor sicknesses will naturally be gradually extinguished. With each peaceful passing day increasing the friendly nations' power to help, how can every day not be newer and more up-to-date? Just because of that, our company produces Ruosu. For those people who have enterogastritis, taking it will regulate the intestines and stomach. Not only can newly ill patients recover, but the quality of intestine and stomach resistance quality will also naturally be increased. This humble opinion is sincerely conveyed to congratulate Manchukuo on its prospects.[98]

The ad features the above congratulatory prose, accompanied by images of a peacock in full plume, a (presumably) rising sun, and other information detailing the origins and composition of the supplement and instructions on where to purchase it. The healthy development of the state and its survivability are attributed to political doctrine, participation of the people, international co-operation, and the latest in scientific knowledge. The Kingly Way is credited with a gradual extinguishment of "various kinds of minor sicknesses." *Shengjing shibao* ads often referred to Ruosu as a "Kingly Way medicine," linking its efficacy with Manchukuo's Confucian monarchical ideology, which supporters hoped would transform the region from a troubled warlord state into

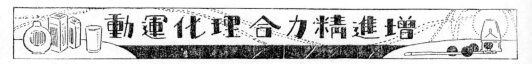

25 "A Rational Movement to Promote Energy." *Source: Shengjing shibao* [Shengjing times], 26 November 1932, 8.

a progressive modern one.[99] Just as the Kingly Way could "fully develop" the people, Ruosu could regulate its consumers' bodies, enhancing their own survivability.

Two months later, on 26 November 1932, a full-page promotion of Ruosu was featured in the *Shengjing shibao* under the heading "Zengjin jingli hulihua yundong" (A Rational Movement to Promote Energy) (see Figure 25).[100] At the top of the page, the title is bracketed by drawings: on the right is an opium pipe with three balls of opium, and on the left is a glass, two small boxes, and a bottle – suggesting medicines to counter the use of opium. Smoke from the pipe spirals across the top of the page, weaving through the words of the title. The page is divided into short essays on Ruosu, with the bottom left-hand quarter devoted to an explicit advertisement for Ruosu; the latter features oversized characters for Ruosu and the image of a bottle of Ruosu, with the name Wakamoto and the shot-putter image clearly visible. The product is identified as foreign in origin, with importers based in key Manchukuo cities such as Changchun, Fengtian, Harbin, and Dalian, as well as in Shanghai, Hankou, Beiping, Tianjin, Qingdao, and other cities – linking local cities with Chinese cities elsewhere on the mainland. These connections were no doubt intended not only to provide consumers with information but also to add lustre to the product's image and to appeal to consumers beyond the Great Wall, who continued to look south for cultural cues. Thus, despite official stress on the independence of Manchukuo (and its "Manchoukuoan" subjects), Ruosu was advertised in ways that drew attention to the interconnectedness of Chinese populations and their shared culture.

The short essays relate Ruosu's various benefits. In "Ruosu zhi renshou fangfa" (Ruosu's Workforce Method), farm, factory, and commerce workers are encouraged to consume Ruosu in order to produce healthy bodies and clear, intelligent minds that will strengthen the country.[101] The essay "Ruosu chengfen you tianran zucheng" (Ruosu Ingredients Are Natural Compositions) lists its contents, including deer penis, seagull kidney, and fish liver, which are argued to maximize human absorption by imitating the performance of testicles and prostate glands.[102] American, European, and Japanese pharmaceutical makers and their effusive praise for the revolutionary nature of their newest scientific discoveries (such as the use of cow and goat testicles) are belittled by description of the Chinese millennia-long use of seal and tiger testicles, deer penis, and chicken liver in medicines and sexual stimulants; the foreigners "try to be clever only to end up with a blunder" *(nong qiao cheng zhuo).*[103] The essays stress the progressive, "rational," essentially Chinese nature of the science behind the nutritional claims and the naturopathic benefits afforded by fish-liver extracts, which are praised for balancing the body and enhancing sexual activities.[104] The essays outline the effectiveness of Ruosu in restoring one's immune system and reversing signs of aging by replicating vitamin D, asserting that consuming it is as effective as nude exercise or sunbathing. Ruosu was promoted as useful to consume at the same time as opium in order to minimize damage.[105] The supplement was prescribed especially for "disciples of Li Bai" (Li Bai *zhi tu*) to cure hangovers if consumed before or after drinking alcohol. Ruosu was advertised as a cure-all that blended age-old traditional Chinese medical rationality with the latest foreign advances.

By the mid-1930s, Ruosu promotion had brought treatment of the poisons related to opiates, alcohol, and overconsumption of food to the fore. Treating addiction was recognized as a painful and time-consuming process, and the supplement was promoted as being able to painlessly remove poisons while restoring cells to their original state.[106] Although alcohol, food, and opium were argued to have medical, physical, and spiritual benefits, habitual overconsumption violated understandings of "proper" nutrition, destroyed health, and shortened lives.[107] Excessive consumption was blamed for creating addictions by producing acids and ulcers that damaged innards and led to loss of appetite, internal bleeding, and in extreme cases, death. The reputed curative powers of Ruosu extended to every aspect of nourishment and health.[108] In an essay titled "Yan, jiu, cha yu jiankang de yinxiang" (The Influence of Tobacco, Alcohol, and Tea on Health), consumption of each is cited as being among the general public's "favourite hobbies."[109] They are recognized for their popularity and their potential danger – especially ethyl alcohol, which is argued to reduce life spans. Li Bai's "negative inheritance" is noted, again, for making alcohol "popular throughout the entire country," pointing to and criticizing the Chinese identities that many officials in Manchukuo sought to erase. The harm that derived from such "hobbies" necessitated consumption of Ruosu, a "holy medicine" *(sheng yao),* to guarantee health during "Holy War" *(shengzhan).* The supplement was promoted as frontline health protection, with micro-organisms that reproduced the benefits of fresh fruit and vegetables in order to combat disease and enable middle-aged, overweight people to better manage their metabolism.[110] Consumption of Ruosu would provide the physical strength necessary to survive opium withdrawal and wartime exigencies.[111]

Ruosu was promoted not only for adults but also for children as a means to reduce childhood deaths and raise healthier citizens.[112] To promote consumption by the young, references in texts to childhood health increased in number, pictures of healthy, happy children at school and at play started to be featured in ads, and cartoons with children began to appear. Direct targeting of children was central to two major advertising campaigns. In one, children were invited to mail in photographs of themselves and their friends for promotional use by the company. In another, children were encouraged to collect and mail to the company labels from Ruosu bottles in return for educational materials that would be supplied for the children's school (see Figure 26).[113] Thus parents and children were urged to take active roles in securing their own individual health while contributing to the education and advancement of society as a whole.

In both the *Shengjing shibao* and *Qilin*, the efficacy of Ruosu was popularized in comics, as in the 1940 *Shengjing shibao* series "Huo baobei" (Live Baby). In the first frame of "Tianmi de wen" (Sweet Kiss), an instalment of this series, a man seeks recognition from a woman (see Figure 27).[114] She rebuffs him in frame two. In frame three, her attitude is changed when the man reveals that his bottle contains Ruosu. The fourth frame depicts the sweet kiss of the title. In "Xin sheng qu" (New Life Melody), a 1944 full-page comic in *Qilin*, Ruosu's benefits are even more forcefully underlined (see Figure 28).[115] The first frame, "self-ashamed of being sloppy," shows a man sadly bent over behind a couple of marching people. The second frame, "grey-coloured memory," features the bedraggled man surrounded by a haze of alcohol, a woman's face, a pair of lips, a cigarette, and a book. In frame three, the man is "pitifully sick." Frame four, "try it out," shows the man taking a dose of Ruosu. In frame five, "the result is gradually effective," the man is newly invigorated, standing tall under the sun with his arms spread outward and upward. Frame six, "be a more productive hero," demonstrates his newly found strength, allowing the man to march upright like the couple in frame one. In frame seven, an untitled scene, the man is shown with a woman and a dream of a baby. The transformation of the man is shown to be complete in terms of his physical appearance, his ambitions, and even his clothing, which changes from Chinese-style dress to a uniform. Ruosu is credited with helping consumers to attain the health, happiness, and virility that supporters of the regime identified with the Kingly Way.

Ruosu remained a prominent feature in popular media throughout the Manchkuo period. During Holy War, ads shrank in size but continued to

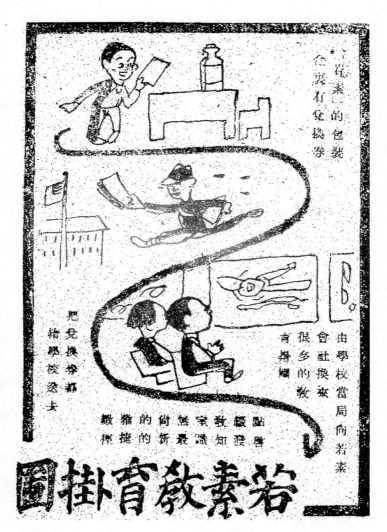

26   Ruosu child's ad. *Source: Qilin* [Unicorn], September 1944, 12.

aggressively assert the supplement's power to protect against general physical weakness and tuberculosis and to aid women in recovery after giving birth.[116] From 1942, *Shengjing shibao* ads even more fervently appealed to consumers to fulfil their public duties by enhancing their physical strength for the sake of the state.[117] Ads in *Qilin* primarily featured pictures and text relating to personal health, anti-aging, and the weather. In both publications, Ruosu was a prominent presence. Although it is difficult to gauge the extent to which Ruosu actually assisted addicts in ending opium use, the good nutrition that

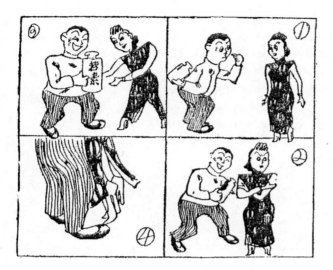

27 "Sweet Kiss."
Source: Shengjing shibao [Shengjing times], 28 June 1940, 5.

28 "New Life Melody." *Source: Qilin* [Unicorn], July 1944, 22.

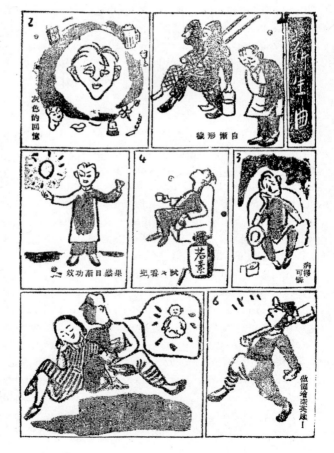

it could provide was generally recognized as helpful in withdrawal programs. For those who attempted domestic withdrawal bolstered by products such as Ruosu, success rates cited in the *Shengjing shibao* in 1941 averaged 40 percent, and those at Healthy Life Institutes were higher, at 50 percent.[118] These rates may appear dubious or low, but they were considered adequate to employ in lauding improvements to addiction treatment. Through the end of Manchukuo, Ruosu remained one of the most visible consumer products to treat addiction and restore health – a reflection of the company's commitment to supporting local health practices and official policies as well as an indication of the continued viability of the consumer market for relatively inexpensive products that promised good health.

For those who preferred professional assistance in quitting, or who had no choice in the matter, a wide range of institutions existed. Zhang Jiyou cautioned that domestic withdrawal left the addict too vulnerable to temptations, arguing that hospitals enabled professionals to control external contacts. Zhang and Xiang Naixi, especially, promoted "psychiatric hospitals" *(jingshenbing bingyuan)*, which specialized in a "supervise and prohibit method" *(jianjin zhi fa)* that separated addicts from all external contact during withdrawal.[119] Believing that if recovered addicts smoked just once or twice, they would turn into addicts again, Jin Long agreed that institutionalization was best since it enabled them to avoid other smokers and smoking areas as well as friends and brothels.[120] In 1940, in his position as director of the Opium Administration in the Opium Prohibition Department, Yong Shanqi stressed that domestic withdrawal was rarely successful and that all addicts would benefit from the services of state-funded Healthy Life Institutes (see Figure 29).[121] Admitting that facilities in the past had been underfunded and understaffed, he argued that his administration was striving hard to make conditions more acceptable.[122] He stressed that even greater focus was being placed on skills training so that recovered addicts could return to society with marketable skills. Yong defended the government's progress on treating addiction, noting that 36 million yuan had been spent on rehabilitation facilities and even more on hiring local doctors and relocating addiction specialists from Japan.[123] Yong admitted difficulties that his department faced with rising food and medicine costs but insisted that the state-funded institutions were capable of effectively treating addicts.

State-run institutions competed with privately run clinics and hospitals, and all advertised their withdrawal programs, which ranged from first- to third-class and from fast to slow.[124] Specialists in morphine replacement included Harbin's Huaying Clinic and Liaoning's Xinmin yiyuan (New People) Hospital.[125] Liaoning's Dongbei jieyan yiyuan (Northeast Quit Smoking)

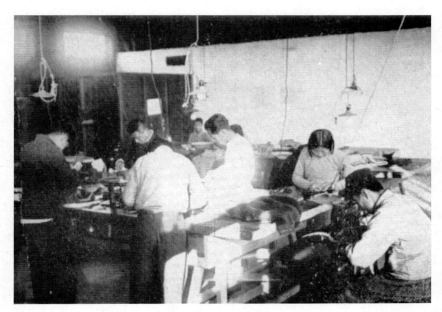

29 "Addicts and cured smokers of opium receive manual and vocational training in the training schools maintained by the Government of Manchoukuo. This is a representative picture showing the type of training that cured addicts and addicts receive." *Source:* T. Nagashima, "Opium Administration in Manchoukuo," *Contemporary Manchuria* 3, 1 (1939), 35.

Hospital advertised its services (including those free of charge) for addicts who wanted to quit opium, heroin, morphine, or barbiturates. Fengtian's Zhenhua yiyuan (China Rise with Force and Spirit) Hospital offered safe, painless withdrawal methods for old and young, with admittance daily from 8:00 a.m. to 6:00 p.m.; nurses were in attendance for programs that ranged from two to seven days.[126] Interested parties were invited to send stamps to the hospital for educational materials. In Xinjing, Daqian yiyuan (Boundless) Hospital advertised procedures to quit opium, morphine, and heroin that were painless, guaranteed, and based on the latest physiological studies, as introduced by the director, Dr. Guan Yunzhang. Patients lived in a hospital dorm for 30 yuan per week, inclusive of medical fees.[127] Another promotional tool in the *Shengjing shibao* was columns of thanks, in which recovered addicts thanked the institutions and their staff. Two institutions in Fengtian were regularly featured, namely the Zhenhua yiyuan and Boji (Abundant Aid) Hospitals. Zhenhua yiyuan, for example, was thanked by Shi Xichen, who praised the staff for employing the most modern methods to help him and his brother end years of addiction in eight and nine days, respectively.[128] Boji received similar commendation, as Wan Hongkui thanked hospital staff and director Luo Rong'ge for painlessly curing him in seven days.[129] Regardless of whether Shi and Wan were in fact addicts who recovered in the institutions or whether any advertised treatments were in fact painless, these columns, as well as the ads and articles describing the institutions, demonstrated a commitment to securing positive reputations and attracting clients. The prominent discussion of medical doctors and their professional opinions and activities suggests that the institutions were not driven solely by financial considerations or by the more diabolical ambitions that have been attributed to them – and that the general public was expected to respond favourably to them.

State-sponsored Healthy Life Institutes, from their inception, were promoted as ideal addiction-treatment institutions where rehabilitation programs ranged from withdrawal and harm reduction to skills training. By 1939, 46 institutes (each with a capacity of 2,672 patients) had been established in accordance with provisions of the Opium Law.[130] In 1940 there were 159 Healthy Life Institutes, and plans were drawn up to bring the total to 219.[131] These operated in addition to already existing private or state-sponsored institutions, with the intent of increasing the numbers of addicts who could be rehabilitated. On average, treatments were supposed to last for fifty days at a cost of 800 yuan to the institution (which was mostly funded by the state), money that Yong Shanqi argued needed to be raised by banning private trade in its entirety and taxing legal sales until opium was no longer a social problem.[132] In 1941 the director of the People's Livelihood Department, Lin Quanqing, praised ongoing rehabilitation developments, noting that addicts were not being punished or executed, as in the Republic of China, but were being rehabilitated, often at the expense of the Manchukuo government.[133] Underlining the progressive nature of adjustments to programs, in 1944 Healthy Life Institutes joined forces with the Morality Society to improve women's chances of successful withdrawal by having women members who were former addicts visit and talk with patients, providing them with female rather than male role models, who till then had tended to dominate examples of successful recovery.[134]

By the early 1940s, promotions for Healthy Life Institutes had become regular features of the newspapers *Datong bao (Great Unity Herald)* and *Shengjing shibao* in ads and articles that praised rehabilitation treatments and achievements. A 1941 ad for Healthy Life Institutes in the *Datong bao* exemplifies the official stance toward the institutions (see Figure 30).[135] A woman holds a banner that beseeches, "Give up opium and morphine medicine." She towers over a number of faceless bodies that raise their arms upward. The caption at the side reads, "Opium dens guide you into hell, Healthy Life

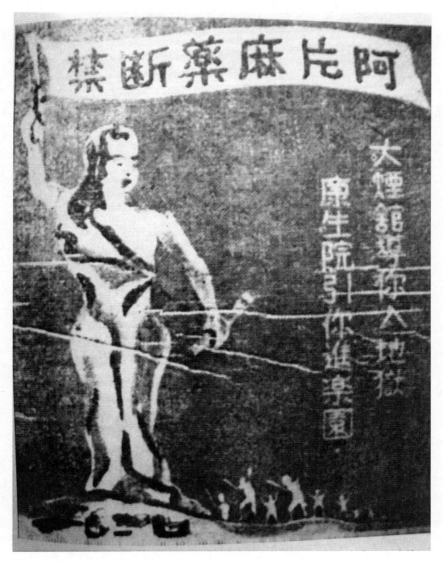

30 "Healthy Life Institutes Lead You into Paradise." *Source:* Kangsheng yuan [Healthy Life Institute] ad, *Datong bao* [Great unity herald], 6 December 1941, 4. Original producer: Manchukuo Opium Monopoly, company defunct.

Institutes lead you into paradise." Drawing on depictions of Manchukuo as a "paradise land" *(letu),* Healthy Life Institutes were meant to symbolize the state's benevolence and to achieve one of the primary goals identified by officials. The female figure melds the nurturing nature of rehabilitation programs with the ideal of the "good wife, wise mother" *(xianqi liangmu)*, through which conservatives sought to modernize women of the region.[136] The figure appears vital and the addicts enthusiastic. But the rehabilitation of all addicts exceeded even the abilities of state-funded institutions, and despite all efforts, private facilities were still necessary and operated through the end of Manchukuo.

Perhaps the most impressive Healthy Life Institute was described by Xu Bochun in his article "Tiantang de kangsheng yuan" (The Heavenly Healthy Life Institute). The Fengtian Healthy Life Institute was established at Beiling (the Qing Dynasty's "Northern Tombs"), a compound then about sixteen kilometres to the west of the city, a spot noted for its beauty and peace.[137] The state reportedly spent 40,000 to 50,000 yuan furbishing the facilities, which featured a courtyard of over nine square metres set amid several bright buildings. The first director, Xiang Naixi, was a medical doctor and enthusiastic anti-opium reformer whose writings on addiction are cited earlier in this chapter; he supervised construction and initial program offerings. His successor, Tsuru Kunitake, was a Japanese medical specialist in addiction. Journalist Xu Bochun described the institute as ideal, with clean bedding and clothes for patients, who, he wrote, spent their days talking, playing chess, and sitting in the sun reading magazines and newspapers. He characterized the institution as more of a country club than an addiction-treatment facility. Xu noted that conditions at Beiling were far more favourable than those at other facilities he had visited, which featured stern staff working in decrepit conditions. Xu defended Manchukuo's Opium Law, stating that the earliest versions were drafted to ensure morality and justice but that by the early 1940s it had become more urgent to affirm the country's fate and the economy, which suggests even greater emphasis on the efficacy and reputation of Healthy Life Institutes. Xu acknowledged critics of the institutions but dismissed their derisions as excuses for continuing their own self-destructive and suicidal addictions, which made them willing to ridicule the efforts of others who were engaged in battling addiction on a daily basis. Despite his recognition of critics, Xu's effusive praise for the Fengtian Healthy Life Institute's accomplishments was likely dismissed by many readers as sycophantic or naive and regarded as revealing little about what addiction treatment actually entailed while admitting how inadequate other addiction treatment facilities were, with their stern staff and decrepit conditions.

Proceedings from the Exultant Forum provide a more likely description of the experiences of seven patients at Healthy Life Institutes; these were published in a series of eight articles in the *Shengjing shibao*.[138] Xing Canlü noted that the pain lasted for a week but was worth it for the full recovery achieved.[139]

Zhang Lin'ge stated that the treatment of patients was attentive and conducted without discrimination, whether they arrived of their own volition or not. Chen Yuxin agreed, adding that treatment was fast, despite the fact that she stayed for two months to achieve her full recovery; she noted that the only difference in treatment among patients of many nationalities and backgrounds was the food, as only Japanese were served white rice.[140] Chen recounted how her treatment was divided into three stages.[141] During the first week, physical withdrawal was most painful, but by the tenth day, the physical pain had generally dissipated. The second stage focused on psychological treatment since even though her body had been weaned off opium, spiritual issues remained. The third stage was departure from the hospital, commonly after twenty days – not the fifty days described by officials. By the end of treatment, she argued, temptations could still exist, but the physical compulsions for opium were gone, and the spirit was being restored as energy, appetite, and interest in sex returned.[142] Jin Chengrong concurred, noting, too, that throughout his withdrawal he did not think about food or sex or experience any pain but for the most part was numb and obsessed with the need to obtain morphine.[143] These testimonies stressed physical and spiritual hardships endured under the watch of professional staff in reasonably comfortable conditions.

An even less flattering view of the rehabilitation institutes can be found in a revealing article in the academic journal *Dongfang yixue zazhi (Far Eastern Medical Journal)*. Xiang Naixi provided reputedly verbatim interviews with four Japanese women (only their surnames were provided) who sought assistance for their morphine addiction.[144] All of the women had entered hospitals or clinics and there experienced the pain of withdrawal and neglect or abuse from the staff. Ms. Ōto recounted her eight-month stay at a hospital where she was given injections containing opiates of some form for the first month, during which the doctors manipulated morphine content, presumably to monitor her withdrawal process.[145] While undergoing treatment, Ōto and another patient began injecting and smoking heroin purchased for them by workers at the facility and smuggled in – and they smoked it for seven months, despite being seen by nurses, until they were discharged. Ms. Nakayama also recounted secretly injecting heroin while under medical care – noting that her kimono kept her arms covered – until the doctor discovered what she was doing and confiscated her needles and drug supply.[146] Several of the women described treatments of questionable efficacy with injected medicine or a placebo; the former included Kraepelin, Pantopon, and Scoporamin (i.e., Scopolamine), whereas the latter contained varied degrees of opiates and/or salt water. All of the women, Xiang noted, relapsed. Xiang, a physician

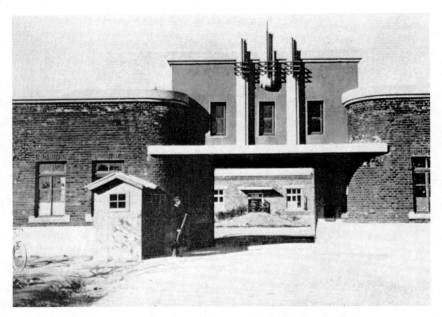

31 "An infirmary operated by the Hsinking Special Municipality." *Source:*
T. Nagashima, "Opium Administration in Manchoukuo," *Contemporary Manchuria* 3,
1 (1939), 25.

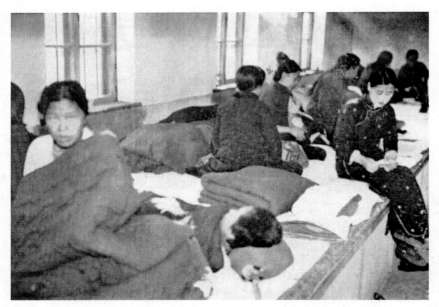

32 "Interior of an infirmary. Women addicts receiving medical attention."
Source: T. Nagashima, "Opium Administration in Manchoukuo," *Contemporary
Manchuria* 3, 1 (1939), 25.

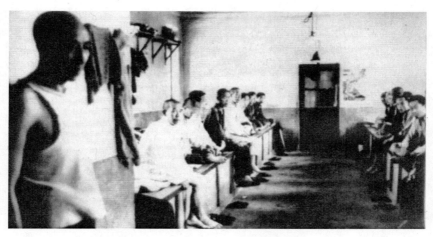

33 Interior of the Hsinking State Infirmary for Opium Addicts. *Source: Progressing Manchoukuo* (Dalian: The Manchuria Daily News), 58.

committed to battling opiate addiction, thus pointed to systemic problems in the institutions as well as to the difficulties of treating addiction in a journal aimed at highly educated readers, most of whom were undoubtedly involved in medical practice.

In the popular press, Healthy Life Institutes were frequently lauded by reporters and former addicts (see Figure 31). In 1940 a new director for the Jilin Healthy Life Institute arrived from Andong province and made headlines for encouraging doctors and staff to be more sympathetic and caring toward their charges.[147] The enthusiasm with which he approached his position was starkly contrasted with that of his predecessor and co-workers, whom he had inspired with the introduction of new treatment programs that involved injections and physiotherapy (including steam baths, sunbathing, outdoor exercise, and skills training) and that were said to achieve withdrawal in six days for light addiction and in ten days for heavy addiction. Every day there were lectures on individual health and its relevance to the state. Entertainment included radio, chess, and magazines. Other institutions featured faith-based religious treatment, offered by the Buddhist or Taoist Red Swastika Society or by the Christian Salvation Army.[148] In Fengtian and Kaiyuan, especially, centres were lauded for training patients in specific skills, such as printing, papermaking, and matchbox construction.[149]

Former addict Chen Li described a schedule of work that was established for him when he entered a Healthy Life Institute in Baiquan county (Heilongjiang) in 1941.[150] On registration, he was introduced to the Japanese director, who escorted him to a room dominated by a *kang* (a heatable brick bed) and occupied by other patients at various stages of recovery (see Figures 32 and 33). Each patient was set various tasks to complete each day, creating a sense of responsibility and achievement – and no doubt defraying costs of operating the Healthy Life Institute. Meals for Chinese patients consisted primarily of *gaoliang* (Chinese sorghum) and tofu.[151] In the evenings, the director and doctors told stories, especially about the dangers of opium. Chen recovered in two months and left. Similarly, Bai Yu, who blamed his addiction on stress caused by the death of his father, family issues, and business failings, checked himself into Tieling city's Healthy Life Institute, which he noted was built in a peaceful location on a mountain.[152] Bai described the institution as so impressive that on recovery he underwent training and joined its workforce. Liu Jingliang, in response to pleading from his son, entered Liaoyang city's facility, which he praised as an angel that had returned human happiness to him.[153]

Not all entered Healthy Life Institutes of their own free will.[154] In "Tiantang de kangsheng yuan" (The Heavenly Healthy Life Institute), Ma Ji recounted how he had been ordered institutionalized by the state and had subsequently come to credit the institution with saving his life.[155] Ma described his doubts and fears before his arrival, when he believed Healthy Life Institutes to be no more than jails for addicts. Once inside, his worries disappeared. The staff members were comforting and kind, and the facilities were clean and comfortable, providing patients with what he described favourably as a "middle-class" experience. In Xinjing, in 1941, Wei Yonggui's addiction to opium caused family distress and forced his son Chaochen to quit school.[156] Chaochen tried to persuade his father to quit. When he did not, Chaochen went to the police and informed them that his father was secretly smoking opium. He begged them to intervene and send his father for treatment. The police did not blame Chaochen for betraying his father, a cardinal sin in the eyes of conservative Confucianists, but rather called him a "little hero" *(xiao yingxiong)* and fulfilled his wish by institutionalizing his father and ridding him of his addiction.

How should one evaluate these testimonies? Should they be taken at face value or dismissed as no more than propaganda? Such positive tributes appeared in the Manchukuo press as frequently as post-Manchukuo condemnation of the institutes. Praise for the institutions during Manchukuo and condemnation of them afterward were encouraged by officials. Both the praise and condemnation served multiple purposes. During Manchukuo, the praise explicitly supported anti-opium policies while implicitly creating a far from flattering portrait of contemporary society, one that paved the way for postwar condemnation. Although the testimonies did praise the achievements of some Healthy Life Institutes, their facilities, and their staff, they also pointed out insufficiencies in others, as attested to by professionals such as Xiang Naixi and Yong Shanqi, the director of the Opium Administration in the Opium Prohibition Department. Further, most described pain and hardship during the early days of withdrawal, undermining other forms of advertising that stressed the painless nature of withdrawal. The contradictions inherent in the testimonials undermined the work of anti-opium activists; how could they insist the people quit using when they could not agree on how, where, or if it could be accomplished? Even in the most positive contexts, rehabilitation was controversial: sudden withdrawal could result in death, and harm reduction raised cries of addiction enabling. In a colonial context, rehabilitation through labour or "skills training" bore a distinctively negative tone. To make matters worse, rehabilitation proved elusive: according to the state's own statistics, up to 70 percent of patients relapsed.[157] Healthy Life Institute staff faced the unenviable task of applying inadequate funding to treatments that were made more controversial simply by nature of their foreign influences. Officials conceded that the Healthy Life Institutes were "far from satisfactory in point of scale and equipment" yet still insisted that they could effectively treat patients.[158] Accomplishments of the Healthy Life Institutes were hampered as state resources were stretched thin by other demands, including the quelling of domestic disorder, industrial development, and Holy War. Post-occupation condemnations make clear that the centres were not all they were advertised to be, but they also suggest that on some level the population expected the institutions to deliver what they promised. Wang Xianwei, for example, denounced the institutions for "trying to pawn off something inferior to what it purports to be" *(gua yangtou mai gourou).*[159]

Methods created to treat addiction were not only controversial but also of questionable value. No consensus existed on best treatments. Some institutions, like the one at Beiling, had optimal facilities, whereas others struggled with conditions that even the Healthy Life Institute enthusiast Xu Bochun described as decrepit. Some offered skills training and others hard labour. All of the institutions had to raise money or cut corners to continue operations, thereby creating the need to embellish the truth or to lie, which ultimately undermined their legitimacy. As Holy War demands accelerated, and the need for more workers and soldiers increased, the institutions found themselves forced into doing more with less, without treatments that could offer less painful means to end addiction. Techniques such as "supervise and prohibit" only aroused suspicions even if the sheltering of addicts from temptation and from family and friends was for their own good. Some products to treat addiction were nutritious and contributed to good health practices. Others, despite their claims, killed consumers. None of the products, not even Ruosu, could cure addiction for all those who sought help.

In the post-Manchukuo period, Healthy Life Institutes were widely condemned as "fraudulent" *(qipian)*.[160] Many were argued to be no more than drug-distribution centres or labour camps; Mark Driscoll notes a post-Manchukuo recounting of a 1944 campaign during which rehabilitation centres reportedly served as fronts for hard-labour recruitment, as registrants were shuttled directly out the back doors.[161] Unknown numbers of addicts were said to have entered rehabilitation and lost their lives along with their addictions; post-Manchukuo memoirs argued that the Chinese mocked Healthy Life Institutes as "Cheating Life Institutes" (Kengsheng yuan).[162] That most addicts arrived at Healthy Life Institutes as a last resort guaranteed that some would not survive withdrawal. The institution at Fengtian's Beiling Northern Tombs, so praised by Xu Bochun, was condemned for its isolated location, which made many question what went on behind its high red walls. Outrage over the failings of state-sponsored rehabilitation to achieve optimal results led locals to ridicule the centres as "Raising Resistance Institutes" (Shengkang yuan).[163] The "resistance" that such centres inspired is suggested by accounts of the murders of Healthy Life Institute directors by enraged locals on the collapse of Manchukuo in 1945.[164] However, not all met this fate. Xiang Naixi, for example, who directed rehabilitation centres, including the Beiling Healthy Life Institute, continued a prestigious career after 1945, teaching in the People's Liberation Army and later in the Medical College at Tianjin Normal University.[165] However, even the well-intentioned efforts of professionals such as Xiang appear to have enflamed anti-Manchukuo sentiment. Part of the anger no doubt resulted from despair that even the most modern, scientific knowledge and techniques seemed inadequate to end the scourge of opium. Most of this anger was inspired by the hypocrisy of an Opium Monopoly that was created to eradicate, but seemed only to simultaneously promote and demonize, recreational opium use and addiction.

Products to treat addiction were popular but seemingly no more successful at battling addiction than the institutions. Ruosu may have fostered good nutrition, but it proved inadequate to fully treat opium addiction. Nonetheless, the product became one of the most popular consumer products of its day, and it remains a big seller in Japan; as of March 2005, the company was valued at 3.395 billion yen.[166] Significantly, the history section on the company's current website makes no reference to business activities outside of Japan in the 1930s and 1940s, despite Ruosu's marked popularity in China and Manchukuo. The company's stated mission, in 2010, was to contribute to the creation and development of a healthy and affluent society through the research and development, production, and supply of pharmaceuticals. We have contributed to the health and welfare of human beings by improving a variety of non-prescription drugs and ethical drugs produced thanks to longstanding accumulation of fermentation and culture techniques and research results from the latest biotechnology.[167]

These longstanding techniques and research results were employed on the Asian mainland in the mid-twentieth century, bolstered by similarly themed promotional campaigns that mirror the company's product promotion today:

We can help to create a happy society for people all over the world who wish to live a healthy and prosperous life. In order to realize this, we pride ourselves and take responsibility for contribution to society from the joy in seeing smiles on the face of as many patients as possible and through maintaining high ethical standards as a life and health-related company.[168]

In terms of guaranteeing good health and the highest ethical standards, the promotion of Ruosu today echoes the advertising of decades ago, although any reference to treating opium and alcohol addiction has disappeared, along with any reference to connections to Manchukuo and the larger Japanese Empire.

In the early to mid-twentieth century, a sizable anti-opium movement developed in Manchuria to stigmatize recreational opium use and to try to explain and treat addiction. Rana Mitter has noted that the region's largest newspaper, the *Shengjing shibao,* was "by no means a crude propaganda organ for the Japanese presence in the region."[169] Coverage of the opium question, and of addiction and its treatment, underscores Mitter's observation: the health professionals, officials, and addicts cited in this chapter held critical stances toward opium and addiction. Their attitudes toward official policies and treatments ranged from support to outrage and were reported in earnest in media such as the *Shengjing shibao.* Supporters of the Japanese Empire often associated it with "modernity and newness," and the attempted solutions to the opium problem and addiction were no exception.[170] Eradication of recreational opium use and addiction was considered an essential element of Japan's "civilizing mission" on the mainland. Popular anger toward Healthy Life Institutes, Manchukuo, and more generally the Japanese Empire testifies to the long-term dominance of Japanese in the intoxicant industries, both in their promotion and censure, and to the difficulties of treating addiction even with the most modern scientific methods. Try as they might, Manchukuo's anti-opium activists were incapable of eradicating addiction or altering dominant perceptions of the regime as a narco-state. Not even support from the Opium Monopoly, the subject of the following chapter, could accomplish these goals.

8 The Opium Monopoly's "Interesting Discussion"

In 1942, Manchukuo's Yapian zhuanmai gongshu (Opium Monopoly; henceforth Monopoly) issued a collection of fourteen short stories and documents titled *Qu tan conglin, di'yi ji (Interesting Discussion Thicket, Volume Number 1)*. The richly illustrated book was printed in Fengtian by publisher Arai Chōjirō at the Xing Ya yinshua zhushi huishe (Rising Asia Printing Company). Distributed free of charge, it was produced by the Monopoly's Jin yan zongju (Ban Smoking Central Office) under the direction of Kakegawa Akikuni. The volume promotes the Monopoly's prohibitionist platform by outlining a brief history of opium in China and by describing the causes and effects of addiction, the means by which the Monopoly sought to reduce and eventually eradicate opium addiction in Manchukuo, and the difficulties of achieving this goal. This chapter focuses attention on *Qu tan conglin* to highlight Monopoly officials' attempts to control opium, namely how it was understood and consumed. The Monopoly's narrative of the history of opium in China, the focus of two chapters, attributes central roles to the Japanese Empire's enemies – England and the United States – with no acknowledgment of Asian complicity in the trade. A brief description of the two official documents in the volume, the 1932 Ahpian fa bugao (Opium Law Proclamation; henceforth Opium Law) and a 1937 Guowuyuan bugao (State Proclamation), illustrates the significance that the state attributed to the Monopoly's work and to the eventual eradication of recreational opium consumption, which was so prominently advocated. Most of the eleven short stories detail the heavy cost of addiction. These provide the background for works that centre on the travails of overcoming addiction, especially in state-sponsored Healthy Life Institutes. Finally, the difficulties of achieving eradication are addressed through two fictional accounts of drug dealers. Together, the works in *Qu tan conglin* propagate the Monopoly's main policies and underline a serious, yet flawed, effort to raise public consciousness of the dangers of drugs.

From the first chapter, blame for China's opium problem is placed squarely on England. In "Jinlin de Zhao laoyezi" (Neighbour Master Zhao), the ninety-year-old Master Zhao, whose family moved to Jilin in 1860 to escape invading

British troops during the Second Opium War (1856-60), shares his interpreta-
tion of the modern history of China and, especially, Manchuria with a young
boy while they peruse an illustrated history book.[1] Zhao tells of the dramatic
changes that have shaped China since he was a child. He compares the ten-
year-old "happy country" *(xingfu guojia)* of Manchukuo, described as "politically developed, [with] no internal turmoil, many schools, and a progressive
culture," with the tumultuous Qing Dynasty's decline, dated to the Taiping
rebels and their uprising (1850-64), which reversed longstanding power relations between the Qing and foreign states.[2] The latter Qing rulers, facing
constant pressure from within and beyond their borders, hesitantly allowed
formal, mass migration to their Manchurian homeland in order to block
Russian imperialist expansion.[3] Han Chinese migrants poured in, eager to
pioneer the land and help the local people to, as Zhao terms it, "become
civilized" *(kai hua)*.[4] But, as he sadly observes, the Chinese took with them
their habit of using opium recreationally, which had not previously been a
local custom.[5] Master Zhao describes how late Qing efforts to ban such consumption were met with indifference from a population that ignored court
edicts, paid hefty taxes, and, on occasion, suffered legal punishments. In the
post-Qing order, warlords manipulated and magnified the opium trade to
raise funds for their armies. Opium flooded the land, turning the region into
a "frightening human hell" *(kepa de renjian diyu)*,[6] as illustrated by the three
male smokers trapped in the spider's web in Figure 34.[7]

   Zhao recounts that when Manchukuo was established in 1932, there were
an estimated 1 million addicts in the region, although by 1942, after ten years
of implementation of the Opium Law, addict numbers had been reduced
by half, with officials predicting that only ten more years were necessary to
achieve a total ban on recreational opium use.[8] Zhao singles out the end of
addiction as the inspiration for Japan and Manchukuo to work together
to fulfil the promise of a Greater East Asia Co-Prosperity Sphere. The story
ends with the old man exhausted from describing such a turbulent history.
In "Jinlin de Zhao laoyezi," Zhao depicts a Qing Empire led by well-meaning
but incompetent rulers who faced an ignorant public, obstructive officials,
and Anglo-American imperialists. Ultimately, Qing rulers were replaced by
Chinese warlords whose depravity knew no bounds. The joy with which the
warlords Zhang Zuolin and Zhang Xueliang engaged in the opium trade is
illustrated in Figure 35.[9] They stand, smiling, among poppy flowers, towering
above the blackened figures of opium users writhing in agony. Master Zhao
explains that, in response to the unending turmoil inflicted on the mainland
by warlords and foreigners, the Japanese, as fellow Asians, felt compelled to
rescue the Chinese people.[10] Zhao provides a sympathetic portrait of Qing

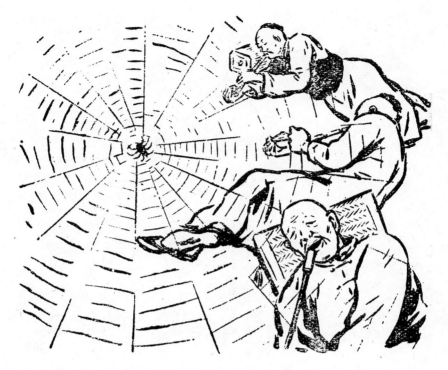

34 "Frightening human hell." *Source:* "Ahpian zhanzheng yu Yinguo de dong Ya qinlüe" [Opium War and England's East Asia aggression], in Kakegawa Akirashū, ed., *Qu tan conglin, di'yi ji* [Interesting discussion thicket, volume number 1] (Fengtian: Xing Ya yinshua zhushi huishe, 1942), 35. Original producer: Manchukuo Opium Monopoly, company defunct.

rulers, from whom the Manchukuo royal family descended. He also correctly points to early English involvement in the opium trade and to foreign aggression during which Beijing was occupied and the Summer Palace destroyed in a savage act of barbarity. There should be little doubt that, as Zhao argues, some Japanese felt compelled to protect other Asian peoples from such foreign intrusions, if only for their own salvation. But Zhao's narrative is weakened by his failure to account for the late 1920s strengthening of the Chinese Republican regime, which had begun to revoke the most egregious terms of the unequal treaties, for the heavy-handed Japanese military aggression that forced Manchuria into the fold of the Japanese Empire, and for Japanese involvement in the drug trade in any capacity besides seeking its termination.

Chapter 5, "Ahpian zhanzheng yu Yinguo de dong Ya qinlüe" (Opium War and England's East Asia Aggression), provides an even more in-depth description of England's crimes against the Chinese people. The English are blamed

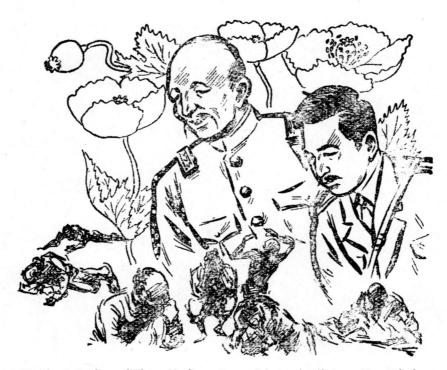

35   Zhang Zuolin and Zhang Xueliang. *Source:* "Ahpian zhanzheng yu Yinguo de dong Ya qinlüe" [Opium War and England's East Asia aggression], in Kakegawa Akirashū, ed., *Qu tan conglin, di'yi ji* [Interesting discussion thicket, volume number 1] (Fengtian: Xing Ya yinshua zhushi huishe, 1942), 42. Original producer: Manchukuo Opium Monopoly, company defunct.

for secretly transporting opium into China, which involved relying on their government's military strength to "knowingly violate" *(ming zhi gu fan)* Qing prohibitions.[11] Once the masses began to emulate elite consumption practices, sales of opium soared, and as England benefited from the illicit trade, Qing society declined. In response, the Daoguang emperor (1782-1850) proscribed recreational opium use, but officials could not, or would not, fully enact his edicts. Finally, the patriot Lin Zexu (1785-1850) was sent to Guangdong to implement the law. He famously confiscated and burned 20,283 chests of the English traders' opium, and shortly thereafter the First Opium War (1839-42) began.[12] The Qing military was defeated by England, and the first unequal treaty, the Nanjing Treaty, was forced on the humbled state. The chapter argues that the treaty irreparably weakened the Qing and made importation even easier for the English. In the early twentieth century, England's imperialist aggression transformed China into an opium hell.[13] In the post-Qing era,

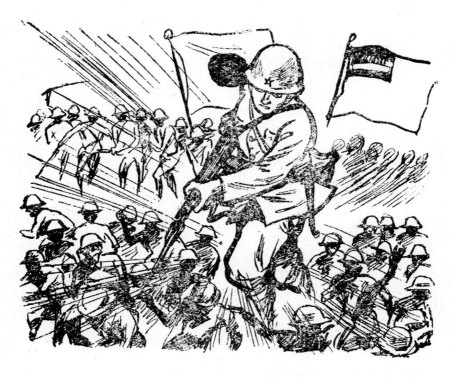

36 Japan protects Asia. *Source:* "Zhengyi Riben de fenqi" [The righteous Japanese rise with force and spirit], in "Ahpian zhanzheng yu Yinguo de dong Ya qinlüe" [Opium War and England's East Asia aggression], in Kakegawa Akirashū, ed., *Qu tan conglin, di'yi ji* [Interesting discussion thicket, volume number 1] (Fengtian: Xing Ya yinshua zhushi huishe, 1942), 44. Original producer: Manchukuo Opium Monopoly, company defunct.

warlords sank profits from drug sales into European weaponry that Chinese then used against other Chinese, further weakening the whole. In this historical account, ceaseless warlord violence and what was believed to be widespread opium addiction compelled the "righteous" *(zhengyi)* Japanese to intervene and establish Manchukuo on behalf of the suffering Chinese masses, as illustrated in Figure 36, in which a soldier is shown to defend the territories of Japan and Manchukuo.[14]

The twin goals of curbing violence and recreational drug use are described as the "foundation of establishing the country" of Manchukuo.[15] On 30 November 1932 the Opium Law was proclaimed. With the foundation of the new state and a body of laws regulating opium use, Japan had moved decisively to avenge the Chinese and liberate them from hateful England's "Caucasian colony" *(baizhongren de zhimindi).*[16] On 7 December 1941 the Japanese military smote American imperialists at Pearl Harbor and then continued to tear

England's empire assunder by liberating Hong Kong and Singapore. The chapter accords blame for China's degradation into drug addiction and warlord rule to England and, less clearly, to the United States, while commending Japanese liberation of Asia from Western colonization and drug addiction. This popular-history approach was meant to foster feelings of patriotism among readers, an aspiration that was no doubt hampered by the absence of any acknowledgment of Chinese, Japanese, or Korean involvement in the drug trade, an issue that would have been glaringly obvious to most, if not all, readers and one that detracts from the chapter's legitimate arguments regarding China's treatment by the Western powers. And although much of Chinese society was touched by imperialist aggression, China could never have been considered a "Caucasian colony," even if Caucasians did for a long time play central roles in the opium trade while violating local laws and customs with impunity under the protection of extraterritoriality and "gunboat diplomacy." Both of the historical accounts in *Qu tan conglin* attempt to construct coherent interpretive frameworks, but they are weakened by their overly subjective position. *Qu tan conglin* was published in 1942 during the first year of Holy War, when it was more politically expedient to stress the evils of the Japanese Empire's enemies, most notably England and the United States, than to expose internal ones. It does bear noting, however, that the narratives in this volume are hardly more biased than contemporary American and English popular histories explaining the Second World War to readers in those countries.[17]

As stated repeatedly in *Qu tan conglin,* a key legitimizer of Manchukuo was the Opium Law, which was proclaimed on 30 November 1932. The law decried the "daily habit" *(richang xiguan)* of recreational opium use for weakening the people, draining the economy, and humiliating the nation on the international stage.[18] Through the eventual eradication of recreational opium consumption, the Opium Law promised to construct a new, ideal state and society and to protect addicts' health through supervised sales, on condition of their registration and commitment to eventual rehabilitation. The seriousness of Manchukuo's control of drugs is illustrated in Figure 37, as the hand of the state takes firm hold of an opium smoker.[19] Five years after establishing the Opium Law, in 1937, the State Proclamation repeated the basic arguments contained in the law, stressing that recreational consumption of opium and morphine caused harmful "addiction" *(shi),* which destroyed individuals, families, and the nation by transforming ordinary people into criminals.[20] The peace attained in the empire of Manchukuo was praised for enabling the application of laws to stop recreational drug use and reverse the tide of addiction. As a moral exemplar for the general public, government workers who

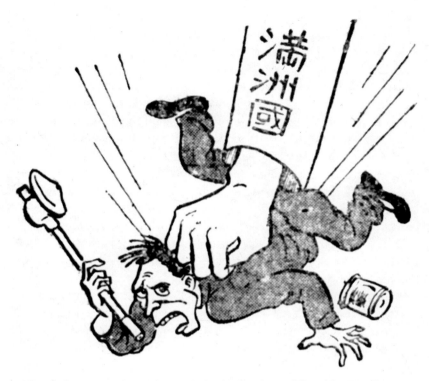

37 Manchukuo government. *Source:* "Jinlin de Zhao laoyezi" [Neighbour Master Zhao], in Kakegawa Akirashū, ed., *Qu tan conglin, di'yi ji* [Interesting discussion thicket, volume number 1] (Fengtian: Xing Ya yinshua zhushi huishe, 1942), 7. Original producer: Manchukuo Opium Monopoly, company defunct.

continued to smoke opium were ordered to immediately stop. Both the Opium Law and the State Proclamation echoed arguments made in the above two historical accounts by stressing that people who recreationally consumed opium were "weak-willed" *(yizhi boruo)* and inflicted on themselves a "chronic poisoning disease" *(manxing zhong du de bing)*.[21] Those who used opium were warned that they had only one fate in store: to be "poor quickly, die early" *(qiong de kuai, si de zao)*.[22]

The weakening and poisoning of the people are the subject of Chapter 6, "Xiguan wu" (Custom Error). This essay argues that despite widespread belief to the contrary, illness was not the leading cause of addiction to opiates since, it is reasoned, most addicts were between thirty and fifty years old, when physical health should be most robust.[23] If illness were the cause, why, the essay questions, would addiction occur at the strongest period in one's life? Also, arguing that only about 20 percent of addicts were women, the essay raises the issue of gender disparity. If opium addiction were because of illness, wouldn't the numbers of female and male addicts be more equivalent? Thus medical reasons are not argued to be responsible for high levels of addiction but rather the erroneous customs surrounding opium use. Opium was traditionally consumed to treat stomach ache, coughing and other breathing difficulties, diarrhea, and insomnia. People may have believed that opium had curative powers, but it only numbed the pain and did not cure the condition. So, when the drug's effects wore off, the original condition persisted, yet the patient mistakenly believed that more opium would keep the illness under control. Over time, poisons developed in the body as it grew accustomed to the drug, and increased amounts were necessary to achieve the initial pain-free condition.[24] With consistent use, addiction resulted. This essay stresses the need for Manchukuo to unite with Japan and save the people of East Asia by eradicating such "custom errors," which caused unsuspecting citizens to needlessly poison themselves by consuming a nonmedicinal drug that did nothing more than assuage pain.

Perhaps the most disheartening story in the collection, Chapter 11, "Gu bei tan" (Sigh for an Age-Old Stele), describes the dissolute descendants of the Qing general Mutushan (d. 1886). To honour his decades of loyal service to the dynasty, including a prominent role in the Sino-French War (1884-85), the Guangxu emperor (1871-1908) inscribed two stone tablets, which graced the entrance to a park in his hometown, Qiqihaer's Longsha Park.[25] In striking contrast to his father, Mutushan's son devoted his life to smoking opium, an activity that the narrator argues was possible because Qing prohibitions against the use of opium were no more than "an empty show of strength" *(xu zhang shengshi)*.[26] His addiction influenced the rest of his family; his wife and concubine also smoked opium. The narrator criticizes the "so-called Chinese big family-ism" *(suowei Zhongguo de dajia zhuyi)*, referring to the tendency of blood and adopted relatives to turn to more successful family members for support and to follow the example of the family elder.[27] Mutushan's son, sinking into addiction, paid no attention to increasingly weighty family matters, and as his wife and concubine fought, his hands never left his pipe. Before long, his addiction and financial pressures led him to completely dismantle the family: he sold the belongings in the home and then the house, the wife, and the concubine. After they were gone, he sold the land of his father's tomb, in violation of the most basic norms of filial piety. When he attempted to sell the Guangxu-inscribed stone tablets, the municipal government intervened and purchased them for the park. At the conclusion of the story, the narrator observes that addicts are like "horse ears in the east wind" *(ma'er dong feng)*, unable to hear or recognize anything.[28] Addiction is depicted as completely overwhelming its victims, and, the narrator argues, for many like Mutushan's son, there is no medicine that can save them from a fate of homelessness and death in the jaws of wild dogs. This story is the sole work in the volume that argues that some addicts are unsalvageable.

The heavy toll of addiction is further recounted in Chapter 7, "Mayao yinzhe de wang'en" (The Ingratitude of Anaesthetic Addicts), a fictional account of a man who is cured of heroin addiction. Liu Enhui was the scion of a wealthy family, which had prospered in official, artistic, and business capacities. When Enhui graduated from school, he was hired to assist his father in managing the affairs of another wealthy family. One day after his father died, he took heroin to treat severe stomach pain. Mistakenly, he thought heroin was a cure for his ailment, whereas it actually only temporarily reduced the pain. Believing heroin to be a "wonderful medicine" *(miao yao),* he was unaware of its side effects and injected it increasingly often.[29] As he was the head of the family, no one dared to confront him. Once he had assumed his father's position, he drained the wealth of both families to try to satisfy his cravings for heroin. The physical damage caused to Enhui is described by the narrator as a "minor matter" *(xiao shi)* in comparison to its destructive impact on his conscience, echoing a Chinese adage that had long been applied to women as an encouragement to maintain their chastity: "To starve to death is a small thing, but to lose one's integrity is a great one."[30] Addicted, humiliated, and impoverished, Enhui eventually entered a Healthy Life Institute, where the staff members were shocked by his appearance because of repeated injections, with rusty needles, of heroin mixed with dirty water: his lower limbs, shoulders, chest, and stomach were all deeply scarred. Despite the odds, he was cured in three months and released to reconcile with the two families that he had bankrupted. This story has a troubled ending, as Enhui is left wracked with guilt over his earlier behaviour, and it is unclear whether he will be welcomed back into his family and community.

The fearful consequences of addiction are coupled with a more promising rehabilitation in Chapter 2, "Tang Xinji de shi gong" (Tang Xinji's True Confession). The story begins as Xinji is being beaten by his father for becoming addicted to opium. His father, a sixty-year-old former police officer, cries as he berates his son. His father curses such suicidal behaviour, and Xinji submits so that they may be reunited. In flashback, it is revealed that Xinji's father has sacrificed everything for his son's happiness and education. After Xinji's mother died of pneumonia, Xinji's schooling was interrupted. Unable to bear seeing his father bereft and struggling as a single parent, Xinji persuaded his father to remarry. The woman he married was less than half his age, a beautiful young woman from the capital, Xinjing. Since Xinji wanted to go there for to further his education, she soon hatched a plan to accompany the nineteen-year-old, "thin-skinned" *(lianpi bo)* Xinji back to her hometown so that his father would not worry about his inexperienced son.[31] Thus Xinji's downfall appears to begin with family breakdown, exacerbated by his relationships with women – his dead mother, an unfaithful stepmother, and a Korean waitress, with whom he commiserated and drank in a bar.

When Xinji and his stepmother first arrived in the capital, Xinji was happy in what he perceived to be an exotic (primarily Japanese) environment, although he was scandalized by his stepmother's living arrangements. They settled in a brothel, and her behaviour immediately changed as she began wearing pretty clothes and makeup. Xinji was afraid to tell his father because he did not want to hurt his father's feelings and, without money of his own, he relied on her. To cope with the stress of quietly bearing this humiliation, he began to drink on a daily basis. Xinji went to a bar where he was comforted by a Korean waitress, with whom he became "degenerate" *(duoluo)*.[32] Their intimate, although alcohol-centred, relationship is shown in Figure 38, with Xinji and the waitress in the bar, surrounded by Western furnishings and images and by bottles of alcohol.[33] Xinji soon quit school and left town to visit his friend Wang Jun in Mudanjiang. Jun told Xinji that heroin was a good medicine that could help him overcome his grief over his father and the course of his own life; Xinji decided to try it. Intoxicated, he forgot his father, stepmother, and school, and he decided to stay and get a job in the factory where Jun worked. When he was working or when he was using heroin, Xinji forgot his anxieties. But working all day and using drugs all night exhausted him. In less than a week, Xinji lost his job. Then he turned to morphine, which was even cheaper and caused graver consequences.

In the section "Yinzhe de xinli" (Psychology of an Addict), Xinji is shown to have lost his conscience and sense of morality in the attempt to satisfy his cravings.[34] He sold everything he had, aged prematurely, and did anything to get money, even losing fear of the police. Scavenging for food in the garbage, subconsciously looking for a place to die and end his misery, he thought he had hit rock bottom when he witnessed a group of wild dogs attacking a dying addict who had fallen down and was too weak to get back up. Terrified of this fate, he hurriedly sold the Western-style clothes he had borrowed from Jun and bought more heroin. After the drugs wore off, scared, broke, and having sold most of the clothes on his back, Xinji walked home. When his father saw how much his son had changed in only two years, he blamed himself for spoiling his son and making his character weak. The narrator concurs, arguing that the person most responsible for Xinji's addiction is his father for not making his son stronger. Through the police, Xinji is sent to a Healthy Life

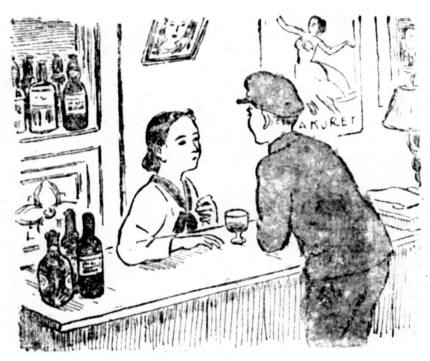

38 Xinji at the bar. *Source:* "Tang Xinji de shi gong" [Tang Xinji's true confession], in Kakegawa Akirashū, ed., *Qu tan conglin, di'yi ji* [Interesting discussion thicket, volume number 1] (Fengtian: Xing Ya yinshua zhushi huishe, 1942), 15. Original producer: Manchukuo Opium Monopoly, company defunct.

Institute. In two months, he recovers and returns home. The story concludes as the reader is told that Xinji found a job in a factory where he worked so effectively that he was promoted to division head. The moral of Xinji's story is that "addiction can be stopped, only through consciousness" *(yin fei bu neng jie, yao zai neng juewu er yi)* – that is, by developing a strong will and character, which is difficult when parents spoil their children or families split up.[35] Xinji's path to ruin is linked more firmly with his early childhood and the way that his parents raised him than with the later disruptions and temptations for which he was inadequately prepared.

In Chapter 4, "Chun guang zailai" (Spring Scenery Returns), another young man, Elder Brother, leaves his family and later returns home to his village after rehabilitation in a Healthy Life Institute. His father initially refuses to allow him in the house, despite pleading by his wife and daughter. Elder Brother explains to his sister how he was led astray by a man wearing Western-style clothes. Initially suspicious of the well-dressed stranger, he was lured by the promise of a good job in the big city. In pursuit of his dreams, he ended up working for a pittance, barely covering daily expenses. After he heard that a friend had won money gambling, he tried his hand and in short order lost even his meagre savings. To console himself, he went with a friend to get drunk, which then led him to even stronger intoxicants. Driven to despair and misery by the need for money, but unable to do anything but barely scrape by, one day he tried opium, an inexpensive drug that, his friend promised, with one puff would make him "immediately able to travel to the Kingdom of Heaven" *(like neng youli tianguo).*[36] In short order, he became an addict, lost his job, and lived on the streets, picking through garbage. Eventually, Elder Brother was taken to a Healthy Life Institute, where he recovered in two months. With his health fully restored, he returned to his family. His father was moved to see his son drug-free and allowed him to stay so that he could once again "make friends with the soil" *(yu nitu wei you).*[37] Elder Brother, like Xinji, left the safety and security of his family and moved to a big urban centre, where out of despair he started to drink alcohol, which served as a gateway drug for opium. Both were saved by treatment in a Healthy Life Institute and then restored to their families.

The most inspiring rehabilitation in *Qu tan conglin* can be found in Chapter 12, "Zhang Dexin xiansheng" (Mr. Zhang Dexin), the story of a fifty-five-year-old man from Jiutai village, Jilin province, who became a director of Xinjing's Morality Society (Daode hui). His father, Zhang Yu, had been an upright official who one day after retiring treated a cough with opium. In front of his son's eyes, he wasted away in addiction. Terrified, Dexin vowed never to use opium. On graduation, Dexin was not able to find a job in the city and moved his family to the countryside. There, he lived a comfortable but uneventful life. At the age of thirty-two, he began to smoke opium, realizing a folk adage cited by the narrator: "being full and warm leads to trouble" *(bao nuan sheng xianshi).*[38] Soon afterward, his wife, son, two daughters, and daughter-in-law all began to follow his example. As their smoking increased, the family's wealth dissipated. When Dexin was thirty-eight, they turned to morphine – because it was a cheaper, less time-consuming intoxicant. But, as with Tang Xinji, morphine proved even more devastating than opium. Dexin argued that every five minutes it was necessary to use it or the cravings "could not be tolerated" *(bu neng zhi chi le).*[39] For six years, they injected morphine until their skin was so badly disfigured that the whole family had "human faces and snake bodies" *(ren mian she shen).*[40] Dexin shows his body's disfigurement to dismayed onlookers in Figure 39.[41] Eventually, Dexin sold their land and moved the family to Changchun. There, they heard a speech by Li Huaiyuan, a lecturer from the Morality Society, who sought to help addicts to stop using

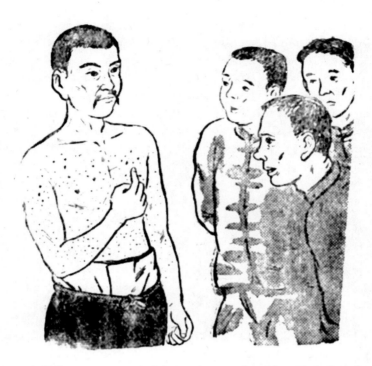

39 Dexin's disfigurement. *Source:* "Zhang Dexin xiansheng" [Mr. Zhang Dexin], in Kakegawa Akirashū, ed., *Qu tan conglin, di'yi ji* [Interesting discussion thicket, volume number 1] (Fengtian: Xing Ya yinshua zhushi huishe, 1942), 99. Original producer: Manchukuo Opium Monopoly, company defunct.

morphine.[42] As he lectured about the unfilial nature of the self-inflicted physical abuse caused by addiction, Dexin decided to quit out of respect for his ancestors. Dexin recounts the extreme pain of withdrawal, arguing that the extent of the physical and spiritual pain cannot be described in words. After losing consciousness several times, in four or five days he succeeded in overcoming the worst of his addiction. Then his resolve grew stronger to the twentieth day, when his addiction had waned. From his own personal experience, he came to believe that opiates could be quit with personal resolve and "resolute belief in the teachings and decrees of sages and men of virtue, divinities, and Buddha" *(shenxin shengxian shen fu zhi jiao zhi).*[43] Considering himself to have been reborn, he showed his gratitude by taking a prominent position in the Morality Society and making speeches about his personal triumph.

In 1932 a director of the Morality Society, Wang Shangren, encouraged Dexin to fully dedicate himself to social reform. Dexin first followed his advice by emulating his grandparents and established a home school to emphasize moral education. Women were taught to become "good wives, wise mothers" so that they could raise their children accordingly. That same year, he helped to establish branches of the Morality Society in Changchun and Harbin, supported by the incomes of hundreds of acres of rice fields.[44] In 1933 a Xinjing Morality Society headquarters was established, and Dexin was hired to direct its rehabilitation class. Later, branches were established in other Manchukuo locations, including Yushu county, Jilin city, Guojiadian, and Gongzhuling. After his own salvation from drug addiction, which it should be noted came in the wake of the founding of Manchukuo, Dexin was driven by a religious fervour to help others and become part of the establishment that had assisted him in restoring his drug-free life. Dexin admitted that rehabilitation was a painful process, an assertion that countered advertising claims of pain-free cures in other media. His example was provided in *Qu tan conglin* to convince readers that addiction could be overcome, that meaningful lives could be achieved after withdrawal, and that not all involved in the rehabilitation business were interested in torturing or otherwise harming those afflicted with addiction.

Unlike Zhang Dexin, not all could overcome their addictions without official or medical intervention. Such help was available through the sale of products for home use or in clinics and hospitals as well as in state-funded Healthy Life Institutes, the latter of which are featured in several *Qu tan conglin* stories. In "Tang Xinji de shi gong," as Xinji lay on his deathbed, his father called the police to transport his son to rehabilitation.[45] His father's love and Manchukuo's virtuous government are credited with his recovery in a Healthy Life Institute. Through rehabilitation, Xinji learned he could overcome his addiction if he came to terms with the difficulties of his life.[46] In "Chun guang zailai," Elder brother expressed his gratitude to the Healthy Life Institute, which he regarded as his "benefactor" *(en ren)* for rescuing him from a premature death.[47] In "Mayao yinzhe de wang'en," Healthy Life Institute staff feared that Liu Enhui had damaged his body beyond repair. Despite their reservations, the skilled doctors saved his life, and after three months in rehabilitation, he recovered his health and conscience. All of these men sought rehabilitation, or were sent for it, as their addictions pushed them to the edge of death. Intervention by the state-funded institutions saved their lives.

Two accounts of experiences in Healthy Life Institutes are provided to counter the fear with which many viewed the institutions. In "Qin'ai de Liu Zheng xian di" (Dear First Brother Liu Zheng), Liu Shaoxian reveals in a letter

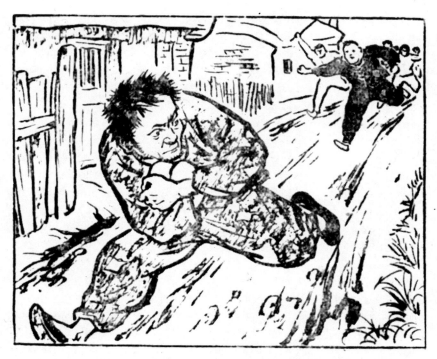

40 Shaoxian on the run. *Source:* "Qin'ai de Liu Zheng xian di" [Dear first brother], in Kakegawa Akirashū, ed., *Qu tan conglin, di'yi ji* [Interesting discussion thicket, volume number 1] (Fengtian: Xing Ya yinshua zhushi huishe, 1942), 107. Original producer: Manchukuo Opium Monopoly, company defunct.

to his brother why he left his hometown five years before.[48] As a high school student, Shaoxian had dreamed of becoming a world-famous researcher, but his plans were stymied when his family could not afford to send him to university. Instead, they arranged an unwanted marriage for him and set him to work managing the farm. One day, a tenant who was delinquent in rent convinced an exhausted and unhappy Shaoxian to try opium. His immediate enjoyment of the drug led to an addiction so heavy that all he wanted to do was to use opium. Intoxicated, Shaoxian forgot his former dreams of university and his current despair. One day, he absconded with 5,000 yuan to spend on opium. Shaoxian's experience taught him that all addicts are the same; whether they are men or women, old or young, poor or rich, there is no difference: with opium as the centre of their lives, they have no way to survive in the "so-called chaotic world of animals" *(suowei wu zhixu de dongwu shijie).*[49] Figure 40 shows a desperate Shaoxian being chased by outraged townspeople, from whom he has stolen to support his habit.[50] Shaoxian warns that all addicts inevitably end up on the streets, where they will either die or be incarcerated by the authorities. Those who have the strength can try to evade the police, but most curl up where they lie and are apprehended and sent to a Healthy Life Institute.

Shaoxian notes that addicts are scared of Healthy Life Institutes because they believe the institutes are worse than jail, like hell. But Shaoxian writes that once an addict is admitted, a truer perspective can be attained. The day that he was taken in during a police crackdown, he had nothing to eat or drink and was very weak. The group of addicts was taken to the countryside in a vehicle that stopped in front of a foreign building with a wide courtyard. As they got out, they were met by fourteen or fifteen workers, who sent the police away, greeted the new arrivals, and then walked the group inside to see the director. The director addressed them thus:

> This here is called a Healthy Life Institute. Gentlemen, this Healthy Life Institute, perhaps you think this is the most terrifying place. But it is absolutely a good place to live. After residing here two or three days, gentlemen, you will naturally understand. To conclude, this is not a prison, it is a large household. I am this household's master, and you from today on should count yourselves as family members. Since you have come here, we are all family, please everyone feel at ease. Today, gentlemen, you all look exhausted. So first, please eat. Then after that, go for a haircut and take a bath.[51]

The depiction of the Healthy Life Institute as a large household dominates the rest of the account, as Shaoxian and the others are repeatedly told to view the institution as their home. Shaoxian describes the institution in glowing terms, writing of the spacious eating hall and good food. While the others ate their first meal, Shaoxian drank only a cup of tea since his addiction had left him with no appetite. Lunch was followed by a rest, haircuts, and the assigning of new, clean, and comfortable white clothing. Accommodations were Chinese-style, with a *kang* (a heatable brick bed) per room, each capable of hosting eight people. The newly arrived were placed among others already in recovery, doubtless to inspire the newcomers and to remind the nearly rehabilitated of the pain that they had survived. As directed, they arranged their quilts and lay down. On the edge of sleep, Shaoxian suddenly had a craving for opium. Thinking about his addiction, Shaoxian decided he had to deal with it one step at a time and to just put it out of his mind that night. Later, the courtyard nurse came to take the patients' temperatures and pulses.

The next morning, patients were awakened by a bell, and the nurse returned to take temperatures, pulses, and urine tests. Then all went outside to stand at attention, salute the Japanese and Manchukuo flags, and sing the national anthems. This was followed by exercise and cleaning duties, with each person assigned work in the office, dining area, lounge, toilet, or outside the house. Tasks completed, they washed their faces and went for breakfast. The meal was followed by a short rest and a visit to the clinic. The director supervised as nurses reported on results of urine tests, from which three levels of addiction were distinguished – heavy, medium, and light – each to be treated differently. During inspections, which occurred every three days, the director returned. He rarely spoke, but Shaoxian notes that his professionalism was comforting to the patients. After lunch, "light" addicts and those who had been resident for several weeks accompanied the director and staff out to the courtyard to play ball games and sports together. After dinner, Japanese lessons lasted for fifteen minutes, during which the patients were taught the Japanese and Manchukuo national anthems as well as general vocabulary.

On the second night, the staff told the patients to stay in the classroom for a speech from the director. Each person was given a cup of tea and, those who smoked, a cigarette. The director asked for their opinions of the Healthy Life Institute and told them that if they all worked together, they could live happily and peacefully. It was their responsibility to take care of and watch over each other; if one person was lazy, that would affect the whole family. Everyone had to participate in work. Men and women cooked together, washing vegetables, peeling peas, or preserving vegetables, often while singing songs. Men also engaged in heavier labour and helped with transportation, and women attended to sleeping furniture and clothing. In the winter, indoor exercises and weekly entertainment meetings were held; some would dance, and others would sing or recite poetry. When rehabilitation was complete, those with family left. Many of them later returned with gifts, including chickens, pears, eggs, or pork; the narrator compares them to new brides returning home to see their mothers.[52] Several of the rehabilitated with no family opted to stay and work at the Healthy Life Institute for room and board. Volunteers were given some spending money and were allowed out to shop but only during the daytime. Some chose never to go out. Shaoxian argues that only in a Kingly Way *(Wangdao)* country could such a nurturing and supportive environment have been created, echoing the director's insistence that Healthy Life Institutes should not be regarded as jails but rather as large households.[53] Rehabilitation, Shaoxian reckons, transforms addicts' lives by making the lazy hardworking, liars honest, the bad-tempered kind, and the poor rich.⁵⁴ Working together, the community of 120 staff and patients created an environment where they could respect each other and gain satisfaction and self-worth from their work. Although the volunteers did not earn much money, it was a job that guaranteed food, shelter, clothing, and distance from temptations to use drugs. This chapter describes hardworking, dedicated staff who oversee patients as they happily complete chores and other responsibilities as part of a rehabilitation treatment that was difficult but a far cry from the imprisonment and torture charged by critics.

A similar depiction of a Healthy Life Institute from a different perspective is provided in "Qingtian zai lai di shang" (Sunny Days Come Again to the Land), a story told from the perspective of a female nurse who supervises the rehabilitation of her patient Sun Jun. She has worked in Healthy Life Institutes for three years, and Jun is the first to express heartfelt gratitude for her assistance in restoring him over the course of a month to a potentially "bright life" *(minglang de shenghuo)*.⁵⁵ When Jun arrived at the institute, like other addicts, he had trouble breathing and was close to death. Lying on a bench, he could barely move. He would alternately fall into a deep sleep or suddenly violently awake, screaming, "This can't be done, this time I am really being tortured. Yesterday I was thrown out by my parents; my suffering, I can't bear it anymore."⁵⁶ Or he yelled, "Old Liu, what have you done? Already spent over 300 yuan. Whatsoever, you have to smoke another puff. You are afraid of the police."⁵⁷ The hallucinations and pain were so unnerving that the nurse believed that his was the most serious addiction that she had ever seen. After two weeks, he had passed through the worst pain and physical effects. The nurse was well aware that it was not easy to quit drugs, but she believed it possible if one had the "willpower" *(yizhi li)* to change into an "upright person" *(zhengren)*.⁵⁸ Since, she believed, all forms of rehabilitation necessarily involved some degree of pain, addicts had to work hard to regain their health, and their success depended on willpower. Pleased that Jun had survived withdrawal, she asked him why he had started using.⁵⁹ Jun responded that it stemmed from social reasons, namely his use of opium for "social intercourse" *(ying chou)*.⁶⁰

These two fictional accounts of Healthy Life Institute experiences stress the pain that addicts on the edge of death had to endure during treatment. This helps to explain why the state-funded institutes were so unpopular, especially when compared with the promises of pain-free commercial formulas for domestic treatment. But although withdrawal pain is explicitly discussed, neither account mentions patients dying or relapsing – outcomes that vexed addicts, their families and friends, health practitioners, and officials. Since Opium Monopoly officials themselves observed that up to

70 percent of addicts relapsed,[61] some recognition of this issue would have imparted a greater veneer of truthfulness to the accounts. The reader is also left wondering why Jun was the first person in three years to express such gratitude to the nurse. The repeated stress on Healthy Life Institutes as large households, and explicitly not jails, capable of curing even the most hopeless addicts suggests the degree to which officials had to combat popular, negative perceptions of the institutions. If they had been generally accepted, there would have been little need to exaggerate their efficacy and repeatedly deny that they were jails. Nor would staff have needed to be depicted as unilaterally conscientious and whole-heartedly devoted to patients who sang happy songs while working. Ultimately, the one-dimensional praise for Healthy Life Institutes attributed a naiveté to readers that many would have found offensive and that detracted from appreciation for whatever merits the institutions actually did have.

Similarly flawed accounts of law enforcement can be found in two stories that detail the criminal behaviour linked with the drug trade. "Xiaozhang xiansheng" (Mr. Principal) tells the tale of principal Yamada, who was stationed in a village on Manchukuo's border with Korea and who aimed at the moral cultivation of the community. During the early twentieth century, it is recounted, many Korean farmers had migrated across the border. Local Chinese who were unhappy with the new migrants confiscated the farmlands that they had cleared for planting.[62] Displaced, the Koreans had to find another way to make a living or return home; many turned to the opium trade on both sides of the border. In the 1920s, the narrator explains, the warlord government did not enforce opium laws, and officials made money selling opium. After Manchukuo was established, ethnic relations improved as Manchurian and Korean people began working co-operatively and in law-abiding ways to create a community and country in the spirit of Manchukuo's Kingly Way. Some Koreans, however, continued the private selling of opium. Principal Yamada, intent on fully implementing the Opium Law in his community, ran into trouble with a local group of Korean dealers. Their first appearance in the story takes place in a bar, where they commiserate over the principal's determination to destroy their livelihoods. The four ruffians, who started drinking early in the evening, are surrounded by fifteen or sixteen empty alcohol bottles as they discuss how they should deal with Yamada, as illustrated in Figure 41.[63] Despite recognizing the positive changes he has introduced, including encouraging children to be frugal and community-minded, they argue that he has exceeded his authority by dictating the end of their business. They defend their work by reasoning that it was a sanctioned business practice long before Yamada arrived.

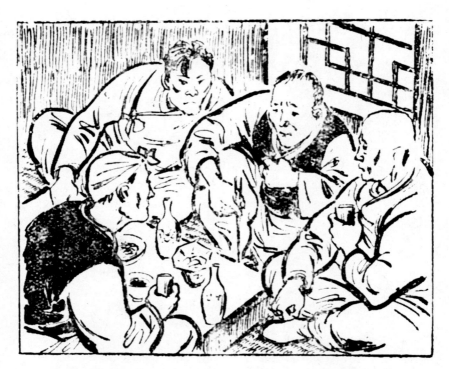

41   Korean dealers. *Source:* "Xiaozhang xiansheng" [Mr. Principal], in Kakegawa
Akirashū, ed., *Qu tan conglin, di'yi ji* [Interesting discussion thicket, volume number 1]
(Fengtian: Xing Ya yinshua zhushi huishe, 1942), 59. Original producer: Manchukuo
Opium Monopoly, company defunct.

In the face of their intransigence, Yamada suggests to his supportive community members a three-pronged approach to ending the opium trade.[64] First,
a private seller should be revealed to him so that he can discreetly intervene
and reason with the person. If this person is caught a second time, then the
trader will be publicly exposed to the community, and all profits from drug
dealing will be confiscated. If caught a third time, the person will be expelled
from the community and sent to the police. Yamada approaches his intervention into the drug trade with great enthusiasm, spending much time collecting
evidence, even on winter nights in weather of minus thirty degrees Celsius.
One night, on his rounds, he is attacked by the conspiring Korean dealers.
The next day he goes to work with his head bandaged but spirits high, telling
people that he expects no less in his line of work and that he will not be de-
terred. Yamada's attitude increases public sympathy for his crusade. One day,
a former drug dealer, Mr. Lin, visits the principal to report on his trip to Korea
to attempt to convince a major dealer there to quit. During this trip, Lin was

thrown into a hold for several weeks, with nothing to eat, until he managed to dig a hole and crawl out and over to the dealer's house, where he again pleaded with him to stop selling opium. The dealer was impressed by his determination and vowed to stop. The dealer has accompanied Lin back to Manchukuo, where he asks Yamada for forgiveness for hurting people in Manchukuo and ruining the name of the Korean people. The chapter ends with a postscript stating that principals Haseda (in Tonghua) and Ichimaru (in Tieling) also behave like Yamada, striving to stop the private opium trade and to help Koreans better integrate into Manchukuo society. This depiction of Koreans deeply involved in the drug trade mitigates the refusal in other chapters of *Qu tan conglin* to recognize non-Anglo-American complicity. However, the appearance of the Korean leader in Manchukuo to apologize for his behaviour stretches credibility. Further, the citing of only Japanese principals underlines Japan's supposed benevolent mission in the region, but it is insulting and patronizing to other ethnic groups whose members were also prominently committed to eradicating recreational opium use.

In Chapter 10, "Yu shaonian de qi ji" (Young Yu's Surprise Plan), the criminality linked with the drug trade is shown to extend far beyond it. The richest man in the village, Mr. Yu, is kidnapped by a band of opium dealers for his role in enforcing Manchukuo's anti-opium laws. Yu's work deprived the gang of their leader, seventeen or eighteen colleagues, and most of their livelihood. His family is told that they must pay a ransom of 50,000 yuan, or their house will be burned down and Mr. Yu will never be seen again. Yu's thirteen-year-old son searches for his father and eventually finds him with the bandits at their campsite deep in the forest. When the son arrives, he discovers that the gang has been drinking alcohol all night while holding Yu hostage. The son is told by their intoxicated leader that he has three days to return with the ransom money. The boy appears to return with the cash and approaches the gang. However, on his signal, ten police leap out of their hiding places, turning the forest into a battlefield as the twenty or thirty hooligans are all arrested.[65] Yu is rescued, the dealers are defeated, and the determination of the son to vanquish them and restore justice to the community is celebrated.

These two stories describing criminal behaviour associated with the opium trade highlight the collateral damage that was caused by drug dealing as individuals, families, and communities found themselves hostage to criminal elements who, as long as they sought to live off opium earnings, acted with impunity to beat, kidnap, and otherwise hurt law-abiding citizens. The successful conclusions of the stories – Yu's timely rescue and Yamada's transformation of a community and toppling of a major Korean drug dealer – are optimistic, but they do not represent how most of the opium trade was handled in Manchukuo, as private sales persisted to the end of the occupation. Further, as discussed in Chapter 2, the opium trade in Manchukuo was dominated by Japanese, who in this volume do not appear in any criminal capacity. Instead, they are assigned roles as doctors, principals, and law enforcement officials. In 1942, when *Qu tan conglin* was published, censorship restrictions prohibited negative depictions of Japanese, so readers were probably not surprised by such characterizations. But one has to wonder about the degree to which such distortion diminished popular perceptions of this collection. Although this cannot be known with certainty, several aspects of *Qu tan conglin* signal its significance as a historical document.

Much of *Qu tan conglin* is dedicated to decrying the recreational consumption of opium, heroin, and morphine. So, too, is alcohol use criticized. In keeping with the prohibitionist tendencies of wartime Manchukuo officialdom and media, most stories depict alcohol as a gateway drug or as an accompaniment to other drugs. Together, the stories of addiction and its terrible costs for users and their families and friends highlight the widespread problems that the Monopoly was officially established to battle. For the most part, the focus is on male addicts, with women relegated to secondary positions: they lead men to become addicts, they become addicts because of the men in their lives, or they serve as nurses in men's rehabilitation. The volume illustrates that for men and women addiction was a problem and that some Monopoly officials, at least, viewed it as such. The writings in *Qu tan conglin* celebrate victories over addiction as well as the creation of communities and patriotic citizens. These depictions tend to be overly simplistic, one-sided characterizations of questionable value. Were Anglo-American imperialists solely responsible for China's opium problem? Did the Japanese act only as saviours? Were the Chinese all victims? And were all addicts lazy, liars, bad-tempered, and poor? *Qu tan conglin* inadvertently highlights these questions that its producers failed to address adequately. The volume may have violated censorship regulations that forbade negative depictions of Manchukuo to appeal to readers and get its basic message across, but its single-minded focus on convincing readers of the Japanese pursuit of opium eradication would have alienated significant portions of the population who were well aware of the greater complexity of the issue. Many were doubtless sympathetic to popularizing the dangers of drugs and blaming Anglo-American imperialists for an opium problem that was exacerbated by their actual, historically documented aggressive and greedy behaviour. But the singular focus on the Japanese as the saviours of the Chinese does little to enhance the volume's credibility. Perhaps the most enduring contributions of *Qu tan conglin* are the insistence that recreational drug use was devastating and that rehabilitation was a positive yet painful process that brought relief for those with willpower and stamina, two characteristics for which the people of China's Northeast had long been known and that throughout the twentieth century became ever more ingrained in understandings of their character.

Conclusion

In the Chinese-language culture of Manchukuo in the early 1940s, Chinese, Japanese, and Manchu health professionals, officials, social commentators, and writers engaged in a battle against recreational intoxicant consumption. Dark portraits of addiction and its high costs to the wartime society were featured in a wide variety of media in order to reflect official efforts, and failures, to realize the state's anti-intoxicant platform. The expansion of hostilities across the mainland, Holy War, and increasingly oppressive socioeconomic conditions altered individual, industrial, and state priorities and generated more sinister understandings of alcohol consumption, equating it with opium and other drugs. As living standards dropped precipitously and officials appropriated ingredients and machinery used to produce alcohol, advertisements that once hailed alcohol declined, factories closed, and its use was decried across popular culture, foregrounding negative narratives that reflected beliefs dating back hundreds of years and that articulated the demands of an austere wartime regime. Consumers were told to overcome their addictions by strengthening their resolve to toughen up and abandon inappropriate, outdated customs. With the collapse of Manchukuo in 1945, Japanese dominion over the alcohol and opium industries ended.[1] The Russian intrusions and civil war that ensued were marked by a proliferation of opium throughout the region as it was stripped of regulatory controls and as stock from the defunct Opium Monopoly issued into the markets.[2] Ironically, the turmoil that immediately followed the collapse of Japan's empire accentuated the relative stability of Manchukuo.

Chinese Communist Party (CCP) victories through the late 1940s brought significant changes to the region's intoxicant industries: opium was prohibited, and alcohol was again placed under state control. One goal that successive regimes had professed to seek for decades was achieved under early socialist rule: the end of recreational opium use. Cultivation was strictly prohibited, and recreational use disappeared, during the Maoist era at least, as strict enforcement policies accompanied rehabilitation projects, which contributed to the legitimization of CCP rule. Alcohol continued to be produced and consumed even though prices had skyrocketed during the civil war.[3] In the 1950s recreational use of opium could not be seen, but alcohol production rebounded under state direction, until the Great Leap Forward began in 1958, when communes were allowed to produce their own alcohol; restrictions were reintroduced in the early 1960s in response to the devastating national famine. In 1966 the Cultural Revolution swept government control to the sidelines and caused declining official production until 1970. The passing of the Maoist era has brought about a resurgence of both intoxicants, marked by government regulations, licensing and foreign partnerships for alcohol, and underground markets for opiates and other drugs.

For hundreds of years, alcohol and opium have flourished in the area now known as China's Northeast. Both were mainstays of the regional economy. Opium was instrumental in enticing waves of Han migration that enabled Chinese governments to claim the Manchu homelands for their own. Lucrative opium industries encouraged Han settlement of the region, pre-empting late-nineteenth and early-twentieth-century Japanese and Russian territorial ambitions as successive regimes lost the ability to secure the region. In the 1920s both alcohol and opium produced major revenues for economic and military development, funding first Zhang Zuolin's national aspirations and later the Japanese occupation. Despite the circulation of arguments that Europeans and Japanese drank alcohol, whereas Chinese smoked opium, both intoxicants were popular with a wide range of consumers. Alcohol and opium provided leisurely diversions to combat the rigours of life in the frontier region and to pass the long winter months. In the 1930s they appeared, often together, in cultural productions that depicted local social conditions. In the 1940s both were regularly blamed for ruining lives and weakening the nation.

To contemporary observers, and not a few scholars, intoxicants appeared to bolster Japan's imperial ambitions in Manchuria.[4] The reverse was true. The inability of officials to actualize the prohibition policies that they so publicly promoted, and that were echoed by enthusiastic supporters across the Chinese-language culture, helped to undermine whatever legitimacy Manchukuo may have had. Under early Japanese dominion, intoxicant industries expanded. Dominion over intoxicants brought wealth and prestige to the Japanese who controlled them and to their partners, but the industries disheartened those who sought, for whatever reason, an intoxicant-free society. Manchukuo's Opium Law was undermined by minimal actual restrictions on the production and distribution of opiates. Rehabilitation programs failed to win popular support because even the most well-intentioned efforts were defeated by officials who wearied of consigning resources to an endeavour of questionable efficacy that did not directly contribute to their own enrichment, economic development, or Holy War. Healthy Life Institutes engendered greater fear in the populace than did addiction, partly because the institutions' reputations kept those who needed them most from entering until they were on the verge of death, which mitigated the possibility of successful rehabilitation. The failings of the Opium Monopoly created the impression that it was no more than a façade for Japanese drug dealing, which made the regime appear to be not only ruthlessly parasitic but also impotent to effect the social change advocated by officials and critics alike.

The changes the Japanese were most able to implement occurred in the alcohol industry, in which they amalgamated businesses by ejecting Chinese, Russian, and other ethnic groups from control and by extending Japanese ownership and practices of product promotion. The industry grew by leaps and bounds in the early 1930s through the promotion of products that consumers were told were both good and good for them. Ads for a remarkably wide variety of alcohol products contributed to the look and content of the most popular journals and newspapers, underlining retailer-driven connections between product consumption and Chinese culture. Alcohol's status as a nutritious, essential part of Manchukuo life was touted, for example, in Red Ball (Chi yu) advertisements to attract consumers through imagery and text that underscored the state's multiculturalism and modernity and the traditions of its subjects. Beer was "fashionable." Writers boasted of drinking and of getting drunk. But by the early 1940s, Holy War demands had forced production to contract according to state dictates, and the product promotion that had once been so prominent had begun to disappear. Alcohol joined opium as an intoxicant that, critics warned, if not controlled, would poison the population and lead the empire to ruin.

Intoxicants held as prominent a position in the Chinese-language culture of Manchukuo as they did in official policies. The popularity of social realism and the ambition of Chinese writers to raise the consciousness of the masses made literature an ideal vehicle for battling addiction. The anti-intoxicant narratives pursued by writers such as Li Zhengzhong, Mei Niang, Xiao Jun, and Zhu Ti bolstered Manchukuo's prohibitionist platform and warned of the potential dangers of drugs to the exclusion of positive references to their recreational use. By the 1940s, at least, popular literature tended to promote prohibition and thus allowed for critical reflection on the nature of Manchukuo society. Since the Japanese were officially prohibited from using opiates, Chinese criticism of opiate addiction was not perceived by officials to be critical of the Japanese per se but rather of Chinese weakness and wilful disobedience to the law, discourses they also promoted. Chinese writers decried elite indulgence in, or profit from, opium while the lower classes groaned under the weight of addiction, poverty, and subjugation. In the 1940s, too, alcohol was increasingly depicted as a gateway drug to life-crippling addiction, and thus the writers supported official priorities in describing tragic Chinese and Russian attempts to overcome melancholy and alienation from the state through alcohol consumption. Such depictions reflected newspaper reports that consistently warned Japanese that they risked their leading role in Asia if alcohol use was not brought under control.

In Manchukuo's Chinese-language culture, little sympathy was extended to addicts, or "ghosts," a term that accentuated the "half-death" nature of addiction in these portraits. Alcohol and opium may have been considered requirements of polite society before foreign occupation, but during the Manchukuo era they assumed a sinister nature that was denounced throughout popular culture. Consumption was linked with weak wills, the lack of courage to face rehabilitation, and a subjugated people. In the intoxicant narratives that emerged, a critical disjuncture attested to contemporary gender constructs. Both men and women condemned addiction for its destructive nature, but men tended more explicitly to link this destruction with society or the nation, whereas women associated it with the family, especially its patriarchal foundations – the source of women's tragedy. These narratives not only underlined traditional Confucian maxims that consigned women to the domestic sphere but also reflected deep-seated anxieties over the health, status, and self-identities of the Chinese in Manchukuo – not the economic obsessions that came to dominate official rhetoric.

Perhaps nowhere was concern over gender more deeply expressed than in the heated debate over the position of women working in opium retail outlets. From its first appearance as a marketing ploy, the hostess profession was controversial and, for some women and business owners, lucrative. Women worked as hostesses for various reasons, all of which they were criticized for, whether independence, love, money, or drugs motivated their desire to be professional women working beyond the domestic sphere. Criticism was even more severe, and rightfully so, if they were forced unwillingly into the position. Critics saw intoxicants as a troubling condition of their working environment, but newspaper reports, especially, suggest that many of these critics were concerned more with the women themselves and the potential for independence (economic, sexual, or otherwise) that their jobs represented than with questions of addiction. Women who appeared to live like "Kings of Fengtian" *(Fengtian wang)* were a prime target for criticism, as they earned their incomes from an industry that most viewed as morally suspect in a larger environment where notions of women's "proper behaviour" were greatly contested.

Those who condemned the recreational consumption of intoxicants did so because such a stance appealed to them as well as to officials. Many officials treated intoxicants and Chinese popular culture with a similar disdain, contending that both required supervision, and laws were drafted to control them, but Manchukuo officialdom never mustered the willpower or the resources necessary to bring either fully to heel: legal and illegal alcohol and opium sales continued to the end of the occupation and, despite the odds, a vibrant Chinese culture was created. The intoxicants were too lucrative and officials, even if willing to enforce the law, found themselves impotent to implement it in a manner that produced significant change. At the same time, cultural producers, social commentators, and health professionals did not simply parrot official policies but also actively moulded them to suit their own purposes and in the process delegitimized Manchukuo. Dark portraits of addiction, poverty, and individual subjugation were implicitly critical of contemporary society. The failure of Manchukuo officials to achieve the eradication of recreational intoxicant consumption, identified as key to their Kingly Way modernization, fuelled Chinese alienation through constant reiteration of anti-addiction rhetoric that highlighted, if not magnified, the severity of the problem. This alienation is one of the intoxicants' most significant contributions to the history of the region. Anti-intoxicant reformists, anti-Japanese activists, and Western critics condemned the regime, claiming that it aimed for the destruction of local Chinese society. The chorus of condemnation stigmatized intoxicant consumption and turned the Manchukuo regime into a lightning rod for criticism due to its inability to effect the social change that it so loudly trumpeted. Ironically, the "truly terrifying" costs of addiction decried by Li Xianglan and others wreaked havoc in their own lives. In post-occupation society, each of them suffered the burden of their success in Manchukuo. Li Xianglan went into self-imposed exile after 1945, but most of the Chinese writers discussed in this study stayed within China to endure decades of persecution for their presumed traitorous relations with the colonial state; each of the writers was silenced by the political movements that swept China in the Maoist era.

The consumption of alcohol in Manchuria during the first half of the twentieth century mirrors that in other "frontier" and colonial arenas, including Canada and the United States, where alcohol was also prominently used. Cheryl Warsh has noted that economies such as these, often based on subsistence agriculture and rootlessness, tend to promote consumption.[5] The wave of migration to Manchuria in the early part of the twentieth century constituted one of the largest in modern history, yet the experiences of these pioneers remain hardly known, partly because of the Manchukuo legacy. The difficulty of establishing lives in the "frontier" region was exacerbated by agricultural or other migratory work that in the 1930s and 1940s was often at subsistence level, especially during the war. Rootlessness was endemic. Many believed alcohol and opium necessary to survival in what was widely regarded as a harsh environment. To this day, alcohol famously remains a distinctive element of Northeast living. Feng Qi has noted that Northeast-erners "drink habitually and excessively" *(haoyin)*, especially with close friends.[6] Such drinking customs in the Northeast reflect those in surrounding societies.

In the Russian Far East, alcohol has long been used by inhabitants to pass the long winters, although the Russian ability to drink alcohol has been dis-missed by Northeasterners, who brag that Russian consumption simply cannot compare with theirs.[7] Indeed, Chi Xiucai argues that of one of Harbin people's "three great oddities" *(san da guai)* is to "drink beer like irrigation" *(he pijiu xiang guanggai).*[8] In Korea alcohol is considered a necessary means of promot-ing social communication.[9] As in China, Confucian moral ethics discourage excessive exhibition of drunken behaviour while not denouncing consumption altogether. In Japanese "popular culture, drinking is constructed as a vehicle for the expression of individuality and, particularly, masculinity."[10] Stephen Smith's 1988 study on alcohol in Japanese society argues that the amount or frequency of alcohol consumption has not been considered symptomatic of alcoholism or problem drinking; rather, intoxication is seen to be a problem when it gives rise to public conflict or disruption.[11] Descriptions of problem-atic recreational alcohol consumption by writers and officials in Manchukuo reflect this concern as well as the Confucian stress on ritual and order.

In *The Alcoholic Republic,* W.J. Rorabaugh applied Donald Horton's thesis that drinking, through its sedative qualities, encourages social peace. Rorabaugh argues that "a high level of drunkenness is likely in cultures that are anxiety-ridden, structurally disintegrating, or incompetent in providing individuals with a sense of effectiveness. Such societies are most likely to be found under conditions of stress, when the social order has been wrenched either by contact with alien cultures or by internal dislocations caused by changes in ideology, institutions, structure, or economy."[12] Cheryl Krasnick Warsh also argues that "drinking is a function of a culture's social organiza-tion," but if a social system fails to fulfil individual needs, alcohol consumption tends to increase.[13]

Rorabaugh and Warsh could be describing Manchukuo, but they are not. They are explaining North American conditions that seemingly have more universal application. In a similar vein, Tsung-Yi Lin and David Lin have argued that when Chinese adopt Western lifestyles, or when there is a break-down of traditional Chinese social organizations, or when both occur in combination, problematic alcohol consumption results.[14] Catherine Carstairs, too, has noted that heavy drug use is often found among people "who have relatively few opportunities due to lack of education, racial discrimination, and poverty."[15] These scholars point to conditions that predominated in China's Northeast in the first half of the twentieth century. The Manchukuo years were marked by stress, internal dislocations, disintegration of the region's nascent urban consumer culture, and perhaps most fatefully, the racial dis-crimination enforced by officialdom. The tone and extent of the campaigns against recreational intoxicant consumption suggest that use was widespread, costly, and difficult to sustain as war spread across Asia, devouring lives, labour, and resources.

This study demonstrates that despite widespread belief to the contrary, alcohol has played significant and varied roles in Chinese history. It continues to do so. The contradictory ways that alcohol is viewed are clearly expressed by Gong Li in *Yin jiu shihua (History of Wine Drinking):*

> Wine, a magic spirit, presents as fire sometimes and then ice. It is sometimes like a lingering dream, a piece of soft silk and then poses as the evil and a sharp sword. It is actually mighty and presents everywhere. With it, you may get unfettered to display your genius in full blossom; you may also become un-scrupulous and degenerate into abysm.[16]

Alcohol has inspired cultural production, yet it is alleged to have contributed to the death of China's greatest poet, Li Bai. Alcohol has played roles in spiritual activities and funded brutal military campaigns. The positive and negative beliefs concerning alcohol consumption derive from Chinese and foreign influences – whether they be Confucian teachings, Silk Road travels, Yuan monopolies, or Japanese advertising – and they represent the long-term ability of Chinese culture to integrate local and foreign practices. In recent decades, policies of the post-Mao reform era have once again turned a spot-light on alcohol and its presence in China. Alcohol's significance within China is increasingly being recognized, as are China's achievements in alcohol markets at home and abroad. China is now the largest producer of beer in the world.[17] A beer from the Northeast, Xuehua (Snow), established in 1964,[18] currently ranks second in the world in sales; it is 49 percent owned by the South African–based company SABMiller, demonstrating ongoing local-foreign connections in China's alcohol industry. Every year, Harbin hosts the

Harbin Summer International Beer Festival, one of the three most popular in China (all of which are in China's north).[19] Chinese are said to now consume one-quarter of the global supply of cognac.[20] Chinese wines regularly win awards in international competitions and have been doing so since the Wujiapi brand won a gold medal in Singapore over 100 years ago in 1873.[21] Annual production of Kweichow Maotai, one of the most popular Chinese wines, is in the millions of tons, and it is now argued to be the most popular alcoholic beverage in the world.[22] These commercial achievements and a plethora of new publications on the subject all point to the need for a deeper understanding of alcohol, its place in Chinese cultures, and the ways that relationships between consumption and national or cultural identities are forged.[23]

To date, opium has held a pre-eminent position in the modern history of China and in how it has been understood. The beginnings of the modern era are routinely traced to the Opium War. Opium has influenced understandings of individual health, local society, and foreign relations. Opium has been omnipresent in modern historical narratives even though it was not recreationally consumed during the Maoist era. The reform-era resurgence of the recreational use of opiates and other drugs in China will doubtless lead to new understandings of usage and addiction. This time, far fewer foreigners are involved in the illegal trade, and those who are caught are punished according to Chinese laws. Although such drugs do not appear to be as prevalent in the Northeast as in the Southwest, consumption still garners critical attention, although nowhere near as much as it did during the 1930s and 1940s. And despite decades of research, the treatment of addictive behaviours still remains dishearteningly elusive, yet the programs today, as well as the sales of intoxicants, are not regularly associated with foreign designs to destroy society. In the past, alcohol and opium were used as recreational products and, eventually, as indices to gauge the state of the nation. Through their promotion or prohibition, intoxicants have helped to shape the ways that individuals perceive their own health, the society in which they live, and their history. In the Northeast of China, they play these roles still.

Glossary

Abe Tomoji	阿部知二	
ahfurong	阿芙蓉	opium
ahmulu	阿木魯	a (Manchu) mountain grape wine
ahpian	阿片	opium
Ai Jingpu	艾景璞	
Aibiaosi	愛表斯	Ebosi
Aisin-Gioro Puyi	愛新覺羅 溥儀	
Anqimaoqin	安其毛沁	
Ao Shuang'an	傲霜俺	
Arai Chōjirō	新井長治朗	
Asahi	旭	Brilliance of the Rising Sun
Ba bu	八不	Eight Abstentions
Bai Chun	白純	
Bai Lang	白朗	
Bai Linfu	白林富	
bai tu	白土	white mud
bai yao zhi zhang	百藥之長	the oldest of a hundred medicines
Bai Yu	白玉	
baigan jiu	白乾酒	white dry liquor
baijiu	白酒	distilled alcohol
baimian	白面	white flour/heroin
baimianr	白面兒	white flour/heroin
baizhongren de zhimindi	白種人的植民地	Caucasian colony
Bao jing	寶鏡	Precious Mirror
Bao Kun	寶崑	
bao nuan sheng xianshi	飽暖生閒事	being full and warm leads to trouble
bianzhi	變質	degenerate
Bin Tou	繽頭	
bixu de wupin	必須的物品	essential article

Boji yiyuan	博濟醫院	Abundant Aid Hospital
bu liaojie zui de ren shi bu liaojie rensheng de a	不了解醉的人是不了解人生的啊	to not understand an intoxicated person is to not understand life
bu neng zhi chi le	不能支持了	could not be tolerated
Cai Weijian	蔡維儉	
Cao Cao	曹操	
Changshi hui	常識會	Common Sense Society
chao xi yi bei you yu bai yao	朝夕一杯優于百藥	one cup in the morning and evening surpasses one hundred medicines
Chen Li	晨黎	
Chen Yuxin	陳玉新	
Chi yu pai putaojiu	赤玉牌葡萄酒	Red Jade Brand Grape Wine
Chikamori Kansuke	近森勘助	
Chuan tu	川土	Sichuan mud
chun yixue de jingshen	純醫學的精神	pure medical spirit
chun zhi yu tai	春之育胎	early-stage development foetuses
ciji	刺激	stimulation
Cui Yu	翠玉	
cuguang	粗獷	tough
da guo qi yin	大過其癮	enjoying the addiction
da jiujiazhe	大酒家者	big drinker
da mianbao xiang guogai	大麵包像锅盖	bread as big as a lid
Da Riben maijiu zhushi huishe	大日本麥酒株式會社	Dai-Nippon Breweries
Da yang	大陽	Big Sun
Da Yong	大庸	
da zui	大醉	very drunk
dabingzi chi zai wai	大餅子吃在外	eat big pancakes outside
dadi	大敵	archenemy
Daji	妲己	
Dalasuo	達拉索	Dariasha
damafengr	大麻風兒	drug addict
Daode hui	道德會	Morality Society
Daqian yiyuan	大千醫院	Boundless Hospital
dayan	大煙	big smoke/opium
dayan gui	大煙鬼	opium ghost
Deng Yujiao	鄧玉嬌	
dineng	低能	mentally deficient
Dixin	帝辛	

Doihara Kenji	土肥原賢二	
Dong Guxuan	董古軒	
dong tu	東土	Eastern mud
Dongbei fang	東北坊	Northeast Mill
Dongbei jieyan yiyuan	東北戒煙醫院	Northeast Quit Smoking Hospital
Dongguang ji	東光劑	Eastern Light Agent
dou jiangzhe dazhong de yuyan	都講著大眾的語言	all speaking the language of the masses
dou jiu shi bai pian	斗酒詩百篇	produce 100 poems after drinking a whole *dou* (about ten litres) of wine
Du Fu	杜甫	
Du Kang	杜康	
duanjin zhengzhuang	斷禁症狀	stop and ban symptom
duli	獨立	independent
duoluo	墮落	degenerate
duoluo chenlun	墮落沉淪	sink into degeneracy
dusi	堵死	suffocate to death
dute de jiu wenhua	獨特的酒文化	unique alcohol culture
e pi	惡癖	loathsome addiction
e shehui de xunran	惡社會的熏染	gradual corrupting influence of evil society
e xi	惡習	loathsome habit
e zui	惡醉	evil intoxication
Eguo ren quan shi shihao yin jiu de!	俄國人全是嗜好飲酒的	Russian people all love to drink!
Eiyō to ikuji no kai	栄養と育児の会	Society for Nutrition and Raising Children
en ren	恩人	benefactor
er	餌	bait
er ru mu ran	耳濡目染	imperceptibly influenced by what one constantly sees and hears
Fan Ying	范瑩	
fangdang	放蕩	dissolute
fangdang de xingge	放蕩的性格	dissolute nature
fangren	放任	indulgent
fei jiu wu yi cheng li	非酒無義成立	without wine, there is no etiquette
feng jiu ze zui de qingxiang	逢酒則醉的傾向	tendency to get drunk when coming upon alcohol
Feng Qi	馮啟	
Feng Sen	逢森	
Feng Shuo	馮朔	

fenghua	風化	morals and manners
fengliu yuan shi	風流怨事	dissolute, resentful matters
Fengtian wang	奉天王	Kings of Fengtian
fengtou	風頭	trendy
fengyue	風月	Temptress Moon
Fu Chen	拂塵	
Fu Shen	福神	Good Fortune Spirit
Fujī Kyūta	藤井久太	
Fujita Osamu	藤田修	
funü de kunnan	婦女的困難	women's difficulty
Furen jiao feng hui	婦人矯風會	Married Women's Rectify Customs Society
furong	芙蓉	opium
fuza	複雜	complicated
Gangyao yiwen zhidao	綱要藝文指導	Summary of Guidelines to Art and Literature
gaoliang	高粱	Chinese sorghum
gaoliang jiu	高粱酒	distilled alcohol (made primarily from Chinese sorghum)
gongkai de mimi	公開的秘密	open secret
Gotō Shinpei	後藤新平	
Gu Ding	古丁	
gu yan	菰煙	wild rice smoke/opium
gua yangtou mai gourou	掛羊頭賣狗肉	trying to pawn off something inferior to what it purports to be
guan tu	官土	official mud/opium
Guan Yunzhang	關韻章	
Gui pai haomeng putaojiu	龜牌好萌葡萄酒	Soft-Shell Turtle Brand Grass Grape Wine
gulu gulu de guan yi qi	咕嚕咕嚕的灌一氣	pour it gurgling in, in one breath
guo chan	國產	national product
guo fen de canbao	過份的殘暴	excessive brutality
Guobuluo Wanrong	郭布羅 婉容	
Guowuyuan bugao	國務院佈告	State Proclamation
Hachijirushi Kozan Budoshu	蜂印香竄葡萄酒	Fragrant Wine
hailuoyin	海洛因	heroin
hailuoying	海洛英	heroin
Han Hu	韓護	
Han Kunjin	韓崑津	
Han Wenming	韓文明	

Hanjian	漢奸	traitor to China
hao jiu de ren	好酒的人	person who is fond of alcohol
hao yin jiu	好飲酒	fond of drinking alcohol
haojie zhi hao jiu	豪傑之好酒	people of exceptional ability are fond of alcohol
haoqi wanpiao	好奇玩票	curious and do it just for fun
haoyin	豪飲	drink habitually and excessively
Haseda	長谷田	
he jiu	喝酒	drink alcohol
he jiu shi Dongbei ren zui zhongyao de goutong fangshi	喝酒是東北人最重要的溝通方式	drinking alcohol is Northeasterners' most important means of connecting
he jiu yu han	喝酒御寒	drink alcohol to resist the cold
he pijiu xiang guan'gai	喝啤酒像灌溉	drink beer like irrigation
he yu	喝欲	urge to drink
He Yujie	何玉潔	
Hei	黑	Black
hei ya	黑鴉	black opium
hei jinzi	黑金子	black gold/opium
Hei'ermisi	黑兒眉斯	Hermes
heyi jie you, wei you Du Kang	何以解憂, 唯有杜康	to relieve worries, only Du Kang will do
Higashimoto Hide	東本秀	
Hong Nian	鴻年	
hong pizi	紅皮子	red leather
hong tu	紅土	red mud
Hong xing	紅星	Red Star
hongwan	紅丸	red pills
Hoshino Naoki	星野直樹	
Hua Jiangrong	花江容	
hua yan guan	花煙館	flower opium den
Huai Yin	懷音	
huangjiu	黃酒	yellow wine
Huaying yishi	華英醫室	Huaying Clinic
Hugu Huashe yaojiu	虎骨花蛇藥酒	Tiger Bone, Flower Snake Medicinal Wine
huibi	迴避	avoidance
humei shouduan	狐媚手段	trick and bewitch by cajolery
humei shu	狐媚術	skill in bewitching by cajolery
hyakuyaku ni masaru	百薬に勝る	the best of all medicines

Ichimaru	市丸	
Imamura Masu	今村益	
Itō Ryōichi	伊藤亮一	
ji jian fa	急減法	rapid reduction method
ji kexue	極科學	mighty scientific
Jia Xiao	笳嘯	
jian jiao de jindai de nüxing	健腳的近代的女性	healthy-feet modern females
Jian tu	建土	Fujian mud
jian jian fa	漸減法	gradual reduction method
jianjin zhi fa	監禁之法	supervise and prohibit method
Jin Chengrong	金成榮	
Jin he	金鶴	Golden Crane
Jin Long	金龍	
Jin Xiaoru	金小茹	
jin yan	禁煙	ban smoke
Jin yan zongju	禁煙總局	Ban Smoking Central Office
Jin Yin	金音	
jinduan fa	禁斷法	ban and stop method
Jing Chun	精純	
jingji baoguo, pumie anxing	經濟報國, 撲滅暗行	Dedicated Service to the National Economy, Exterminate Dark Behaviour
jingshen	精神	spirit
jingshenbing bingyuan	精神病病院	psychiatric hospitals
jinzhe	進者	progressive
jiu bu zui, bu neng hua	酒不醉不能畫	without being drunk, I can't paint
jiu chang	酒腸	alcohol intestines
jiu chi rou lin	酒池肉林	Wine Pool and Meat Forest
jiu de guxiang	酒的故鄉	birthplace of alcohol
jiu de wangguo	酒的王國	kingdom of alcohol
Jiu keyi shi ni meiyou shenghuo de tongku, jiu ye keyi shi ni meiyou shenghuo de chiru	酒可以使你沒有生活的痛苦, 酒也可以使你沒有生活的恥辱	Alcohol can make you not have the pain of life, alcohol can also make you not have the shame of life
jiu liang	酒量	capacity for alcohol
jiu neng luan xing	酒能亂性	alcohol can disorder one's nature
jiu se wenhua	酒色文化	wine-coloured culture
jiu wei laonianren zhi niuru	酒為老年人之牛乳	alcohol is milk for the elderly

jiu wei wan bing zhi mu	酒為萬病之母	alcohol is the mother of all disease
jiu wei xing Ya zhi di	酒為興亞之敵	alcohol is the enemy of the rise of Asia
jiu wenhua	酒文化	alcohol culture
jiu xian	酒仙	wine immortal
jiu xing zhi bing	酒性之病	diseases of an alcohol nature
jiu yi cheng li, jiu yi zhi bing, jiu yi cheng huan	酒以成禮, 酒以治病, 酒以成歡	alcohol is for ceremonies, alcohol is for curing illness, alcohol is for making merry
jiu yin	酒癮	alcohol addiction
jiu yu tiandi tongshi	酒與天地同時	alcohol and the earth are contemporaries
jiu yu wenhua	酒域文化	alcohol regional culture
jiu zhang wenhua	酒章文化	alcohol regulations culture
jiu zheng wenhua	酒政文化	alcohol political culture
jiu zhong you zhen	酒中有真	in wine there is truth
jiujing hai shen	酒精害身	alcohol harms the body
Ju quan	菊泉	Chrysanthemum Spring
Ju ying lou	聚英樓	Gathered Flowers Building
Jun Jun	君君	
Jun Qing	君清	
kai hua	開化	become civilized
Kakegawa Akikuni	掛川晃洲	
kang	炕	a heatable brick bed
Kangde	康德	
kangdusu	抗毒素	antitoxins
Kangsheng yuan	康生院	Healthy Life Institutes
kangzhan	抗戰	war of resistance
Kawabe Taichi	川邊太一	
Ke Ju	柯炬	
Kengsheng yuan	坑生院	Cheating Life Institutes
kepa de renjian diyu	可怕的人間地獄	frightening human hell
kexue	科學	scientific
kexue de jinbu	科學的進步	scientific progress
Kikuchi	菊池	
Kin Mitsunari	金三成	
Kirin	麒麟	Unicorn
Kishida Kunio	岸田國士	
Kobayashi Hideo	小林秀雄	
Kong Rong	孔融	
Koshio Kanji	小鹽完次	

kuanxin ying shi jiu	寬心應是酒	alcohol should bring relief
Kubota Seikō	久保田晴光	
Kudō Fumio	工藤文雄	
kumen	苦悶	depressed
Kunito Sadao	州人定男	
Kuriyagawa Hakuson	廚川白村	
lajidui de baigu	垃圾堆的白骨	a rubbish heap of bones of the dead
Lan Ling	藍玲	
lan zui ru ni	爛醉如泥	dead drunk, as mud
langman	浪漫	romantic
Lao long kou	老龍口	Old Dragon Mouth
laozao	醪糟	a beverage of fermented glutinous rice
Leng Fo	冷佛	
leshi	樂事	pleasure
letu	樂土	paradise land
li	醴	an early form of beer
Li (Ms.)	李	
Li Bai	李白	
Li Bai *zhi tu*	李白之徒	disciples of Li Bai
Li Qiao	李喬	
Li Shixun	李世勳	
li si bu yuan	離死不遠	not far from death
Li Xianglan	李香蘭	
Li Zhengzhong	李正中	
Lian	廉	
Lian Zhi	蓮枝	
liangqiang zuihan zuo zhao kuang dan de zui yu	踉蹌醉漢作着狂誕的醉語	staggering drunkards making wild and absurd drunken talk
lianpi bo	臉皮薄	thin-skinned
like neng youli tianguo	立刻能遊歷天國	immediately able to travel to the Kingdom of Heaven
Lin (Dr.)	林	
Lin Lu	林鹿	
Lin Quanqing	林泉清	
Lin Zexu	林則徐	
Ling Hua	凌花	
lingmaisuo	零賣所	(opium) retail outlets
ling ren jian er sheng yan	令人見而生厭	cause people to be disgusted by the sight

Lingyiji	靈異劑	Supernatural Pharmaceutical
lishi shang de yi ge kongbu zhi ye	歷史上的一個恐怖之夜	a night of terror in history
Liu Guojun	劉國鈞	
Liu Jingliang	劉景亮	
Liu Lang	六郎	
Liu Ling	劉伶	
Liu Shunyi	劉順義	
Liu Yu'an	劉于安	
Liu Zizhi	劉子吱	
Liubineijia	劉比內加	Liubin'ka
liuxing de yinliao	流行的飲料	fashionable beverage
Lo Cheng-pang	羅振邦	
Lu Xun	魯迅	
Luo Rong'ge	羅榮閣	
Ma (Ms.)	馬	
Ma Ji	馬驥	
ma'er dong feng	馬耳東風	horse ears in the east wind
mafei	嗎啡	morphine
mafei gui	嗎啡鬼	morphine ghost
Manshū	滿洲	Manchuria
Manshū eiga kyōkai	滿洲映画協會	Manchuria Motion Picture Producing and Distributing Company
Mantetsu	滿鉄	South Manchuria Railway
manxing zhong du	慢性中毒	chronic poison
manxing zhong du de bing	慢性中毒的病	chronic poisoning disease
Manzhou jiehe yufang xiehui	滿洲結核預防協會	Manchuria Tuberculosis Prevention Association
Manzhou jiuzao heming huishe	滿州酒造合名會社	Manchuria Wine Producers Alliance
Manzhou maijiu zhushi huishe	滿州麥酒株式會社	Manchuria Ale company
Manzhou yinshi liaopin yanjiusuo	滿洲飲食料品研究所	Manchuria Food and Drink Research Institute
Manzhou yiwen lianmeng	滿洲藝文聯盟	Manchuria Arts Alliance
Manzhou zaojiu zhushi huishe	滿洲造酒株式會社	Manchuria Alcohol Production Corporation
Manzhou zazhi she	滿洲雜誌社	Manchuria Magazine Society
Maotai	茅台	
mazui ji	麻醉劑	anaesthetic pharmaceutical

Mei Niang	梅娘	
Mei Shan	美善	
mei yin bi zui	每飲必醉	every time drinks, must get intoxicated
Meng Zijing	孟子敬	
miao ji	妙劑	wonderful pharmaceutical
miao yao	妙藥	wonderful medicine
mimi wuqi	秘密武器	secret weapon
ming zhi gu fan	明知故犯	knowingly violate
minglang de shenghuo	明朗的生活	bright life
Miura Keiko	三浦系子	
mizui	迷醉	intoxicated/intoxication
moxing nülang	魔性女郎	mystical maiden
Murakami (Chairperson)	村上	
Muto Tomio	武藤富男	
Mutushan (General)	穆圖善	
Nakajima Morinobu	中島守信	
Nakamura Kōjirō	中村剛治郎	
Nakatsukasa Hatsutarō	中務初太郎	
Nakayama (Ms.)	中山	
Nan Man tielu	南滿鐵路	South Manchuria Railway
Naoki Rintarō	直木倫太郎	
Ni Fuzhi	尼負之	
nianlao fan tong zhi li	年老反童之力	power to turn the aged into youth
nianlao maochou	年老貌醜	old and ugly
Nie'ou'moxi'en	聶歐莫稀恩	Neo-Mohyn
Nihon kokumin kinshu dōmei	日本國民禁酒同盟	Prohibit Alcohol Alliance of Japan
Nitan'osa Otozō	二反長音蔵	
Nogi Maresuke	乃木 希典	
nong qiao cheng zhuo	弄巧成拙	try to be clever only to end up with a blunder
nü zhaodai	女招待	hostess
nü zhaodai de shenghuo, yi keyi shuo shi dazhong de shenghuo	女招待的生活，亦可以說是大眾的生活	the life of hostesses could also be said to be the life of the masses
nuoruo nüzi	懦弱女子	weak woman
nüren de beiju	女人的悲劇	women's tragedy
Ōhira Tokuzō	大平得三	
Ōto (Ms.)	大音	

Ōuchi Takao	大内隆雄	
Ouzika gaoliang jiu er'shi wu hao de jiu	歐茲卡高粱酒二十五號的酒	Gaoliang Vodka Alcohol, Brand No. 25
Pei Ru	培儒	
pi	癖	addiction; weakness for
pijiu	啤酒	beer
piaopiao yu xian	飄飄欲仙	floating like celestials high
pijiu zhong zhi bawang	啤酒中之霸王	conqueror of beers
pingmin geming	平民革命	common people's revolution
pirou shengya	皮肉生涯	a skin and flesh career
Puluojiabing	普羅加并	
putao jiu	葡萄酒	grape wine
putian gaidi	鋪天蓋地	blot out the sky and cover up the earth
qi hei jiu bai	棄黑就白	abandoned the black for the white
Qi Jinchang	戚金昌	
Qiao Enrun	喬恩潤	
qinggao	清高	aloof from politics and material pursuits
qinheli	親和力	affinity
qiong de kuai, si de zao	窮的快死的早	poor quickly, die early
qipian	欺騙	fraudulent
Qiu Shan	秋山	
Qiu Ying	秋萤	
Qu Kezhong	曲克中	
qu lang ru hu	驅狼入虎	drive a wolf into a tiger's mouth
quanli	權利	rights
quedian	缺點	shortcomings
ren fei sheng er hao jiu	人非生而好酒	humans are not born to drink alcohol
Ren Ji	人驥	
ren mian she shen	人面蛇身	human faces and snake bodies
renjian shen dan miaoyao	人間神丹妙藥	wonderful, supernatural powder medicine in this world
renrou shichang	人肉市場	a human meat market
rensheng yi chun leshi	人生一樁樂事	a pleasure in life
Riben guomin jinjiu tongmeng	日本國民禁酒同盟	Prohibit Alcohol Alliance of Japan
richang xiguan	日常習慣	daily habit
Riguang	日光	Sunlight
Ru Gai	儒丐	

ru yin	儒飲	scholarly drinking
ruo bu jin feng de guozu guniang	弱不禁風的裹足姑娘	too weak to stand a gust of wind bound-feet girls
Ruo Xue	若雪	
Ruosu	若素	Basic Element
Sakura	櫻花	Cherry
san bei neng he wan shi	三杯能合萬事	three glasses can solve every problem
san da guai	三大怪	three great oddities
San Lang	三朗	
Sapporo	札幌	
Sawamura Makoto	澤村真	
secai banxian wanhuatong	色彩斑斕萬花筒	a very colourful kaleidoscope
sekuang liumang	色狂流氓	sex maniac hoodlums
sha ren bu jian xue	殺人不見血	a bloodless means of killing the people
shanggou	上鉤	hooked
Shao Guanzhi	邵貫志	
shaojiu	燒酒	sorghum or maize alcohol
shaoxing jiu	紹興酒	rice alcohol
shehui gailiang	社會改良	improvement of society
sheji you	設計誘	designs on luring
Shen Kechang	申克常	
Shen rong hugu yanshou jiu	參茸虎骨延壽酒	Ginseng, Antler, Tiger Bone Prolong Life Wine
sheng yao	聖藥	holy medicine
sheng zhan	聖戰	Holy War
Shengkang yuan	生抗院	Raising Resistance Institutes
shengli tiaojian xiangbei	生理條件相背	opposite to physiological conditions
Shenxiao hugu yaojiu	神效虎骨藥酒	Magic Tiger Bone Medicinal Wine
shenxin shengxian shen fu zhi jiao zhi	深信聖賢神佛之教旨	resolute belief in the teachings and decrees of sages and men of virtue, divinities, and Buddha
shi	嗜	have a liking for, be addicted to
shi bei zhong wu	嗜杯中物	addiction to the thing in the cup
shi de	失德	lost virtue
Shi Xichen	史洗塵	
Shi Zhizi	史之子	
Shi Ziheng	史子恒	
shihao	嗜好	addiction/hobby
shijie guan	世界觀	worldview

shimaoren hai shimaobing	時髦人害時髦病	fashionable people suffer a fashionable disease
Shimizu Yasuzo	清水安三	
Shinano Kyōkoku	信浓峡谷	
Shinichi Yamaguchi	伸一山口	
Shinjiro Torii	新次郎鳥居	
Shiozawa ke	鹽澤 家	
shouxu	手續	formalities
Shu Shi	叔石	
shufu	舒服	comfortable
si tu	私土	private mud/opium
Song Jiang	宋江	
songming de yan	送命的煙	life-killing opium
Su Jianxun	蘇建勳	
Su Qiu	素秋	
su zui	夙醉	longstanding intoxication
Sun Hanzhong	孫漢忠	
Sun Ying	孫瑛	
Sun Yushan	孫玉珊	
suowei wu zhixu de dongwu shijie	所謂無秩序的動物世界	so-called chaotic world of animals
suowei Zhongguo de dajia zhuyi	所謂中國的大家注意	so-called Chinese big family-ism
Suzuki Umetarō	鈴木 梅太郎	
Suzuki Saburōsuke	鈴木三郎助	
Tairiku kagakuin	大陸科學院	Institute of Science in China
Taiyang	太陽	Sun
Takase	高瀬	
Takeo Akiyoshi	武夫明良	
Tang Yulin	湯玉麟	
tanlan weishijijiu lie xing	貪婪威士忌酒劣性	greedy for whiskey inferior nature
Tao Yuanming	陶淵明	
taozui	陶醉	intoxicated
te xi	特習	a special habit
tiansheng rouruo	天生柔弱	inherently weak
titai qing wen	體態輕溫	soft and warm posture
Tong chun lou	同春樓	Same as Spring Building
Tsuboi (Dr.)	坪井	
Tsuru Kunitake	都留國武	
tu tan duo liang	徒貪多量	those who are too greedy

tuifei	頹廢	decadent
Wan Hongkui	萬鴻魁	
Wang Chaobin	王朝賓	
Wang Dashan	王達善	
Wang Kexun	王克勳	
Wang Luo	王洛	
Wang Meng	王濛	
Wang Qiuying	王秋萤	
Wang Shaoxian	王绍先	
Wang Shigong	王世恭	
Wangdao	王道	Kingly Way
Wangdao yao	王道藥	Kingly Way medicine
Wanling fenghan hugu jiu	萬靈風寒虎骨酒	Cold Souls Tiger Bone Wine
wanneng zhi yao	萬能之藥	all-purpose medicine
wanyir	玩意兒	toy
Wei Chaochen	魏朝臣	
Wei Cheng	韋成	
Wei Yonggui	魏永貴	
wei'an	慰安	comfort
weisheng	衛生	hygiene
wenhua ren	文化人	cultured people
wen xiang xia ma	聞香下馬	smell the fragrance and get down from the horse
wenqing	溫情	warmth
wenya de goudang	文雅的勾當	refined matter
Wo ji shi jiu xiang de yi ge tuzhu	我既是酒鄉的一個土著	I am a native of alcohol country
Wo shi yi jiu shengcun de, meiyou jiu, jiu meiyou wo de shengming	我是以酒生存的，沒有酒，就沒有我的生命	I use alcohol to live. Without alcohol, I have no life
wu a	烏阿	black opium
Wu Lang	吳郎	
wu xiang	烏香	black fragrance/opium
Wu Ying (cartoonist)	伍盈	
Wu Ying (writer)	吳瑛	
wu you bu guan	無有不慣	there are none who do not indulge
wubi gaoji yinliao	無比高級飲料	incomparable high-class beverage
wuchi er beini de diyu	無恥而卑溺的地獄	shameless and addicted hell
Wujiapi	五加皮	

xi tu	西土	Western mud
Xian you	賢友	Virtuous Friend
Xiang Naixi	項乃羲	
xianqi liangmu	賢妻良母	good wife, wise mother
Xiao Jun	蕭軍	
Xiao Ling	小玲	
xiao men fu lai	笑門福來	laughter in the family brings good fortune
xiao shi	小事	minor matter
Xiao Song	小松	
xiao yingxiong	小英雄	little hero
xiaoqian	消遣	pastime
Xie Jieshi	謝介石	
xiguan	習慣	habit
Xin Jiajun	辛嘉君	
Xing Canlü	刑燦呂	
Xing Ya yinshua zhushi huishe	興亞印刷株式會社	Rising Asia Printing Company
xingfen	興奮	stimulants; stimulation
xingfu guojia	幸福國家	happy country
Xinmin yiyuan	新民醫院	New People Hospital
xiong yin	凶飲	ferocious drinking
xiuli ke ren	秀麗可人	beautiful and pleasant
Xu	旭	Brilliance of the Rising Sun
Xu Bochun	徐柏春	
xu dang zui	須當醉	must get intoxicated
xu zhang shengshi	虛張聲勢	an empty show of strength
Xuehua	雪花	Snow (beer)
xueshu	學術	scientific
xueshu mazui	學術麻醉	scientific anaesthetic
Yamamoto Sanehiko	山本實彥	
Yamauchi Saburō	山內三朗	
Yamazaki Hyakuji	山崎百事	
yan gui	煙鬼	smoke ghosts/opium addicts
yan ji	煙季	smoke season/opium season
yan ji	烟妓	opium prostitute
yan ke	煙客	opium addicts
yan tu	煙土	smoke mud/opium
yan yin	煙癮	opium addict

yan yin shen yu seyin	煙癮甚於色癮	opium addiction is worse than sex addiction
Yang Jun	楊軍	
Yang Xu	楊絮	
yang yan	洋煙	foreign smoke/opium
yang yao gao	洋藥膏	foreign medicine paste/opium
yang yao tu	洋藥土	foreign medicine mud/opium
yang yao yan	洋藥煙	foreign medicine smoke/opium
yanghuo re	洋货热	craving for foreign stuff
Yangming jiu	養命酒	Life Support Wine
Yao Jibin	姚紀彬	
Yao Shi yiyuan	姚氏醫院	Yao Shi hospital
yao tu	藥土	medicine mud
Yao Xia	姚霞	
yaojiu	藥酒	medicinal wine
yaoming de yan yin	要命的煙癮	life-killing addiction
yaoyan	妖艷	pretty and coquettish
yapian	鴉片	opium
yapian wenti	鴉片問題	opium problem
yapian zhi pi	鴉片之癖	opium addiction
Yapian zhuanmai gongshu	鴉片專賣公署	(Manchukuo's) Opium Monopoly
yarong	鴉蓉	opium
yashuang yan	鴉霜煙	frosty smoke/opium
Ye Fengsheng	葉犇生	
ye ji	野妓	wild prostitutes
Ye Li	也麗	
Ye Xing	夜行	
yi	醫	cure
yi bi dai jian	以筆代劍	wielding pens as swords
Yi Chi	疑遲	
Yi Di	儀狄	
yi han you yi zhong duzhi	亦含有一重毒质	they harbour a kind of poisonous nature
yi jie zhi zhu quan wei	醫界之諸權威	number one in the medicine world for everyone
yi jin yiliao zhi nengshi	以盡醫療之能事	fulfil the medical treatment capability
yi jiu shao chou chou geng chou	以酒澆愁愁更愁	to drink alcohol to lessen worries, only makes the worries more worrisome

Yi Mei	依梅	
yi mei zhi ci	溢美之詞	excessive praise
yi paiyintuo	一派因脱	one pint
yi ta heng cheng duan di chi	一榻橫陳短笛吹	once they lie down and play with the flute
Yi Ting	怡亭	
Yi Xi	一西	
yi zhong zhangfu zhi, yi fu nan'er gu	一種丈夫志一副男兒骨	a kind of husband's will and a man's bones
yi zui jie qian chou	一醉解千愁	one intoxication solves 1,000 worries
Yilong quan	意隆泉	Elan Springs
yin	隱	hidden from view
Yin (author)	隱	
yin	癮	addiction
yin fei bu neng jie, yao zai neng juewu er yi	癮非不能戒, 要在能覺悟而已	addiction can be stopped, only through consciousness
yin jiu	飲酒	drink alcohol
yin jiu de bingtai	飲酒的病態	morbid state of drinking alcohol
yin jiu jia	飲酒家	alcohol drinkers
yin le daliang de weishiji	飲了大量的威士忌	drinks a great quantity of whiskey
Yin shi yin. Yin shi ren. Yin shi guanyin.	癮是引. 癮是任. 癮是慣因.	Addiction is attraction. Addiction is waywardness. Addiction is habit.
Yin Zhengping	尹正萍	
Ying	英	
ying chou	應酬	social intercourse
ying chou zhoudao	應酬週到	attentive social intercourse
Yingren de xianhai	英人的陷害	English frame-up
yingyang	營養	nourishment
yinshi	飲食	food and drink
yinshi	癮士	addict
yinzhe	癮者	addict
yinzhen ke	銀針客	silver-needle guests
Yishu yanjiu hui	藝術研究會	Arts Research Association
yizhi	意志	will
yizhi boruo yiran gai shihao	意志薄弱易染該嗜好	the weak-willed easily acquired addiction
yizhi boruo	意志薄弱	weak-willed
yizhi li	意志力	willpower
Yong Boping	雍伯平	
Yong Shanqi	雍善耆	

Yoshimura	吉村	
you bing de	有病的	with an illness
you jia nan ben, you guo nan tou	有家難奔, 有國難投	when families hasten to difficulties, the nation is cast into difficulties
You You	悠悠	
youlingban	幽靈般	ghostly
You'ni'en	優呢恩	Union
yu han	御寒	resist the cold
Yu Li	于里	
yu nitu wei you	與泥土為友	make friends with the soil
Yu Zhizhu	余織竹	
Yuanming yuan	圓明園	(Old) Summer Palace
Yun tu	雲土	Yunnan mud
Zhai Wenxuan	翟文選	
zhanbai	戰敗	defeated
Zhang Chunyuan	張春園	
Zhang Dexin	張德馨	
Zhang Feng	張鳳	
Zhang Guochen	張國臣	
Zhang Haide	張海德	
Zhang Jiyou	張繼有	
Zhang Lin'ge	張麟閣	
Zhang Nianhui	張念會	
Zhang Xinglou	張星樓	
Zhang Xueliang	張學良	
Zhang Zuolin	張作霖	
Zhao Kuiru	趙魁儒	
Zhao Min	兆民	
Zhao Yinglin	趙英林	
Zheng Xiaoxu	鄭孝胥	
Zheng Zhi	正之	
zhengren	正人	upright person
zhengyi	正義	righteous
Zhenhua yiyuan	振華醫院	China Rise with Force and Spirit Hospital
Zhi Jing	止敬	
zhi jiu neng gaosu gei wo shengming shi zenyang jimo de shiti	只酒能告訴給我生命是怎樣一個寂寞的屍體	only alcohol can tell me what kind of lonely corpse life is
Zhi Yuan	支援	

Zhi Xing	之行	
zhiwu zhi shen	植物之神	the god of plants
zhiye	職業	professional
Zhong Xin	中心	
zhong zai hu ni lizhi	終在乎你立志	in the end it is up to your determination
Zhongguo gu yi you zhi guocui de mazuifa, dayue keyi shuo shi yin jiu	中國古已有之國粹的麻醉法,大約可以說是飲酒	It could be said that in ancient China the anaesthesia method that was the quintessence of Chinese culture was drinking alcohol
Zhongguo ren bu shi jiu tuo hun, er zhengfu jiu	中國人不使酒奪魂,而征服酒	Chinese people do not use alcohol to cast off their soul, they conquer alcohol
Zhou Zuoren	周作人	
Zhu Jiqing	朱季清	
Zhu Qinglan	朱慶瀾	
Zhu Ti	朱娣	
Zhuang Kaishui	莊開水	
zhuo jiu	濁酒	turbid alcohol
Zhushi huishe Manzhou yinghua xiehui	株式會社滿洲映畫協會	Manchuria Motion Picture Producing and Distributing Company
zi gu wenren duo'ai jiu	自古文人多愛酒	since ancient times, literati have greatly loved alcohol
zi su	自肅	self-respect
zongfa shehui	宗法社會	patriarchal society
zui gui	醉鬼	drunken ghost
zui ru ni	醉如泥	drunk as mud
Zui xian ge	醉仙閣	Drunken Fairy Pavilion
zui yu bi zhizhong du, you buke buzhi	醉與痺之中毒,尤不可不知	the poison of (being) drunk and numb, especially must be known
Zuo Di	左蒂	
zuosi	作死	seek death

Notes

Introduction

Epigraph: The "Jie yan ge" [Get off opium song] is also known as the "Quit Smoking Song." See "Jie yan ge," words by Li Juanqing, music by Liang Leyin, on *Li Xianglan Collection* (Taipei: Zhonghua Records, 1999).

1 *Yuanjia* means "enemy" or "foe" but is a term that was also commonly used in traditional opera and folk songs in reference to a destined love or sweetheart.

2 Feng Qi, "Jiu ren shuo jiu hua: Dongbei jiu wenhua he xiaofei xiguan yanjiu" [Drinkers talk drink talk: Research on Northeast alcohol culture and consumption habits], http://www.cnbm.net.cn/.

3 For details, see http://sportsillustrated.cnn.com/2011/.

4 Mark Driscoll divides Japanese imperialism into three distinct periods, with the latter (1932-45) titled "necropolitics" for its focus on total war and fascist mobilization. See Mark Driscoll, *Absolute Erotic, Absolute Grotesque* (Durham, NC: Duke University Press, 2010), xii.

5 Ibid., 227.

6 The term "Manchuria" is controversial. The reasons for this are succinctly outlined in Mariko Asano Tamanoi, "Introduction," in Mariko Asano Tamanoi, ed., *Crossed Histories: Manchuria in the Age of Empire* (Honolulu: University of Hawai'i Press, 2005), 2-3.

7 Li is also known as Shirley/Yoshiko Yamaguchi and, since remarriage, as Yoshiko Otaka. Her Japanese-language autobiography was translated into Chinese in 1988. See Li Xianglan, *Zai Zhongguo de rizi: Wo de ban sheng* [Days in China: My half-life] (Hong Kong: Baixing wenhua shirong youxian gongshi, 1988).

8 Contemporary writer Mei Niang argues that Li's Japanese nationality was an "open secret" [*gongkai de mimi*]; Mei Niang, interview by author, Vancouver, 14 February 2004. The extent to which Li "fooled" Chinese audiences is also questioned in Shelley Stephenson, "'Her Traces Are Found Everywhere': Shanghai, Li Xianglan, and the 'Greater East Asia Film Sphere,'" in Yingjin Zhang, ed., *Cinema and Urban Culture in Shanghai, 1922-1943* (Stanford, CA: Stanford University Press, 1999), 222-45.

9 These include "He ri jun zai lai?" [When will my love return?], "Mai tang ge" [The candy selling song], and "Ye lai xiang" [Night fragrance]. Although these songs may have been considered politically incorrect at the time, they remain popular today.

10 Li subsequently starred in several Hollywood movies, appeared on Broadway, and became a television reporter, covering stories in Vietnam, Cambodia, and the Middle East. In 1974 she was elected a Liberal Democratic Party member of the Japanese Parliament (a position in which she served for eighteen years). She is currently vice-president of the Asian Women's Fund, an organization dedicated to securing relief for the "comfort women" of the Second World War.

11 For discussion of drugs and human rights abuses in Unit 731, see Miriam Lynn Kingsberg, "The Poppy and the Acacia: Opium and Imperialism in Japanese Dairen and the Kwantung Leased Territory, 1905-1945" (PhD diss., History Department, University of California at Berkeley, 2009), 314-20.

12 Gong Li, *Yin jiu shihua* [History of alcohol drinking] (Beijing: Zhongguo da bailiao quanshu chubanshe, 2009); Guo Panxi, *Zhongguo yin jiu xisu* [Chinese drinking alcohol customs] (Taibei: Wenhua chubanshe, 1989); Li Zhengping, *Zhongguo jiu wenhua* [Chinese wine culture] (Beijing: Shishi chubanshe, 2006); Xuan Bingshan, *Minjian yinshi xisu* [Popular food and drink customs] (Beijing: Zhongguo shehui chubanshe, 2006).

13 K.C. Chang, *Food in Chinese Culture: Anthropological and Historical Perspectives* (New Haven, CT: Yale University Press, 1977); David T. Courtwright, *Forces of Habit: Drugs and the Making of the Modern World* (Cambridge, MA: Harvard University Press, 2001); John E. Helzer and Glorisa J. Canino, eds., *Alcoholism in North America, Europe, and Asia* (Oxford: Oxford University Press, 1992).

14 David E. Armstrong, *Alcohol and Altered States in Ancestor Veneration Rituals of Zhou Dynasty China and Iron Age Palestine* (Lewiston, NY: Edwin Mellen, 1998).

15 Zhang Huinuan, *Beifang shaoshu minzu de jiu wenhua* [Northern national minority alcohol culture] (Huhhot: Nei Menggu daxue chubanshe, 2008).

16 Originally published in 1975, the essay "Opium" is reprinted in Jonathan Spence, *Chinese Roundabout: Essays in History and Culture* (New York: W.W. Norton, 1992), 229.

17 Timothy Brook and Bob Tadashi Wakabayashi, eds., *Opium Regimes: China, Britain, and Japan, 1839-1952* (Berkeley: University of California Press, 2000); Frank Dikötter, Lars Laamann, and Zhou Xun, *Narcotic Culture: A History of Drugs in China* (Chicago, IL: University of Chicago Press, 2004); Kathryn Meyer, *Webs of Smoke: Smugglers, Warlords, Spies and the History of the International Drug Trade* (Lanham, MD: Rowman and Littlefield, 1998); Yamada Goichi, *Manshukoku No Ahensenbai* [Opium Monopoly in Manchuria] (Tokyo: Kyuko Shoen, 2002); Zheng Yangwen, *The Social Life of Opium* (Cambridge, UK: Cambridge University Press, 2005).

18 Zhou Yongming, *Anti-Drug Crusades in Twentieth Century China: Nationalism, History, and State Building* (Oxford: Rowman and Littlefield, 1999); Alan Baumler, *The Chinese and Opium under the Republic: Worse than Floods and Wild Beasts* (Albany: State University of New York Press, 2007).

19 John M. Jennings, *The Opium Empire: Japanese Imperialism and Drug Trafficking in Asia, 1895-1945* (London: Praeger, 1997); Louise Young, *Japan's Total Empire: Manchuria and the Culture of Wartime Imperialism* (Berkeley: University of California Press, 1998); Lü Yonghua, *Wei Man shiqi de dongbei yandu* [Opium poison in the Northeast during the bogus Manchukuo era] (Changchun: Jilin renmin chubanshe, 2004); Yamamuro Shin'ichi, *Manchuria under Japanese Dominion*, trans. Joshua Fogel (Philadelphia: University of Pennsylvania Press, 2006); Driscoll, *Absolute Erotic*.

20 Ronald Suleski, *Civil Government in Warlord China: Tradition, Modernization and Manchuria* (New York: Bern, 2002); James H. Carter, *Creating a Chinese Harbin: Nationalism in an International City, 1916-1932* (Ithaca, NY: Cornell University Press, 2002); Prasenjit Duara, *Sovereignty and Authenticity: Manchukuo and the East Asian Modern* (New York: Rowman and Littlefield, 2003); Liu Jinghui, *Minzu, xingbie yu jieceng* [Nation, gender, and social stratum] (Beijing: Shehui kexue wenxian chubanshe, 2004); Mariko Asano Tamanoi, ed., *Crossed Histories* (Honolulu: University of Hawai'i Press, 2005); Dongbei lunxian shisi nian shi zong bian shi and Riben zhimin di wenhua yanjiu hui, eds., *Wei Manzhouguo de zhenxiang* [The real truth of the puppet Manchukuo] (Beijing: Shehui kexue wenxian chubanshe, 2010); Blaine R. Chiasson, *Administering the Colonizer: Manchuria's Russians under Chinese Rule, 1918-29* (Vancouver: UBC Press, 2010).

Chapter 1: Alcohol and Opium in China

1   For example, see David T. Courtwright, *Forces of Habit: Drugs and the Making of the Modern World* (Cambridge, MA: Harvard University Press, 2001), 10. Biological and sociocultural views are cited in Eng-Kung Yeoh and Hai-Gwo Hwu, "Alcoholism in Taiwan Chinese Communities," in John E. Helzer and Glorisa J. Canino, eds., *Alcoholism in North America, Europe, and Asia* (Oxford: Oxford University Press, 1992), 214.

2   Tsung-Yi Lin and David T.C. Lin argue that there are three hypotheses for why Chinese do not drink: physiology (sensitivity), substitution (gambling and narcotics), and socioculture (drinking rituals and social factors). See Tsung-Yi Lin and David T.C. Lin, "Alcoholism among the Chinese: Further Observations of a Low-Risk Population," *Culture, Medicine and Psychiatry* 6, 2 (1982): 109.

3   Bai He, "Lun yan jiu zhi hai (xia)" [Discussing the harm of alcohol and opium (second)], *Xin Manzhou* [New Manchuria], June 1939, 39.

4   Li Zhengping, *Zhongguo jiu wenhua* [Chinese wine culture] (Beijing: Shishi chubanshe, 2006), 37.

5   Quoted original text is in English. Gong Li, *Yin jiu shihua* [History of alcohol drinking] (Beijing: Zhongguo da bailiao quanshu chubanshe, 2009), 78.

6   Guo Panxi, *Zhongguo yin jiu xisu* [Chinese drinking alcohol customs] (Taibei: Wenhua chubanshe, 1989), 1.

7   Xu Xiaomin, "Ganbei through the Ages," *Shanghai Star*, 29 May 2003, http://app1.chinadaily.com.cn/.

8   Shenyang shi Lao long kou jiuchang bianzuan bangongshi, ed., *Shenyang shi Lao long kou jiuchangzhi* [Shenyang city's Lao long kou (Old Dragon Mouth) wine factory records] (Shenyang: Shenyang chubanshe, 1993), 335. The Lao long kou company maintains a museum in Shenyang detailing its lengthy history.

9   Wen Long, ed., *Zhongguo jiu dian* [Chinese alcohol code] (Changchun: Jilin chuban jituan youxian guiren gongsi, 2010), 1.

10 Zhou Zuoren, "Tan jiu" [Talk alcohol], in Yi Yuan, ed., *Jiu mo: Jiu fengqing xiaopinji* [Alcohol mystics: Collection of essays on amorous feelings for alcohol] (Taibei: Yeqiang chuban, 1994), 20.

11 Frederick Simoons argues that *jiu*'s original meaning was "beer" or "ale." See Frederick J. Simoons, *Food in China* (Boca Raton, FL: CRC Press, 1991), 448.

12 Zhu Ruimei, *Yin jiu qudian* [Interesting quotations on drinking alcohol] (Taipei: Shixueshe chuban gufen youxian gongsi, 2004), 88; Zhang Huinuan, *Beifang shaoshu minzu de jiu wenhua* [Northern national minority alcohol culture] (Huhhot: Nei Menggu daxue chubanshe, 2008), 2.

13 K.C. Chang, *Food in Chinese Culture: Anthropological and Historical Perspectives* (New Haven, CT: Yale University Press, 1977), 40.

14 Xuan Bingshan, *Minjian yinshi xisu* [Popular food and drink customs] (Beijing: Zhongguo shehui chubanshe, 2006), 89.

15 Ibid., 87.

16 Gong, *Yin jiu shihua*, 85.

17 Chang Chiung-fang, "Two Thousand Years of Tippling," trans. Chris Findler, *Taiwan Panorama*, 7 June 2002, http://www.sino.gov.tw/.

18 Xu Gan Rong and Bao Tong Fa, *Grandiose Survey of Chinese Alcoholic Drinks and Beverages*, http://www.sytu.edu.cn/.

19 Ibid.

20 Quoted in ibid.

21 Jiang Hai, *Jiu de gushi* [The story of alcohol] (Jinan: Shandong renmin yinshuachang, 2006), 5.

22   Ibid., 5.
23   Chu Guoqing, "Nüren yu jiu" [Women and alcohol], in Li Tongfeng and Zou Changshun,
     eds., *Jiu zhi yun* [The charm of alcohol] (Shenyang: Liaohai chubanshe, 2007), 11, 14.
24   See also Li, *Zhongguo jiu wenhua*, 238.
25   Xuan, *Minjian yinshi xisu*, 87.
26   Chang, *Food in Chinese Culture*, 30. In the second century BCE, the writer Zou Yang also
     argued that alcohol was "by definition an indispensable part of the feast"; quoted in ibid.,
     68. Li Zhengping labels the Shang Dynasty a *"jiu se wenhua"* [wine-coloured culture]; see
     Li, *Zhongguo jiu wenhua*, 1.
27   Chang, *Food in Chinese Culture*, 11.
28   Li, *Zhongguo jiu wenhua*, 238.
29   David E. Armstrong, *Alcohol and Altered States in Ancestor Veneration Rituals of Zhou
     Dynasty China and Iron Age Palestine* (Lewiston, NY: Edwin Mellen, 1998), 49.
30   For example, see Xuan, *Minjian yinshi xisu*, 88; Guo, *Zhongguo yin jiu xisu*, 226.
31   For example, see Jianfei Zhu, *Chinese Spatial Strategies: Imperial Beijing, 1420-1911*
     (London: RoutledgeCurzon, 2004), 217.
32   Li, *Zhongguo jiu wenhua*, 152.
33   See Chang-Hua Wang, William T. Liu, Ming-Yuan Zhang, Elena S.H. Yu, Zheng-Yi Xia,
     Marilyn Fernandez, Ching-Tung Lung, Chang-Lin Xu, and Guang-Ya Qu, "Alcohol Use,
     Abuse, and Dependency in Shanghai," in John E. Helzer and Glorisa J. Canino, eds.,
     Alcoholism in North America, Europe, and Asia (Oxford: Oxford University Press, 1992),
     264.
34   Li, *Zhongguo jiu wenhua*, 109.
35   K. Singer, "Drinking Patterns and Alcoholism in the Chinese," in Mac Marshall, ed., *Beliefs,
     Behaviors, and Alcoholic Beverages: A Cross-Cultural Survey* (Ann Arbor: University of
     Michigan Press, 1979), 315; Zhu, *Yin jiu qudian*, 78.
36   Li, *Zhongguo jiu wenhua*, 308.
37   Xu and Bao, *Grandiose Survey*.
38   Guo, *Zhongguo yin jiu xisu*, 221.
39   Xu and Bao, *Grandiose Survey*.
40   Ibid. Jiang Hai dates the popularity of drinking among the masses to the Zhou Dynasty;
     see Jiang, *Jiu de gushi*, 6.
41   Chang, *Food in Chinese Culture*, 119. Li Zhengping labels the Tang Dynasty an "alcohol
     regulations culture" *[jiu zhang wenhua]*; see Li, *Zhongguo jiu wenhua*, 2.
42   Quoted in Simoons, *Food in China*, 450.
43   Xu and Bao, *Grandiose Survey*.
44   Chang Chiung-fang suggests that the Mongols took this technology to Russia, where beets
     were substituted for cereals, thereby inspiring the creation of vodka. See Chang, "Two
     Thousand Years."
45   Chang, *Food in Chinese Culture*, 122.
46   Ibid.
47   Ibid., 120.
48   Xu and Bao, *Grandiose Survey*.
49   Arthur Cooper, *Li Po and Tu Fu: Poems, Selected and Translated* (Harmondsworth, UK:
     Penguin, 1973), 25.
50   Jiang, *Jiu de gushi*, 95.
51   Jiang Hai argues that Liu Ling was the first to be named a "drunken ghost." See Jiang, *Jiu
     de gushi*, 15.
52   Gong, *Yin jiu shihua*, 120.
53   Zhu, *Yin jiu qudian*, 254-55.

54 See Tsai Yu, "Cong yin jiu dao ziran: Yi Tao shi wei hexin tantao" [From Drinking to Nature: A Study on the Poetry of Tao Yuan-Ming], *Taida zhongwen xuebao* [National Taiwan University Chinese Journal] 22 (June 2005): 225.

55 Jiang, *Jiu de gushi*, 90.

56 Li, *Zhongguo jiu wenhua*, 3.

57 Quoted in Chang, "Two Thousand Years."

58 Xu, "Ganbei through the Ages."

59 The other members are Cui Zongzhi, He Zhizhang, Jiao Su, Li Jin, Li Shizhi, Su Jin, and Zhang Xu.

60 One *dou* is about ten litres. Hellen Zhou and Shannon Roy, "New Wine, Old Stories," *Beijing This Month*, 1 August 2004, http://www.btmbeijing.com/.

61 Zhong Xin, "Tan yin jiu" [Discussion of drinking alcohol], *Shengjing shibao* [Shengjing times], 25 August 1935, 5.

62 Xuan, *Minjian yinshi xisu*, 87.

63 Jiang, *Jiu de gushi*, 31.

64 Xu, "Ganbei through the Ages."

65 Ibid.

66 Simoons, *Food in China*, 452.

67 Chang, *Food in Chinese Culture*, 278. In her tour-de-force study of the history of tobacco use in China, Carol Benedict notes that Han Tan had a "national reputation as an ardent smoker and a heavy drinker"; see Carol Benedict, *Golden-Silk Smoke: A History of Tobacco in China, 1550-2010* (Berkeley: University of California Press, 2011), 67. Similar drinking parties occurred in Japan. See Chris Bunting, *Drinking Japan: A Guide to Japan's Best Drinks and Drinking Establishments* (North Clarendon, VT: Tuttle Publishing, 2011), 30-33.

68 Li Zhengping argues that Western efforts at prohibition differed from those of the Chinese due to the West's focus on social improvement and the protection of individual health, whereas Chinese efforts tended to focus on crop availability. See Li, *Zhongguo jiu wenhua*, 153.

69 Xu and Bao, *Grandiose Survey*.

70 Chang, *Food in Chinese Culture*, 10.

71 Li Zhengping labels the Qin and Han Dynasties an "alcohol political culture" *[jiu zheng wenhua]*; see Li, *Zhongguo jiu wenhua*, 2. See also Fang Fei, "Jin jiu jin du" [Ban alcohol, ban gambling], *Shengjing shibao* [Shengjing times], 10 February 1936, 5.

72 Li, *Zhongguo jiu wenhua*, 37.

73 During the Xiaozong reign (r. 1162-89), alcohol taxes were not collected. See Fang, "Jin jiu jin du," 5.

74 Ibid.

75 Xu and Bao, *Grandiose Survey*. Li Zhengping labels the Yuan Dynasty an "alcohol regional culture" *[jiu yu wenhua]*. See Li, *Zhongguo jiu wenhua*, 2.

76 Xu and Bao, *Grandiose Survey*.

77 Simoons, *Food in China*, 451.

78 Frank Dikötter, Lars Laamann, and Zhou Xun, *Narcotic Culture: A History of Drugs in China* (Chicago, IL: University of Chicago Press, 2004), 15.

79 Xu and Bao, *Grandiose Survey*.

80 Ibid.

81 "Xin guomin yundong de quchu yapian zuotanhui" [New Citizens' Movement to Get Rid of Opium Forum], *Xin Manzhou* [New Manchuria], August 1941, 29.

82 Wang Shigong, "Manzhouguo yapian wenti, di'yi: Fengtian shi yishi jiangxihui tebie jianyan yanchi" [The Manchukuo opium question, part one: Fengtian city medical doctor conference special speech draft], *Shengjing shibao* [Shengjing times], 30 December 1936, 5.

83 For example, see Hsin-pao Chang, *Commissioner Lin and the Opium War* (Cambridge, MA: Harvard University Press, 1964); Tan Chung, *China and the Brave New World* (Durham, NC: Carolina Academic Press, 1978); and J.Y. Wong, *Deadly Dreams: Opium, Imperialism and the Arrow War* (Cambridge, UK: Cambridge University Press, 1998).

84 For example, see Timothy Brook and Bob Tadashi Wakabayashi, eds., *Opium Regimes: China, Britain, and Japan, 1839-1952* (Berkeley: University of California Press, 2000); and Kathryn Meyer, *Webs of Smoke: Smugglers, Warlords, Spies and the History of the International Drug Trade* (Lanham, MD: Rowman and Littlefield, 1998).

85 An incisive discussion of the long-term duration of opium in late-imperial China, and the means by which opium came to be demonized, can be found in R.K. Newman, "Opium Smoking in Late Imperial China: A Reconsideration," *Modern Asian Studies* 29, 4 (1995): 765-94.

86 David Anthony Bello, *Opium and the Limits of Empire: Drug Prohibition in the Chinese Interior, 1729-1850* (Cambridge, MA: Harvard University Press, 2005), 38.

87 See James Polachek, *The Inner Opium War* (Cambridge, MA: Harvard East Asian Monographs, 1992).

88 Zheng Yangwen, *The Social Life of Opium in China* (Cambridge, UK: Cambridge University Press, 2005), 154.

89 For discussion of the history of tobacco in Manchuria, see Benedict, *Golden-Silk Smoke*, 22-25.

90 In the early twentieth century, Sakai Kyoshi noted perceived links between opium smoking and the enhancement of sexual pleasure in Shanghai. See Mark Driscoll, *Absolute Erotic, Absolute Grotesque* (Durham, NC: Duke University Press, 2010), 191.

91 Zheng, *Social Life of Opium*, 8.

92 Bai Chun, "Jin yan chuyan" [Brief introduction to ban smoking], *Shengjing shibao* [Shengjing times], 4 May 1941, 8.

93 Miriam Lynn Kingsberg, "The Poppy and the Acacia: Opium and Imperialism in Japanese Dairen and the Kwantung Leased Territory, 1905-1945" (PhD diss., History Department, University of California at Berkeley, 2009), 42-43.

94 Zheng, *Social Life of Opium*, 81.

95 Zhou Yongming, *Anti-Drug Crusades in Twentieth Century China: Nationalism, History, and State Building* (Oxford: Rowman and Littlefield, 1999), 171.

96 Bello, *Opium and the Limits*, 275.

97 "Xin guomin yundong," 29.

98 Madancy credits the efforts of unofficial elite who were reliant on the state's moral and legal authority. See Joyce A. Madancy, *The Troublesome Legacy of Commissioner Lin: The Opium Trade and Opium Suppression in Fujian Province, 1820s to 1920s* (Cambridge, MA: Harvard University Asia Centre, 2003), 9.

99 Bob Wakabayashi cites the "will to empire" as the catalyst for the Japanese trade in drugs and charts three stages through which it developed. See Bob Tadashi Wakabayashi, "'Imperial Japanese' Drug Trafficking in China: Historiographic Perspectives," 5-6, http://chinajapan.org/articles/13.1/13.1wakabayashi3-19.pdf.

100 Meyer, *Webs of Smoke*, 189.

101 Mark Driscoll notes that in 1897 Gotō set opium prices so high that they generated a profit of 2.4 million yen that year, equal to Taiwan's total tax revenues. See Mark Driscoll, *Absolute Erotic*, 31.

102 Gotō's estimate proved prophetic given the collapse of the Japanese Empire in 1945.

103 Meyer, *Webs of Smoke*, 188.

104 Huai Yin, "Junfa yu yapian" [Warlords and opium], *Shengjing shibao* [Shengjing times], 19 November 1924, 1.

105 Ru Gai, "Yu zhi jie yan jingyan" [After quitting smoking experience], *Shengjing shibao* [Shengjing times], 30 November 1930, 7.

106 Dikötter, Laamann, and Zhou, *Narcotic Culture*, 207.

107 Alan Baumler, *The Chinese and Opium under the Republic: Worse than Floods and Wild Beasts* (Albany: State University of New York Press, 2007), 7.

108 Ibid.

109 Major works on anti-opium campaigns do not discuss Japanese prohibitionist agendas on the mainland. For example, see Zhou, *Anti-Drug Crusades;* and Baumler, *Chinese and Opium.*

110 Kunito Sadao cites these consumables as addictive substances. See Kunito Sadao, "Manzhou weisheng xue dayao, qi'san" [Main points of Manchurian hygiene studies, part three], *Dongfang yixue zazhi* [Far Eastern medical journal] 16, 4 (1938): 169.

111 Carol Benedict notes that positive and negative views of tobacco could be held at the same time, depending on individual health; see Benedict, *Golden-Silk Smoke*, 89. In Manchukuo media, tobacco was often recognized for its use in dissipating worries and boredom and in enhancing short-term mental capacity, but the nicotine within was poisonous. The caffeine and other contents in tea could have positive health benefits, but overconsumption would damage digestion and could cause constipation and heart disease. For example, see the Ruosu advertisement "Zhuyi!! Yan du, jiu du, cha du: Yingdang zenyang jiuzhi" [Attention!! You ought to know how to cure tobacco poison, alcohol poison, and tea poison], *Shengjing shibao* [Shengjing times], 5 April 1941, 4.

112 Carol Benedict, citing a Korean source, notes that tobacco use in Fengtian in 1638 was prohibited but that it was still widely popular. See Benedict, *Golden-Silk Smoke*, 24.

Chapter 2: Manchurian Context

1 English-language accounts of the Zhang regimes and the establishment of Manchukuo include Gavin McCormack, *Chang Tso-lin in Northeast China, 1911-1928* (Stanford, CA: Stanford University Press, 1977); Rana Mitter, *The Manchurian Myth: Nationalism, Resistance, and Collaboration in Modern China* (Berkeley: University of California Press, 2000); and Ronald Suleski, *Civil Government in Warlord China: Tradition, Modernization and Manchuria* (New York: Bern, 2002).

2 Li Zhiting, ed., *Zhongguo bianjiang tongshi congshu: Dongbei bianshi* [A complete history of China's borders: Northeast borderland] (Zhengzhou: Zhengzhou guji chubanshe, 2003), 522.

3 Feng Qi, "Jiu ren shuo jiu hua: Dongbei jiu wenhua he xiaofei xiguan yanjiu" [Drinkers talk drink talk: Research on Northeast alcohol culture and consumption habits], http://www.cnbm.net.cn/.

4 This was the case especially with the soil around Antung and Fengtian. See Kathryn Meyer, "Japan and the World Narcotics Traffic," in Jordan Goodman, Paul E. Lovejoy, and Andrew Sherratt, eds., *Consuming Habits: Drugs in History and Anthropology* (London: Routledge, 1995), 197.

5 T. Nagashima, "Opium Administration in Manchoukuo," *Contemporary Manchuria* 3, 1 (1939): 25-26. Lü Yonghua dates opium's arrival to 1863, arguing that by 1878 local production had reached 50,000 kilograms; see Lü Yonghua, *Wei Man shiqi de dongbei yandu* [Opium poison in the Northeast during the bogus Manchukuo era] (Changchun: Jilin renmin chubanshe, 2004), 17.

6 John M. Jennings, *The Opium Empire: Japanese Imperialism and Drug Trafficking in Asia, 1895-1945* (London: Praeger, 1997), 78.

7 During harvest times in Rehe province, for example, gambling, eating, and drinking establishments, hotels, storytelling artists, theatrical troupes, film theatres, and brothels

could double population levels. See Yang Chaohui and An Linhai, "Wei Man shiqi de Rehe yapian" [Rehe opium during the bogus Manchukuo era], in Sun Bang, ed., *Wei Man wenhua* [Bogus Manchukuo culture], in *Wei Man shiliao congshu* [Collection of historical materials on bogus Manchukuo], 10 vols. (Changchun: Jilin renmin chubanshe, 1993), vol. 6, 425-26. Annika Culver argues that "prostitution, hard liquor and opium were often the endpoint of a coolie's hard-earned wages"; see Annika A. Culver, "Two Japanese Avant-Garde Writers' Views of Gender Relations and Colonial Oppression in Manchuria, 1921-31," *US-Japan Women's Journal* 37 (2009): 16.

8   Yin Zhengping, for example, argues that in addition to deaths from overconsumption, over half of those admitted for treatment to Kangsheng yuan [Healthy Life Institutes] died there because of torture; see Yin Zhengping, "'Zui'e zhi hua' zai Dongbei – Riben zai Dongbei shixing de yan du zhengci" [The "pattern of crime" in the Northeast: Japan's implementation in the Northeast of an opium poison policy] (2008), http://www.minge.gov.cn/.

9   Frank Dikötter, Lars Laamann, and Zhou Xun, *Narcotic Culture: A History of Drugs in China* (Chicago, IL: University of Chicago Press, 2004), 82.

10   Yang and An, "Wei Man shiqi," 427.

11   Jennings, *Opium Empire*, 78.

12   Yang and An, "Wei Man shiqi," 425.

13   T. Nagashima, "Opium Administration," *Contemporary Manchuria* 3.1 (1939): 25-26.

14   Zhang Guochen, "Yaowuxue shiye zhong de yapian" [Opium in the view of pharmacology], *Jiankang Manzhou* [Healthy Manchukuo] 3.4 (1941): 6. For an in-depth discussion of heroin composition and quality, see Itō Ryōichi, "Guanyu xi hailuoying (heroin) shi yixing yu yan zhong de youxiao chengfen liang" [Regarding measurements of active ingredients in heroin when smoking], *Dongfang yixue zazhi* [Far Eastern medical journal] 14, 10 (1935): 376-96.

15   Zhang Huinuan, *Beifang shaoshu minzu de jiu wenhua* [Northern national minority alcohol culture] (Huhhot: Nei Menggu daxue chubanshe, 2008), 21.

16   Ibid., 52.

17   Jiang Hai, *Jiu de gushi* [The story of alcohol] (Jinan: Shandong renmin yinshuachang, 2006), 84. Wen Long argues that Han and Manchu drinking practices differed greatly in terms of women's consumption: Manchu women could drink with men and participate in ritual offerings; alcohol also played important roles in the Manchu matchmaking process. For further discussion of Manchu drinking practices, see Wen Long, ed., *Zhongguo jiu dian* [Chinese alcohol code] (Changchun: Jilin chuban jituan youxian guiren gongsi, 2010), 308-9.

18   Ahmulu is also the name of a Northeast brand of wine today.

19   For consistency, present-day Shenyang, also known by its Manchu name, Mukden, is called here by its former Chinese name, Fengtian.

20   For details, see an edited volume inspired by the brand: Li Tongfeng and Zou Changshun, eds., *Jiu zhi yun* [The charm of alcohol] (Shenyang: Liaohai chubanshe, 2007), 1. Lao long kou is also the topic of Zou Changshun's three-volume novel: *Lao long kou: Jiu shang, jiu hun, jiu she* [Old Dragon Mouth: Alcohol vessel, alcohol soul, alcohol god] (2005).

21   Zhang notes, too, that although bars began to be seen in China in the early Zhou Dynasty, they didn't appear in the Northeast until the Han, approximately 2,000 years ago. See Zhang, *Beifang shaoshu minzu*, 92.

22   *Manchuria: Land of Opportunities* (New York: South Manchuria Railway Company, 1922), 43.

23   White Russians evidently found another use for *gaoliang* wine – when mixed with other alcohol, it served as an antifreeze for vehicles in the winter. See John Underwood Jr., *Japanese Armour in Manchuria, 1931-1945* (West Chester, OH: Nafziger, 2001), 26.

24 In a subsequent letter dated 5 November 1906, Fairchild added sherry to the list. See L.N. Fairchild, *Nelson Fairchild* (Boston, MA: Merrymount, 1907), 107, 132.

25 Information on Harbin's early-twentieth-century production can be found in *Ha'erbin shi zhi: Fushi pinshang ye zhi* [Harbin city records: Nonstaple food commodity trade records].

26 In 1908 Harbin's sales of vodka were approximately 1.5 million yuan, of grape wine 800,000 yuan, and of beer 30,000 yuan. Harbin then had factories producing distilled alcohol (three), *baijiu* (nine), beer (five), and yellow wine (nine), in addition to thirty smaller factories producing a variety of alcohol; see *Ha'erbin shi zhi*. For further insight into the multi-ethnic environment in Harbin, see James H. Carter, *Creating a Chinese Harbin: Nationalism in an International City, 1916-1932* (Ithaca, NY: Cornell University Press, 2002), 30.

27 Blaine R. Chiasson, *Administering the Colonizer: Manchuria's Russians under Chinese Rule, 1918-29* (Vancouver: UBC Press, 2010); David Wolff, *To the Harbin Station: The Liberal Alternative in Russian Manchuria, 1898-1914* (Stanford, CA: Stanford University Press, 1999).

28 "The Brewing Industry in Manchoukuo," *Contemporary Manchuria* 3.4 (1939): 71.

29 In 1908 the company was renamed Gulunia, and then in 1932 the brewery was renamed Harbin Brewery Factory. In 1901 a Russo-German enterprise began producing Liujie'erman beer. See Li Zhengping, *Zhongguo jiu wenhua* [Chinese wine culture] (Beijing: Shishi chubanshe, 2006), 119.

30 "Brewing Industry in Manchoukuo," 78.

31 *Ha'erbin shi zhi*.

32 Another alcohol that was popular among Japanese but not Chinese consumers was *taosu*, a drink consumed during New Year festivities. Japanese taosu was noted to be different from the Chinese variety, which dated to the Han Dynasty and was commemorated in poems by Su Dongbo. See Cui Yu, "*Taosu* yu taofu" [*Taosu* and spring festival couplets], *Qilin* [Unicorn], January 1942, 7.

33 "Brewing Industry in Manchoukuo," 71.

34 Cited in Wolff, *To the Harbin Station*, 38.

35 Mark Driscoll argues that the pioneering presence of Japanese sex workers was "indispensable for the spread of related Japanese consumer products: beer, sake." See Mark Driscoll, *Absolute Erotic, Absolute Grotesque* (Durham, NC: Duke University Press, 2010), 62.

36 Penelope Francks, "Inconspicuous Consumption: Sake, Beer, and the Birth of the Consumer in Japan," *Journal of Asian Studies* 68, 1 (2009): 135-64.

37 Further information on the history of sake can be found in Chris Bunting, *Drinking Japan: A Guide to Japan's Best Drinks and Drinking Establishments* (North Clarendon, VT: Tuttle Publishing, 2011), 30-37.

38 "Brewing Industry in Manchoukuo," 63.

39 Frank Dikötter has noted that gin, rum, brandy, whiskey, and other distilled liquors were not popular in imperial China. See Frank Dikötter, *Things Modern: Material Culture and Everyday Life in China* (London: Hurst, 2007), 238. By the 1930s, however, brandy and whiskey had gained considerable popularity in some urban centres.

40 Yu Xuebin, *Dongbei zhaohuang* [Old signboards of the Northeast] (Shanghai: Shanghai shudian chubanshe, 2002), 47.

41 Yu provides details on the symbolism of gourds, which represent honesty and trust – qualities that retailers were eager to link with their establishments; see ibid., 47-48. For classical Chinese literary allusions to alcohol signboards, see ibid., 11-13.

42 Suleski, *Civil Government*, 210.

43 Tim Wright, "The Manchurian Economy and the 1930s World Depression," *Modern Asian Studies* 41, 5 (2007): 1076.

44 In the early 1920s, alcohol taxes were approximately 20 percent; profits averaged 30 percent. See *Ha'erbin shi zhi*.

45 Wright, "The Manchurian Economy," 1075.

46 Suleski, *Civil Government*, 216.

47 Herbert Bix, "Japanese Imperialism and the Manchurian Economy, 1900-31," *China Quarterly* 51 (1972): 430.

48 For information on Japanese management in Guandong, see Jennings, *Opium Empire*, 46-52.

49 The following reductions in sales were reported: *baijiu*, 32.84 percent; beer, 37.77 percent; and wine, 21.43 percent. See *Ha'erbin shi zhi*.

50 For example, see Shenyang shi Lao long kou jiuchang bianzuan bangongshi, ed., *Shenyang shi Lao long kou jiuchangzhi* [Shenyang city's Lao long kou (Old Dragon Mouth) wine factory records] (Shenyang: Shenyang chubanshe, 1993), 5-6. Annual regional production of *baijiu* grew from 47,000 litres in 1905 to almost 240,000 litres in 1916; see ibid., 49.

51 The implementation of standardized taxation is discussed in "Jiu shui fa gongbu" [Alcohol tax law proclamation], *Shengjing shibao* [Shengjing times], 29 July 1935, 2.

52 For further details, see *Ha'erbin shi zhi*.

53 Increases of 10 percent for *baijiu*, 61 percent for beer, and 39 percent for wine were reported. See *Ha'erbin shi zhi*.

54 See "Yu zhi yan jiu jie jiekuan guan" [My point of view on borrowing money for opium and alcohol], *Shengjing shibao* [Shengjing times], 16 September 1919, 1.

55 *Ha'erbin shi zhi* cites the following mid-1920s prices per 500 grams: locally produced *baijiu*, 0.14 yuan; English whiskey, 2.92-5 yuan; French brandy, 3.08-3.5 yuan; French champagne, 5.17 yuan; French red wine, 1.08-4.17 yuan; French sweet wine, 1.67 yuan; French white grape wine, 1-2.5 yuan; Japanese Red Ball grape wine, 1.5 yuan; Japanese sake, 2.2 yuan; Japanese white wine, 1.7 yuan; and Russian vodka, 0.53-0.58 yuan. Prices per bottle included: German black beer, 0.67-1 yuan; and Japanese beer, 0.5 yuan.

56 *Ha'erbin shi zhi*.

57 Suleski, *Civil Government*, 207.

58 Jennings, *Opium Empire*, 79. Responses varied from Zhu Qinglan, under whose rule opium was forbidden, to Zhang Zongchang, who actively encouraged it; see Nagashima, "Opium Administration," 26.

59 Jennings, *Opium Empire*, 80. "Offices" often consisted of just a desk in a corner of a business; see Suleski, *Civil Government*, 171.

60 See Driscoll, *Absolute Erotic*, 233-34.

61 Leng Fo, "Jin yan wenti" [Opium prohibition question], *Shengjing shibao* [Shengjing times], 24 March 1929, 7.

62 Nagashima, "Opium Administration," 26.

63 Ibid.

64 "Yan xun zhifu" [Opium patrol uniforms], *Shengjing shibao* [Shengjing times], 21 August 1927, 5.

65 "Datong gongsuo quan jie yan jiu" [Datong government office persuades to quit smoking and drinking], *Shengjing shibao* [Shengjing times], 5 August 1931, 5.

66 See Lu Shouxin, "Ha'erbin de yapian yandu" [Harbin's poisonous opium smoke], in Sun Bang, ed., *Wei Man wenhua* [Bogus Manchukuo culture], in *Wei Man shiliao congshu* [Collection of historical materials on bogus Manchukuo], 10 vols. (Changchun: Jilin renmin chubanshe, 1993), vol. 6, 445.

67 Dikötter, Laamann, and Zhou, *Narcotic Culture*, 170.

68 Ibid., 187.

69 For more on Harbin's Sino-Russian language, see Olga Bakich, "Did You Speak Harbin Sino-Russian," *Itinerario* 35.3 (March 2012): 29.

70 Dikötter, Laamann, and Zhou, *Narcotic Culture*, 170.

71 "Mafei hai ren" [Morphine harms people], *Shengjing shibao* [Shengjing times], 23 August 1916, 5.

72 Kishi Nobosuke, quoted in Yamamuro Shin'ichi, *Manchuria under Japanese Dominion*, trans. Joshua Fogel (Philadelphia: University of Pennsylvania Press, 2006), 4.

73 Prasenjit Duara, *Sovereignty and Authenticity: Manchukuo and the East Asian Modern* (New York: Rowman and Littlefield, 2003), 75.

74 Liu Guojun, "Jin yan yu juewu" [Ban opium and consciousness], *Datong bao* [Great unity herald], 23 October 1941, 4.

75 Michael A. Barnhart, *Japan Prepares for Total War: The Search for Economic Security, 1919-41* (Ithaca, NY: Cornell University Press, 1987); Alan Baumler, *The Chinese and Opium under the Republic: Worse than Floods and Wild Beasts* (Albany: State University of New York Press, 2007); Miriam Lynn Kingsberg, "The Poppy and the Acacia: Opium and Imperialism in Japanese Dairen and the Kwantung Leased Territory, 1905-1945" (PhD diss., History Department, University of California at Berkeley, 2009); and Yamada Goichi, *Manshukoku No Ahensenbai* [Opium Monopoly in Manchuria] (Tokyo: Kyuko Shoen, 2002).

76 Sun Kungtu and Ralph W. Huenemann, *The Economic Development of Manchuria in the First Half of the Twentieth Century* (Cambridge, MA: Harvard University Press, 1969), 76.

77 Kang Chao, *The Economic Development of Manchuria: The Rise of a Frontier Economy* (Ann Arbor: Center for Chinese Studies, University of Michigan, 1983), 15.

78 Wright, "Manchurian Economy," 1105.

79 Bix, "Japanese Imperialism," 438.

80 Jennings, *Opium Empire*, 83.

81 Lü, *Wei Man shiqi*, 40; Jiao Runming, *Jindai Dongbei shehui zhu wenti yanjiu* [Research on various questions in modern Northeast society] (Beijing: Zhongguo shehui kexue chubanshe, 2004), 283. Kaneda Sei, the Manchukuo vice-minister of welfare in 1944, later at his war crimes trial estimated that there were at most 200,000 opium addicts before the occupation began; he also argued in post-occupation materials that the sale of opium was to weaken and kill the Chinese people; see Driscoll, *Absolute Erotic*, 243, 248.

82 *Manchoukuo Yearbook: 1941* (Hsinking: Manchoukuo Yearbook Company, 1942), 731.

83 Ibid., 728.

84 Levels of use necessitated expanded imports from Korea and Persia. See ibid., 729.

85 The Opium Law allowed for sales only by officially designated agents, government control over cultivation zones, and the licensing and sale of medicinal-use opium. The Opium Law applied to opium, leaving no restrictions on other drugs. The full text of the Opium Law (with 1934, 1935, and 1937 revisions) can be found in Nagashima, "Opium Administration," 38-44.

86 Ten state-sponsored rehabilitation centres were opened in 1933 in Fengtian, Jilin, Qiqihaer, Shanhaiguan, Yingkou, Andong, Harbin, Manzhouli, Xinjing, and Chengde. See "Fengtian jieyansuo fangwen ji" [Notes on an interview at the Fengtian Quit Smoking Centre], *Xin qingnian* [New youth] 8, 5 (1939): 10.

87 Rana Mitter, "Evil Empire? Competing Constructions of Japanese Imperialism in Manchuria, 1928-1937," in Li Narangoa and Robert Cribb, eds., *Imperial Japan and National Identities in Asia, 1895-1945* (London: RoutledgeCurzon, 2003), 156.

88 Ah Ling, "Yinzhe de xin" [An addict's letter], and Yue Ai, "Jin yan lun" [Discussion of opium prohibition], *Shengjing shibao* [Shengjing times], 3 October 1941, 5.

89 Jennings, *Opium Empire*, 82.

90 Nagashima, "Opium Administration," 18.

91 Meyer, "Japan and the World," 197.

92 See Kingsberg, "Poppy and the Acacia," 207. Firms involved in the trade included Mitsubishi and Mitsui, and individuals included Aichi Kiichi; see Bob Tadashi Wakabayashi, "'Imperial

Japanese' Drug Trafficking in China: Historiographic Perspectives," 17, http://chinajapan. org/articles/13.1/13.1wakabayashi3-19.pdf.
93   Meyer, "Japan and the World," 197.
94   Yin, "'Zui'e zhi hua' zai Dongbei."
95   Jennings, *Opium Empire*, 84.
96   *Manchoukuo Yearbook: 1941*, 722.
97   F.C. Jones, *Manchuria since 1931* (London: Royal Institute of International Affairs, 1949), 135.
98   Ibid.
99   Ibid., 132.
100 For details, see "Brewing Industry in Manchoukuo," 63-66. Japanese creation of major beer producers in Manchukuo reflected domestic policies in Japan. For a concise description of beer history in Japan, see Bunting, *Drinking Japan*, 134-41.
101 Beer sales in 1933 were on average 4-10 percent higher than in the previous year. See "Riben pijiu jie: Shengchan jizeng" [Japanese beer world: Production increases], *Shengjing shibao* [Shengjing times], 13 August 1933, 7.
102 "Maijiu shiye zhi hua qi: Nanbei Manzhou zhi daibiao Fengtian ji Ha shi" [Planning stage of the beer business: The representative cities of south and north Manchuria, Fengtian and Harbin], *Shengjing shibao* [Shengjing times], 8 December 1936, 12.
103 "Brewing Industry in Manchoukuo," 74.
104 Taxing Ltd. Brewery was permitted to produce 340,000 cases per year. See "Brewing Industry in Manchoukuo," 74.
105 Ann Rasmussen Kinney, *Japanese Investment in Manchurian Manufacturing, Mining, Transportation and Communications, 1931-1945* (New York: Garland, 1982), 9n9.
106 A case consisted of forty-eight quart bottles; see ibid., 168. Kirin, a leading brand, produced 120,000 cases in 1939; see "Brewing Industry in Manchoukuo," 73-74.
107 These figures can be found in "Brewing Industry in Manchoukuo," 72.
108 "Maijiu shiye zhi hua qi," 12.
109 Ibid.
110 "Niangjiu gongye zhi jingsui" [The quintessence of the fermented alcohol business], *Shengjing shibao* [Shengjing times], 18 June 1936, 13.
111 Jun Qing, "Tan pijiu, shang" [Talking beer, first], *Shengjing shibao* [Shengjing times], 21 August 1937, 4.
112 "Brewing Industry in Manchoukuo," 66.
113 Fengtian was an important centre for the production of *gaoliang* and other distilled liquors. In 1910 there were thirteen *shaojiu* [sorghum or maize alcohol] producers and fifty-four liquor boards. Close to Fengtian, in Qianshan, commercial production began in 1658, and in 1933 there were thirty-five shaojiu producers. See ibid., 68-69.
114 Ibid., 67.
115 Ibid., 68.
116 Ibid., 67.
117 Ibid., 63.
118 Feng Sen, "Yin jiu mantan, yi" [Informal discussion of drinking alcohol, one], *Shengjing shibao* [Shengjing times], 7 July 1937, 9.
119 For further information, see http://www.cnwinenews.com/.
120 For example, see Leng Mei, "Putaojiu" [Grape wine], *Shengjing shibao* [Shengjing times], 1 January 1933, 2.
121 A You, "Putaojiu" [Grape wine], *Shengjing shibao* [Shengjing times], 18 October 1936, 14.
122 Ibid.
123 Feng, "Yin jiu mantan, yi," 9.

124 Feng Sen, "Yin jiu mantan, er" [Informal discussion of drinking alcohol, two], *Shengjing shibao* [Shengjing times], 8 July 1937, 9.

125 Leng Fo, "Shang sheng de jiu" [The harmful nature of alcohol], *Shengjing shibao* [Shengjing times], 30 January 1931, 4.

126 Ibid.

127 "Jiu shui fa gongbu," 2.

128 Ibid.

129 Although Dalian was a colony and not part of Manchukuo, the bar culture in Dalian was representative of developments in neighbouring Manchukuo. Sapporo Bar postcard, author's collection.

130 "Former Friends" Russian postcard, author's collection.

131 Li, *Zhongguo jiu wenhua*, 280, 302.

132 Yang Xu, "Gongkai de zuizhuang" [Open indictment], in *Wo de riji* [My diary] (Xinjing: Kaiming tushu gongsi, 1944), 97.

133 Such discussion of the plight of innocents mirrors that noted by Catherine Carstairs in the writings of Canadian Emily Murphy, who depicted Chinese traffickers as misleading others into trying drugs. See Catherine Carstairs, *Jailed for Possession: Illegal Drug Use, Regulation, and Power in Canada, 1920-1961* (Toronto: University of Toronto Press, 2006), 23.

134 See *Ha'erbin shi zhi*.

135 "Yan jiu qunian shengchan liang" [Last year's production of tobacco and alcohol], *Shengjing shibao* [Shengjing times], 31 March 1937, 7.

136 See *Ha'erbin shi zhi*.

137 "Jiu luo, liang zhang, shui zhong" [Alcohol down, grains rise, taxes heavy], *Shengjing shibao* [Shengjing times], 20 October 1934, 9.

138 *Ha'erbin shi zhi*.

139 Ibid.

140 "Bairi jian jin jiu duanxing: Bin sheng aiguo jingshen zuoxing" [One hundred days' practice of prohibiting alcohol: Patriotic spirits are up in Bin province], *Shengjing shibao* [Shengjing times], 17 February 1938, 9.

141 "Jiu ke wuli nao" [Drunkard is a nuisance], *Shengjing shibao* [Shengjing times], 4 October 1938, 5.

142 Meyer, "Japan and the World," 187.

143 Clandestine operations of the South Manchuria Pharmaceutical Company were reported to have produced 100 kilograms of heroin per night. See Meyer, "Japan and the World," 194, 197.

144 Rates of morphine use ranged from 27 to 44 kilograms per 1 million people. See Motohiro Kobayashi, "Drug Operations by Resident Japanese in Tianjin," trans. Bob Tadashi Wakabayashi, in Timothy Brook and Bob Tadashi Wakabayashi, eds., *Opium Regimes: China, Britain, and Japan, 1839-1952* (Berkeley: University of California Press, 2000), 154.

145 Qu Bingshan, "Yapian zhuanmai yu duhai" [The Opium Monopoly and poison], in Sun Bang, ed., *Jingji lüeduo* [Plundering the economy], in *Wei Man shiliao congshu* [Collection of historical materials on bogus Manchukuo], 10 vols. (Changchun: Jilin renmin chubanshe, 1993), vol. 4, 688.

146 A graphic account of the impact on a community can be seen in Kathryn Meyer, "Garden of Grand Vision: Economic Life in a Flophouse Complex, Harbin, China, 1940," *Crime, Law and Social Change* 36 (2001): 327-52.

147 The children were sold with the wife. See "Mafei zhi hai" [The harm of morphine], *Shengjing shibao* [Shengjing times], 30 December 1933, 4.

148   Mukden is the Manchu name for present-day Fengtian; see Jennings, *Opium Empire*, 85. Figure 7 is from Assemblies of God, Foreign Missions Department, *Gospel Rays in Manchoukuo* (Springfield, MO: Assemblies of God, 1937). Mark Driscoll describes an ash heap at the South Gate near "Japanese shooting galleries" in which users reportedly had ropes tied to their wrists so that if they died they could be more easily removed to the heap; see Driscoll, *Absolute Erotic*, 243.

149   Cited in Timothy Brook and Bob Tadashi Wakabayashi, "Introduction: Opium's History in China," in Timothy Brook and Bob Tadashi Wakabayashi, eds., *Opium Regimes: China, Britain, and Japan, 1839-1952* (Berkeley: University of California Press, 2000), 17.

150   An Longzhen, *Modai de huanghou Wanrong* [The last empress Wanrong] (Beijing: Huaxia chubanshe, 1994), 156.

151   Jennings, *Opium Empire*, 84.

152   Meyer highlights the work of Nitanosa Otozō and Hoshi Hajime. See Meyer, "Japan and the World," 190-91.

153   Losses cited included not only lost work hours and reduced levels of workers' skills but also land lost to opium that could have been mined, used to grow food, and so on; see Jennings, *Opium Empire*, 87. Mark Driscoll notes that "like most of the civilian elite, Hoshino didn't like Chinese people" and was therefore little moved by their suffering; see Driscoll, *Absolute Erotic*, 253.

154   Nine million yuan is cited for the fiscal year 1938-39; see Nagashima, "Opium Administration," 36. Jennings argues that opium revenue was approximately 30 million yuan; see Jennings, *Opium Empire*, 87. In 1949 F.C. Jones argued that the number was 19 million; see Jones, *Manchuria since 1931*, 133. For further discussion of contested numbers, see Driscoll, *Absolute Erotic*, 259-60.

155   One hundred and eighty million yuan was a considerable sum, equal to investment in local private enterprises in 1938. See Louise Young, *Japan's Total Empire: Manchuria and the Culture of Wartime Imperialism* (Berkeley: University of California Press, 1998), 241.

156   Edgar Snow, "Japan Builds a New Colony," *Saturday Evening Post*, 24 February 1934, 84.

157   Ibid., 81.

158   Vespa Amleto, *Secret Agent of Japan: A Handbook to Japanese Imperialism* (London: Victor Gollancz, 1938), 102. "Shops" could be just a hole in the wall: heroin addicts could knock at a door, whereupon a "small peep-hole opens, through which he thrusts his bare arm and hand with 20 cents in it. The owner of the joint takes the money and gives the victim a shot in the arm"; see ibid., 96-97.

159   Ibid., 102. Lu Shouxin asserts that in 1937 there were seventy-seven retail opium outlets in Harbin, a number that accords with Harbin's annual records; see Lu, "Ha'erbin de yapian yandu," 445; and Lü, *Wei Man shiqi*, 142.

160   Quoted in Amleto, *Secret Agent of Japan*, 101. This Japanese Military Command booklet is also cited in Mark Gayn, *Journey from the East* (New York: Alfred A. Knopf, 1944), 418.

161   Alexandre Pernikoff, *Bushido: The Anatomy of Terror* (New York: Liveright, 1943), 105.

162   Ibid., 173.

163   Jones, *Manchuria since 1931*, 134-35.

164   Ibid., 132.

165   Pernikoff, *Bushido*, 106.

166   Jennings, *Opium Empire*, 77, 89.

167   "Chengxiang shu na si yanguan" [Chengxiang office takes firm hold of private opium dens], *Shengjing shibao* [Shengjing times], 4 September 1936, 12.

168   "Shuzhang zhao ji lingmaisuo huiyi" [Director calls for meeting with retail stores], *Shengjing shibao* [Shengjing times], 4 September 1936, 12.

169   Nagashima, "Opium Administration," 21.

170 For details on land, see Lü, *Wei Man shiqi*, 63.

171 "Zhengli yinzhe suqing si yan guan: Wei jin yan zhengci de yaowu, Yu Sheng, weisheng chuzhang fabiao tanhua" [Straighten out addicts, eliminate private opium dens: Important items for the government policies of prohibiting opium, Yu Sheng, section chief of the hygiene department, publishes a statement], *Shengjing shibao* [Shengjing times], 2 September 1941, 11.

172 Two hundred and seventy-two private firms remained in operation. See *Manchoukuo Yearbook: 1941*, 722.

173 Jennings, *Opium Empire*, 101.

174 Ibid.

175 Lo Cheng-Pang, "The Fight against Opium," *Pan Pacific* 3, 4 (1939): 71.

176 "Yinzhe denglu jiang jiezhi" [Addict registry about to be cut off], *Shengjing shibao* [Shengjing times], 11 June 1938, 9.

177 *Manchoukuo Yearbook: 1941*, 722.

178 For example, see Nagashima, "Opium Administration," 20; and *Manchoukuo Yearbook: 1941*, 727, 730.

179 It was estimated that only 2-3 percent of addicts could withstand sustained labour, an intolerable statistic for colonial officials actively engaged in Holy War. See *Manchoukuo Yearbook: 1941*, 727.

180 Wang Shigong, "Manzhouguo yapian wenti, di'yi: Fengtian shi yishi jiangxihui tebie jianyan yanchi" [The Manchukuo opium question, part one: Fengtian city medical doctor conference special speech draft], *Shengjing shibao* [Shengjing times], 30 December 1936, 5.

181 Jing Chun, "Jie yan ge" [Quit smoking song], *Shengjing shibao* [Shengjing times], 10 April 1941, 7.

182 Zhang Nianhui, "Jie yan si ji ge" [Four seasons of quitting smoking song], *Shengjing shibao* [Shengjing times], 20 April 1941, 8.

183 Yong Shanqi, "Jin yan judu zhi juti fangce, si" [Concrete directives for banning smoking and refusing poison, four], *Shengjing shibao* [Shengjing times], 17 October 1940, 5.

184 Yong Shanqi, "Jin yan judu zhi juti fangce, qi" [Concrete directives for banning smoking and refusing poison, seven], *Shengjing shibao* [Shengjing times], 5 December 1940, 8.

185 "Paichu yapian mayao liudu" [Eliminate the pernicious influence of opium and morphine], *Shengjing shibao* [Shengjing times], 27 October 1940, 4.

186 Wang Dashan, "Jin yan ganyan" [Ban smoking heartfelt words], *Shengjing shibao* [Shengjing times], 5 December 1940, 8.

187 "Xin guomin yundong de quchu yapian zuotanhui" [New Citizens' Movement to Get Rid of Opium Forum], *Xin Manzhou* [New Manchuria], August 1941, 28.

188 "Nü yinzhe: Xing xing ba!" [Female addicts: Wake up!], *Shengjing shibao* [Shengjing times], 5 September 1941, 5. Miriam Kingsberg notes that Kō Toriu, a faculty member of the Mukden Medical College of Gynecology, "estimated a female addict community of approximately 170,000, out of a total narcotics consumer population of about one million" in Manchukuo in 1939; see Kingsberg, "Poppy and the Acacia," 139.

189 Wang Shaoxian, "Wo guo jin zheng gaikuang" [Survey of my country's prohibit opium policy], *Shengjing shibao* [Shengjing times], 6 March 1941, 8.

190 "Qudi de juewu" [Understanding the ban], *Shengjing shibao* [Shengjing times], 10 April 1941, 7.

191 Li Shixun, "Jin yan xingzheng zhi zhongdian" [Serious points regarding the official policy of banning smoking], *Shengjing shibao* [Shengjing times], 4 May 1941, 8.

192 "Xin guomin yundong," 26.

193 Ibid., 27.

194 Ibid., 31.

195   Ibid., 30.

196   Ibid., 31.

197   From 1938 to 1940, official statistics suggest a drop in the number of opium and morphine addicts of almost 200,000 – from almost 670,000 to just over 450,000. As cited in "Qudi de juewu," 7, the number of addicts in 1938 was 668,949 (opium, 641,700; morphine, 27,249), in 1939 it was 582,610 (opium, 561,115; morphine, 21,495), and in 1940 it was 452,397 (opium, 436,562; morphine, 15,835).

198   Driscoll, *Absolute Erotic*, 245.

199   Ramon H. Myers, "Creating a Modern Enclave Economy: The Economic Integration of Japan, Manchuria, and North China, 1932-45," in Peter Duus, Ramon H. Myers, and Mark R. Peattie, eds., *The Japanese Wartime Empire, 1931-45* (Princeton, NJ: Princeton University Press, 1996), 138.

200   Kinney, *Japanese Investment*, 140.

201   "Jiu, yanpao, tangtou: Suitong shuilu tigao jiage, ershi ba qian suo zhe buxu zhangti" [Alcohol, tobacco and sugar: Following taxes, prices rise: Those before the 28th are not allowed to raise prices], *Shengjing shibao* [Shengjing times], 28 December 1940, 7.

202   "Wei baoquan jiu lei, shi shi xuke ji" [To protect various kinds of alcohol, implementation of permit system], *Shengjing shibao* [Shengjing times], 28 December 1940, 7.

203   *Ha'erbin shi zhi.*

204   "Xin shui fa shi yi, di'jiu" [New tax laws explanation, part nine], *Shengjing shibao* [Shengjing times], 10 September 1941, 1.

205   Ibid. Tax rates for 1941 are listed per hectolitre *(dan):*

    1   Manufacturing taxes for *shaojiu* (sorghum or maize alcohol): 70 percent volume and higher, 36 yuan; 50-69 percent volume, 21 yuan; less than 50 percent volume, 16 yuan.

    2   Manufacturing tax for *huangjiu* [yellow wine]: 23.5 yuan.

    3   Manufacturing tax for *shaojiu* (rice alcohol): 21 yuan. Tax for leaving the factory: 10.5 yuan.

    4   Tax for leaving the factory: beer, 28 yuan.

    5   Manufacturing tax for sake: 22.5 yuan. Tax for leaving the factory: 11.50 yuan.

    6   Manufacturing tax for Korean medicine wine: 21 yuan.

    7   Manufacturing tax for *zhuo jiu* (turbid alcohol): 10.50 yuan.

206   Ibid.

207   "Pijiu peiji fangfa gaishan: Yi minzhong xuyong wei zhudian" [Beer ration method improvements: The main point is the needs of the common people], *Shengjing shibao* [Shengjing times], 1 July 1941, 5.

208   "Jiu shou wai jiu yingxiang: Jiu jia yi pi zai pi" [Alcohol influenced by nonlocal alcohol: Alcohol prices lower again and again], *Shengjing shibao* [Shengjing times], 20 July 1941, 6.

209   Ibid.

210   For example, see Naotaka Shinfuku, "Japanese Culture and Drinking," in Stanton Peele and Marcus Grant, eds., *Alcohol and Pleasure: A Health Perspective* (Philadelphia, PA: Taylor and Francis, 1999), 113-21; and Bufo Yamamuro, "Notes on Drinking in Japan," in Mac Marshall, ed., *Beliefs, Behaviors, and Alcoholic Beverages: A Cross-Cultural Survey* (Ann Arbor: University of Michigan Press, 1979), 272-73. Chris Bunting argues that prohibitionist movements in Japan were, for the most part, unsuccessful and met with popular resistance. Bunting, *Drinking Japan*, 14-19.

211   Han Hu, "Yan jiu suo hua" [Trivial words about smoke and alcohol], *Qilin* [Unicorn], April 1943, 118-21.

212   By 1944, too, production of *gaoliang* wine stood at one-third of 1936 levels. See *Ha'erbin shi zhi.*

213 Champagne does not appear to have played as central a role in major banquets in Manchukuo as it did in urban China. For discussion of the latter, see Dikötter, *Things Modern*, 237.

214 "Ri jin jiu tongmeng paiyuan lai Man" [The Japanese Prohibit Alcohol Alliance members come to Manchukuo], *Shengjing shibao* [Shengjing times], 8 September 1933, 4.

215 "Jiu wei xing Ya zhi di" [Alcohol is the enemy of a prospering Asia], *Shengjing shibao* [Shengjing times], 2 September 1941, 7.

216 "Fu qiaohui kaishi jin jiu yundong" [Women's society starts a prohibit alcohol movement], *Shengjing shibao* [Shengjing times], 3 September 1938, 5.

217 "Bairi jian jin jiu duanxing," 9.

218 "Zi su ri: Jiu zheng ainao lixing jieyue, yan jin yan jiu du" [Self-respect time: Solemnly encouraging economizing: A serious ban on smoking, alcohol, and gambling], *Shengjing shibao* [Shengjing times], 10 January 1940, 4.

219 For example, see Shenyang shi Lao long kou jiuchang bianzuan bangongshi, ed., *Shenyang shi Lao long kou jiuchangzhi*, 6.

220 For example, see Yin, "'Zui'e zhi hua' zai Dongbei.'"

Chapter 3: Evaluating Alcohol

Epigraph: Quoted in Mei Shan, "Jiu you hai?" [Alcohol has harm?], *Shengjing shibao* [Shengjing times], 17 March 1933, 5.

1 Feng Qi, "Jiu ren shuo jiu hua: Dongbei jiu wenhua he xiaofei xiguan yanjiu" [Drinkers talk drink talk: Research on Northeast alcohol culture and consumption habits], http://www.cnbm.net.cn/.

2 Yang Jun, "Dongbeiren yu dongbei jiu wenhua" [Northeasterners and Northeast alcohol culture], http://tieba.baidu.com/.

3 Shao's argument also included tobacco. See Shao Guanzhi, "Yan, jiu yu renti" [Tobacco, alcohol, and the human body], *Jiankang Manzhou* [Healthy Manchuria] 3.5 (1941): 14.

4 Ren Ji, "Jin jiu zhi yi" [The benefit of banning alcohol], *Shengjing shibao* [Shengjing times], 11 April 1934, 11.

5 Shao, "Yan, jiu yu renti," 14.

6 "Jiu yu yousheng zhi guanxi" [The relationship between alcohol and eugenics], *Shengjing shibao* [Shengjing times], 29 April 1943, 4.

7 "Hao jiu de ren wei shenme bu ai chi tian de?" [Why don't people who are fond of alcohol like to eat sweet things?], *Shengjing shibao* [Shengjing times], 17 January 1937, 5.

8 "Nü shifan chuangban yan jiu zizhi hui zhi xian sheng" [Women's teacher training institute heralds the establishment of a smoke and alcohol self-cure association], *Shengjing shibao* [Shengjing times], 13 April 1916, 4.

9 "Jiu yu yousheng," 4.

10 Zhi Xing, "Jiu yu tianzhen" [Alcohol and innocence], *Shengjing shibao* [Shengjing times], 23 May 1937, 9.

11 Ren, "Jin jiu zhi yi," 11.

12 These translations are from *Han-Ying cidian* [Chinese-English dictionary] (Beijing: Shangwu yinshuguan, 1999).

13 Zhang Feng, "Yin jiu xianhua" [Chatting about drinking alcohol], *Shengjing shibao* [Shengjing times], 6 December 1935, 8.

14 Ibid.

15 Pei Ru, "Weisheng: Wo zhi jin jiu dongji" [Hygiene: My motivation for quitting drinking], *Shengjing shibao* [Shengjing times], 8 February 1923, 5.

16 Yi Mei, "Jiu yu ji" [Alcohol and prostitutes], *Shengjing shibao* [Shengjing times], 11 May 1933, 9.

17   Zhong Xin, "Tan yin jiu" [Discussion of drinking alcohol], *Shengjing shibao* [Shengjing times], 25 August 1935, 5. Carole Benedict notes that seventeenth-century authors in the Qing Empire equated tobacco with alcohol for its "inebriating properties" and called it by various names, including "dry liquor" *[ganjiu]*, "fire liquor" *[huojiu]*, or "smoke wine" *[yanjiu]*; see Carol Benedict, *Golden-Silk Smoke: A History of Tobacco in China, 1550-2010* (Berkeley: University of California Press, 2011), 91.

18   Yin, "Tan yin jiu" [Discussion of drinking alcohol], *Shengjing shibao* [Shengjing times], 29 May 1938, 4.

19   Hong Nian, "Tan yin jiu" [Discussion of drinking alcohol], *Shengjing shibao* [Shengjing times], 26 July 1938, 4.

20   Shao, "Yan, jiu yu renti," 14.

21   Zhang, "Yin jiu xianhua," 8.

22   Yin, "Tan yin jiu," 4.

23   Zhou Zuoren, "Mazui li zan" [Praise for anaesthesia], in Yi Yuan, ed., *Jiumo: Jiu fengqing xiaopinji* [Alcohol mystics: Collection of essays on amorous feelings for alcohol] (Taibei: Yeqiang chuban, 1994), 23.

24   Cited in Lian, "Tan jiu (shang)" [Discussion of alcohol (first)], *Shengjing shibao* [Shengjing times], 24 September 1938, 4.

25   Lian, "Tan jiu (xia)" [Discussion of alcohol (second)], *Shengjing shibao* [Shengjing times], 25 September 1938, 5.

26   Lian, "Tan jiu (shang)," 4.

27   Yi, "Jiu yu ji," 9.

28   Zhi, "Jiu yu tianzhen," 9.

29   Ibid.

30   Yin, "Tan yin jiu," 4.

31   "Jiu lun" [Discussion of alcohol], *Shengjing shibao* [Shengjing times], 9 April 1931, 3.

32   For example, see Ren, "Jin jiu zhi yi," 11; and Zhong, "Tan yin jiu," 5.

33   "Jiu wei xing Ya zhi di" [Alcohol is the enemy of a prospering Asia], *Shengjing shibao* [Shengjing times], 2 September 1941, 7.

34   Zhong, "Tan yin jiu," 5.

35   "Jiu lun," 3.

36   Ibid.

37   For example, see Lin Lu, "Yin jiu you yi tan" [Discussion of the benefits of drinking alcohol], *Shengjing shibao* [Shengjing times], 28 July 1936, 5.

38   "Jiu lun," 3.

39   Ao Shuang'an, "Mei jin jiu gan yan" [Moving words about American Prohibition], *Shengjing shibao* [Shengjing times], 10 March 1922, 1.

40   "Jiu jin kai hou, Mei jing qiguan" [After Prohibition ended, the American environment has strange vision], *Shengjing shibao* [Shengjing times], 18 April 1933, 3.

41   "Meiguo jiujin chong kai hou" [After American Prohibition began], *Shengjing shibao* [Shengjing times], 22 February 1933, 3.

42   Ao, "Mei jin jiu gan yan," 1.

43   Ibid.

44   Zhu Jiqing wrote of Americans finding "inspiration" in whiskey in a report on his visit to Montreal; see Zhu Jiqing, "Canjia Meiguo gonggong weisheng xuehui di'liushi ci nianhui gan yan" [Moving words on participating in the American Public Health Association's 60th Annual Meeting], *Dongfang yixue zazhi* [Far Eastern medical journal] 11, 1 (January 1933): 22. For a discussion of Tijuana, see "Qifo'a'nadunai: Jiu se zhi cheng" [Tijuana: Alcohol-coloured city], *Shengjing shibao* [Shengjing times], 15 May 1937, 6.

45   "Yan, jiu, cha, xiangliao gei ni de haochu?" [Smoke, alcohol, tea, and perfume give you a benefit?], *Shengjing shibao* [Shengjing times], 12 October 1940, 4.

46   "Jiu lun," 3.

47   Feng Sen, "Yin jiu mantan, san" [Informal discussion of drinking alcohol, three], *Shengjing shibao* [Shengjing times], 9 July 1937, 8.

48   Yi Xi, "Jiu de ziwei" [The taste of alcohol], *Shengjing shibao* [Shengjing times], 20 February 1933, 3.

49   Ibid.

50   Zhong, "Tan yin jiu," 5.

51   Hong, "Tan yin jiu," 4.

52   Ibid.

53   Ibid.

54   Ibid.

55   Jia Xiao, "Mantan yan jiu" [Informal discussion of opium and alcohol], *Qilin* [Unicorn], July 1942, 72.

56   Ibid.

57   Han Hu, "Yan jiu suo hua" [Trivial words about smoke and alcohol], *Qilin* [Unicorn], April 1943, 118-21.

58   Ibid.

59   Ōuchi Takao, "Shi jiu ji qi ta" [Poetry, alcohol, and the others], *Xin Manzhou* [New Manchuria], January 1943, 68.

60   Zhi Jing, "Tan yin jiu" [Discussion of drinking alcohol], *Shengjing shibao* [Shengjing times], 30 July 1937, 4.

61   Ibid.

62   Yang Xu, "Zui" [Intoxication], in *Luoying ji* [Collection of fallen petals] (Xinjing: Kaiming tushu gongsi, 1943), 124-25.

63   Nakamura Kōjirō, "Kessenka no sake to tabako" [Sake and tobacco under the condition of total war], *Manshū kōron* [Manchuria debate], March 1945, 58.

64   Naotaka Shinfuku, "Japanese Culture and Drinking," in Stanton Peele and Marcus Grant, eds., *Alcohol and Pleasure: A Health Perspective* (Philadelphia, PA: Taylor and Francis, 1999), 114.

65   Penelope Francks, "Inconspicuous Consumption: Sake, Beer, and the Birth of the Consumer in Japan," *Journal of Asian Studies* 68, 1 (2009): 135-64.

66   Ibid.

67   Ibid.

68   Nakamura, "Kessenka," 58.

69   Ibid.

70   Ibid.

71   Mei, "Jiu you hai?" 5.

72   Ren, "Jin jiu zhi yi," 11.

73   Ibid.

74   Feng, "Yin jiu mantan, one" 9.

75   "Jiu, yanjuan, cha neng qi xueyagao yu jingli: Shenghuo zhi guanxi" [Alcohol, rolled tobacco, and tea can raise high blood pressure and energy: The relationship with life], *Shengjing shibao* [Shengjing times], 31 January 1935, 5.

76   Xiao Ling, "Tan jiu yu tang" [Discussion of alcohol and sugar], *Qilin* [Unicorn], January 1942, 151.

77   "'Yi bei jiu jie qian chou,' danshi zheyang shihou, qing nin bu yao yin jiu" ['One cup of alcohol can relieve a thousand worries,' but in these times please do not drink alcohol], *Shengjing shibao* [Shengjing times], 18 July 1937, 4.

78   Pei Ru, "Weisheng: Wo zhi jin jiu dongji" [Hygiene: My motivation for quitting drinking], *Shengjing shibao* [Shengjing times], 6 February 1923, 5.

79   Xiao, "Tan jiu yu tang," 151.

80 "Jiu yu shensi" [Alcohol and development of the state of mind], *Shengjing shibao* [Shengjing times], 26 February 1941, 3.

81 For example, see "Yan, jiu, cha, xiangliao?" 4; and "Jiu yu shensi," 3.

82 "'Yi bei jiu jie qian chou,'" 5.

83 Yin, "Tan yin jiu," 4.

84 Shao, "Yan, jiu yu renti," 14.

85 Ibid., 15.

86 Ibid.

87 Ibid., 14.

88 Ibid., 14-15.

89 "'Yi bei jiu jie qian chou,'" 5.

90 "Hao jiu de ren wei?" 5.

91 Pei, "Weisheng," 8 February 1923, 5.

92 Pei, "Weisheng," 6 February 1923, 5.

93 "Funü yin jiu yingxiang ertong jiankang" [Women who drink alcohol influence children's health], *Shengjing shibao* [Shengjing times], 29 January 1942, 2.

94 Ibid.

95 Pei Ru, "Weisheng: Wo zhi jin jiu dongji" [Hygiene: My motivation for quitting drinking], *Shengjing shibao* [Shengjing times], 4 February 1923, 5.

96 "Funü yin jiu," 2.

97 Yao Jibin, "Weisheng: Jiu de duhai (xia)" [Hygiene: The poisonous harm of alcohol (second)], *Shengjing shibao* [Shengjing times], 15 March 1935, 9.

98 "Jiu yu yousheng zhi guanxi," 4.

99 Ibid.

100 Ye Xing, "Jiu yu nüren" [Wine and women], *Shengjing shibao* [Shengjing times], 30 November 1941, 7.

101 Ibid.

102 Ibid.

103 Yi Chi, "Guanyu wo de chuangzuo" [Concerning my creative work], in *Hua yue ji* [The flower moon collection] (Xinjing: Yishu yanjiu hui, 1938), reprinted in Zhang Yumao, ed., *Dongbei xiandai wenxue daxi, 1919-49: Sanwen juan* [Compendium of modern northeastern literature, 1919-49: Volume of prose], 14 vols. (Shenyang: Shenyang chubanshe, 1996), vol. 10, 730.

104 Mei, "Jiu you hai?" 5; Shao, "Yan, jiu yu renti," 15.

105 Qi Jinchang, "Jie yan jiu lun" [Discussion of quitting smoking and drinking], *Shengjing shibao* [Shengjing times], 31 January 1942, 2.

106 Pei, "Weisheng," 4 February 1923, 5.

107 Pei, "Weisheng," 8 February 1923, 5.

108 "Jiu zui shenye gui jia: Zhuchu fa qi you nu" [In the deep of the night, a drunk returns home and chases out his original wife and young daughter], *Shengjing shibao* [Shengjing times], 31 May 1937, 3.

109 "Thing in the cup" is an allusion to a Tao Yuanming poem. For other means of referring to alcohol, see "Jiu zhi bie ming kao" [Different names for alcohol test], *Shang gong yuekan* [Commerce and industry monthly] 7 (1942): 66.

110 For example, see the case of Zhang Haide, recounted in "Jiu hou wude, ou bi renming" [After drinking, no morality, beats and drives out person], *Shengjing shibao* [Shengjing times], 7 October 1936, 12.

111 Yao, "Weisheng," 9.

112 For example, see "Wuye gong yin jiuzui dongwu" [Drinking until midnight, start a fight], *Shengjing shibao* [Shengjing times], 10 January 1935, 4.

113 "Jiu yu fang die zhi guanxi" [Relationship between alcohol and guarding against espionage], *Jian'guo jiaoyu* [Building the country's education] 9, 11 (1943): 47.

114 For Bai's court case, see "Jiu hou wude hu qiangqiang hu: Bai Linfu chu tuxing shi nian" [After drinking, no morality rob by force: Bai Lingfu sentenced to prison for ten years], *Shengjing shibao* [Shengjing times], 12 November 1937, 2.

115 For example, see "Nü shifan chuangban yan jiu," 4.

116 "Nüren de nashou shiqing" [Women's expertise matters], *Qilin* [Unicorn], August 1941, 59.

117 "'Ci Liu Ling': Zui jiu shou fu chi yi nu jiu huazuo diaosigui" ['Female Liu Ling': Intoxicated and reprimanded by husband, suddenly angry and becomes a hung dead ghost], *Shengjing shibao* [Shengjing times], 27 February 1942, 4.

118 Wu Ying, "Jiu li chunhou" [Alcohol's strength is rich], *Qilin* [Unicorn], September 1942, 26.

119 Da Yong, "Shuang zhi yan" [A pair of swallows], *Qilin* [Unicorn], December 1941, 26.

120 "Jiu wei xing Ya zhi di," 7.

121 Ibid.

122 Ibid.

123 Nakamura, "Kessenka," 59.

124 Ibid., 60.

125 Ibid., 61.

126 Ibid.

127 For example, see "Jiu wei xing Ya zhi di," 7.

Chapter 4: Selling Alcohol, Selling Modernity

1 Karl Gerth, *China Made: Consumer Culture and the Creation of the Nation* (Cambridge, MA: Harvard University Press, 2003), 3.

2 Shao Guanzhi, "Yan jiu yu renti" [Tobacco, alcohol, and the human body], *Jiankang Manzhou* [Healthy Manchuria] 3.5 (1940): 14.

3 Jiao Runming, *Jindai Dongbei shehui zhu wenti yanjiu* [Research on various questions in modern Northeast society] (Beijing: Zhongguo shehui kexue chubanshe, 2004), 256.

4 For details, see Norman Smith, *Resisting Manchukuo: Chinese Women Writers and the Japanese Occupation* (Vancouver: UBC Press, 2007).

5 Prasenjit Duara, *Sovereignty and Authenticity: Manchukuo and the East Asian Modern* (New York: Rowman and Littlefield, 2003), 69.

6 Yang Xu, "Zui" [Intoxication], in *Luoying ji* [Collection of fallen petals] (Xinjing: Kaiming tushu gongsi, 1943), 124-25.

7 Yi Chi, "Guanyu wo de chuangzuo" [Concerning my creative work], in *Hua yue ji* [The flower moon collection] (Xinjing: Yishu yanjiu hui, 1938), reprinted in Zhang Yumao, ed., *Dongbei xiandai wenxue daxi, 1919-49: Sanwen juan* [Compendium of modern northeastern literature, 1919-49: Volume of prose], 14 vols. (Shenyang: Shenyang chubanshe, 1996), vol. 10, 730.

8 Jiao, *Jindai Dongbei shehui,* 257.

9 Ibid.

10 Ibid., 258.

11 Kawabe Taichi, "Kunao zhi weichang shuairuo" [The distress of gastrointestinal weakness], Yangming jiu [Life Support Wine] ad, *Shengjing shibao* [Shengjing times], 4 October 1935, 3.

12 See Hei'ermisi [Hermes] ads, *Shengjing shibao* [Shengjing times], 18 May 1918, 8, and 25 June 1919, 6.

13 Ouzika gaoliang jiu er'shi wu hao de jiu [Vodka Gaoliang Alcohol, Brand No. 25] ad, *Shengjing shibao* [Shengjing times], 12 February 1935, 3.

14 Xian you [Virtuous Friend] and Ju quan [Chrysanthemum Spring] ad, *Shengjing shibao* [Shengjing times], 20 June 1934, 8.
15 Ibid., 24 July 1934, 3.
16 Bao jing [Precious Mirror] ad, *Shengjing shibao* [Shengjing times], 13 November 1937, 11. For discussion of Republican China, see Gerth, *China Made*.
17 For example, see Hugu huashe yaojiu [Tiger Bone, Flower Snake Medicinal Wine] ad, *Shengjing shibao* [Shengjing times], 6 October 1937, 6; Shenxiao hugu yaojiu [Magic Tiger Bone Medicinal Wine] ad, *Shengjing shibao* [Shengjing times], 19 October 1911, 6; and Shen rong hugu yanshou jiu [Ginseng, Antler, Tiger Bone Prolong Life Wine] ad, *Shengjing shibao* [Shengjing times], 21 July 1938, 3.
18 Wanling fenghan hugu jiu [Cold Souls Tiger Bone Wine] ad, *Shengjing shibao* [Shengjing times], 8 December 1922, 8.
19 For details on Dai-Nippon's history, see http://www.asahibeer.co.uk/.
20 Asahi [Chinese: Xu; English: Brilliance of the Rising Sun] and Sapporo [Zha huang] ad, *Shengjing shibao* [Shengjing times], 15 February 1907, 1.
21 Asahi [Chinese: Xu; English: Brilliance of the Rising Sun] ad, *Shengjing shibao* [Shengjing times], 11 June 1909, 1.
22 Asahi [Chinese: Xu; English: Brilliance of the Rising Sun] and Sapporo [Zha huang] ad, *Shengjing shibao* [Shengjing times], 23 April 1908, 6.
23 For Riguang [Sunlight], see Asahi [Chinese: Riguang; English: Sunlight] ad, *Shengjing shibao* [Shengjing times], 19 June 1912, 8; and for Taiyang [Sun], see Asahi [Chinese: Taiyang; English: Sun] ad, *Shengjing shibao* [Shengjing times], 1 June 1915, 4.
24 Asahi [Chinese: Riguang; English: Sunlight] ad, *Shengjing shibao* [Shengjing times], 19 June 1912, 8.
25 Asahi [Chinese: Xu; English: Brilliance of the Rising Sun] ad, *Shengjing shibao* [Shengjing times], 11 June 1909, 1.
26 Asahi [Chinese: Taiyang; English: Sun], Fu shen [Good Fortune Spirit], and Sapporo [Zha huang] ad, *Shengjing shibao* [Shengjing times], 6 June 1920, 8.
27 Sapporo and Asahi ad, *Manchuria*, 1 November 1937, 759.
28 Da yang [Big Sun] ad, *Shengjing shibao* [Shengjing times], 18 May 1925, 8.
29 Hong xing [Red Star] ad, *Shengjing shibao* [Shengjing times], 18 July 1937, 8.
30 Kirin [Unicorn] ad, *Shengjing shibao* [Shengjing times], 20 June 1934, 3.
31 Ibid., 11 May 1911, supplement.
32 Ibid., 6 May 1937, 6.
33 Ibid., 10 July 1933, supplement.
34 Sakura [Cherry] ad, *Shengjing shibao* [Shengjing times], 2 September 1915, 4.
35 Manshū [Manchuria] ad, *Shengjing shibao* [Shengjing times], 26 June 1920, 8; Sakura [Cherry] ad, *Shengjing shibao* [Shengjing times], 16 June 1936, supplement.
36 You'ni'en [Union] ad, *Shengjing shibao* [Shengjing times], 17 July 1921, 3; Hei (Black) ad, *Shengjing shibao* [Shengjing times], 17 July 1921, 3.
37 Ibid., 16 May 1926, 8.
38 "The Brewing Industry in Manchoukuo," *Contemporary Manchuria* 3.4 (1939): 66.
39 For information on the origins of Akadama wine, and Japanese grape wine more generally, see Chris Bunting, *Drinking Japan: A Guide to Japan's Best Drinks and Drinking Establishments* (North Clarendon, VT: Tuttle Publishing, 2011), 196-99.
40 For details, see http://www.ibo.or.jp/. Information on the origins of whisky in Japan can be found in Chris Bunting, *Drinking Japan: A Guide to Japan's Best Drinks and Drinking Establishments* (North Clarendon, VT: Tuttle Publishing, 2011), 162-67.
41 Jiao, *Jindai Dongbei shehui*, 225.
42 "Putaojiu yu putaojiu zhi shuo" [Grape wine and talk of grape wine], *Shengjing shibao* [Shengjing times], 30 April 1939, supplement.

43 Shi Zhizi, "Ou'gan ou'ji bingyu tan" [A discussion of occassional feelings, occassional memories], *Xin qingnian* [New youth] (October 1937), reprinted in Qian Liqun, ed., *Zhongguo lunxianqu wenxue daxi: Pinglun juan* [Compendium of the literature of China's enemy-occupied territories: Volume of commentary] (Nanling, Guangxi: Guangxi jiaoyu chubanshe, 2000), 390.

44 Chi yu [Red Ball] ad, *Shengjing shibao* [Shengjing times], 16 November 1917, 8.

45 Ibid.

46 "Pang!" [Fat!], *Shengjing shibao* [Shengjing times], 22 April 1938, 3.

47 "Putaojiu yu putaojiu zhi shuo," supplement.

48 "Pang!" 3.

49 Chi yu [Red Ball] ad, *Datong bao* [Great unity herald], 3 March 1939, 7.

50 For example, the ads use representations of arms or torsos instead of entire bodies. Sherman Cochran analyzes changing advertising practices in *Chinese Medicine Men: Consumer Culture in China and Southeast Asia* (Cambridge, MA: Harvard University Press, 2006).

51 Chi yu [Red Ball] ad, *Shengjing shibao* [Shengjing times], 10 September 1921, 3.

52 Chi yu [Red Ball] ad, *Datong bao* [Great unity herald], 26 March 1939, 4.

53 Chi yu [Red Ball] ad, *Shengjing shibao* [Shengjing times], 27 August 1919, 8.

54 "Jingli de yuanquan" [Source of energy], *Datong bao* [Great unity herald], 3 November 1941, 4.

55 Gui pai haomeng putaojiu [Essence of Turtle] ad, *Jiankang Manzhou* [Healthy Manchuria] 1, 4 (1939): back outside cover.

56 "Fasheng xing Ya zhi zhuangli" [Strong prosperous Asia], *Jiankang Manzhou* [Healthy Manchuria] 2, 2 (1940): back outside cover.

57 Yangming jiu [Life Support Wine] ad, *Shengjing shibao* [Shengjing times], 19 December 1935, 13.

58 Yangming jiu [Life Support Wine] ad, *Qilin* [Unicorn], August 1943, 4.

59 Yangming jiu [Life Support Wine] ad, *Shengjing shibao* [Shengjing times], 20 June 1937, 12.

60 Ibid., 4 October 1935, 3.

61 Yangming jiu [Life Support Wine] ad, *Qilin* [Unicorn], August 1943, 4.

62 Yangming jiu [Life Support Wine] ad, *Shengjing shibao* [Shengjing times], 20 June 1937, 12.

63 Ye Fengsheng, Yangming jiu [Life Support Wine] ad, *Shengjing shibao* [Shengjing times], 19 February 1941, 5.

64 Kin Mitsunari, Yangming jiu [Life Support Wine] ad, *Qilin* [Unicorn], September 1941, 4.

65 Fujī Kyūta, Yangming jiu [Life Support Wine] ad, *Qilin* [Unicorn], April 1942, 4.

66 Imamura Masu, Yangming jiu [Life Support Wine] ad, *Qilin* [Unicorn], October 1942, 4.

67 Miura Keiko, Yangming jiu [Life Support Wine] ad, *Qilin* [Unicorn], January 1943, 8.

68 Ibid.

69 Higashimoto Hide, Yangming jiu [Life Support Wine] ad, *Qilin* [Unicorn], December 1942, 4.

70 Jiao, *Jindai Dongbei shehui*, 225.

71 "Pohuai jiankang de si da dusu: Bianbidu, jiehedu, jiudu, yandu" [The four big poisons that destroy health: Constipation, tuberculosis, alcohol, and smoking], *Jiankang Manzhou* [Healthy Manchuria] 2, 5 (1940): 36.

72 Ibid.

73 Ibid.

74 Ibid.

75 Ruosu [Basic Element] ad, *Shengjing shibao* [Shengjing times], 28 June 1940, 5.

76 Ibid.

77 Ibid.

78 http://www.tsingtao.com.cn/.

79 http://en.radio86.com/.

80 Karl Gerth, *As China Goes, So Goes the World: How Chinese Consumers are Transforming Everything* (New York: Hill and Wang, 2010), 129.
81 http://english.caijing.com.cn/.

Chapter 5: Writing Intoxicant Consumption

Epigraph: San Lang, "Zhuxin" [Candlewick], in San Lang and Qiao Yin, *Bashe* [Trek] (Harbin: Wuri huakan yinshuashe, 1933), reprinted in Liang Shanding, ed., *Zhuxin ji* [Candlewick collection] (Shenyang: Chunfeng wenyi chubanshe, 1989), 18. San Lang and Qiao Yin are names used by Xiao Jun and Xiao Hong, respectively.

1   For a more detailed analysis of Manchukuo's literary world, see Norman Smith, *Resisting Manchukuo: Chinese Women Writers and the Japanese Occupation* (Vancouver: UBC Press, 2007), 41-60.
2   Ke Chang, "Zhou Zuoren Xiansheng yulu" [Quotations of Mr. Zhou Zuoren], *Qilin* [Unicorn], March 1943, 84-85.
3   Prasenjit Duara, *Sovereignty and Authenticity: Manchukuo and the East Asian Modern* (Oxford: Rowman and Littlefield, 2003), 145.
4   Jie Xueshi, "Ri Wei shiqi de wenhua tongzhi zhengce" [State policies of cultural domination during the Japanese occupation], in Feng Weiqun, Wang Jianzhong, Li Chunyan, and Li Shuquan, eds., *Dongbei lunxian shiqi wenxue guoji xueshu yantaohui lunwenji* [Collection of papers from the International Symposium on Literature of the Enemy-Occupied Northeast] (Shenyang: Shenyang chubanshe, 1992), 190-91.
5   San, "Zhuxin," 17.
6   Bai Lang was born Liu Donglan. Her pen names also included Yi Bai and Liu Li. She left Manchukuo for Shanghai in 1935. See Bai Lang, "Panni de erzi" [Rebellious son], in Liang Shanding, ed., *Changye yinghuo* [Fireflies of the long night] (Shenyang: Chunfeng wenyi chubanshe, 1986), 37-50.
7   Ibid., 41.
8   Ibid., 43.
9   Ibid., 46-47.
10 Shinichi Yamaguchi, "Contemporary Literature in Manchuria," in Manchuria Daily News, ed., *Concordia and Culture in Manchoukuo* (Xinjing: Manchuria Daily News, 1938), 27.
11 "Patient" is a compound of two characters, *qiu* (to seek) and *zhen* (needle). The couple, however, is not seeking a needle but rather drugs that they can more easily share. See Mei Niang, "Zuihou de qiuzhenzhe" [The last patient], in *Di'er dai* [The second generation] (Xinjing: Wencong han xinghui, 1940), 87-92.
12 Ibid., 88.
13 Ibid., 89.
14 Ibid.
15 Elder Brother aspires to buy thirty to forty ounces of opium at a time. See Mei Niang, "Bang" [Clam], in *Yu* [Fish] (Beijing: Xinmin yinshuguan, 1943), reprinted in Liang Shanding, ed., *Changye yinghuo* [Fireflies of the long night] (Shenyang: Chunfeng wenyi chubanshe, 1986), 165.
16 Ibid.
17 Ibid., 166.
18 Wu Ying, "Gui" [Deceit], in *Liang ji* [Two extremes] (Xinjing: Wenyi conghan hanxinghui, 1939), 93-105.
19 Ibid., 94.
20 See Smith, *Resisting Manchukuo*, 82-83.
21 Li Qiao is considered Manchukuo's foremost Chinese playwright. See Li Qiao, *Xue ren tu* [Bloody sword scheme], *Wensuan* [Literary collective] 2 (1940), reprinted in Zhang Yumao,

ed., *Dongbei xiandai wenxue daxi, 1919-1949: Xiju juan* [Compendium of modern north-eastern literature, 1919-49: Volume of plays], 14 vols. (Shenyang: Shenyang chubanshe, 1996), vol. 13, 237-80.

22 Ibid., 242.

23 Ibid., 252-53.

24 Ibid., 256.

25 Ibid., 241.

26 Ibid., 247.

27 Ibid., 246.

28 Ibid., 242.

29 Ibid., 277.

30 Wu Lang, "Women de wenxue de shiti yu fangxiang" [The substance and direction of our literature], *Daban Huawen meiri* [Chinese Osaka daily], 15 January 1941, reprinted in Qian Liqun, ed., *Zhongguo Zhongguo lunxianqu wenxue daxi: Pinglun juan* [Compendium of the literature of China's enemy-occupied territories: Volume of commentary] (Nanling, Guangxi: Guangxi jiaoyu chubanshe, 2000), 395.

31 The Eight Abstentions can be found in Yu Lei, "Ziliao" [Data], *Dongbei wenxue yanjiu shiliao* [Historical research materials of northeastern literature] 6 (1987): 181.

32 For the Arts Guidelines, see ibid., 174-78.

33 Xu Naixiang and Huang Wanhua, *Zhongguo kangzhan shiqi lunxianqu wenxue shi* [History of the literature of the enemy-occupied territories during China's war of resistance] (Fuzhou: Fujian jiaoyu chubanshe, 1995), 267.

34 Ibid., 269.

35 Ibid., 266.

36 This novel was originally published under the pen name Qiu Ying. See Qiu Ying, *He liu de diceng* [The bottom of the river] (Dalian: Shiye yanghang chubanbu faxing, 1941), reprinted under name of Wang Qiuying, in Kong Fanjin, ed., *Zhongguo xiandai wenxue buyi shuxi* [Addendum of modern Chinese literature series], 8 vols. (Jinan: Mingtian chubanshe, 1990), vol. 5, 720-849.

37 Ibid., 834.

38 Ibid., 742.

39 Ibid., 721.

40 Ibid., 811.

41 Ibid., 805.

42 This novel was published under the pen name of Ke Ju, one of over fifty pen names for author and calligrapher Li Zhengzhong, who is now one of the most renowned calligraphers in the Northeast. See Ke Ju, *Xiang huai* [Homesickness] (Xinjing: Zongdai shusuo, 1941), 3-4.

43 Ibid., 4.

44 Ibid., 23.

45 Ibid., 19.

46 Ibid., 27.

47 Ibid., 20.

48 Ibid., 42.

49 Ibid., 61.

50 Ibid., 61.

51 Ibid., 72.

52 Ibid., 74.

53 Ibid., 5.

54 Ibid., 7.

55 Blaine Chiasson discusses sympathetic portraits of Russians in the local Chinese press. See Blaine R. Chiasson, *Administering the Colonizer: Manchuria's Russians under Chinese Rule, 1918-29* (Vancouver: UBC Press, 2010), 96.
56 Fan Ying, "Beidi lian'ge" [Northern love story], *Qilin* [Unicorn], October 1941, 82-87.
57 Ibid., 83.
58 Ibid., 85.
59 Ibid., 83.
60 Ibid.
61 Zhi Yuan is a pen name of Zhi Zhenyuan, who was born in Hebei. He worked at Chengde's post office until 1939, when he was transferred to manage Harbin's post office. There, he began his writing career. From 1940 to 1941, he edited the literary section in the *Binjiang ribao* [Binjiang daily]. Avoiding arrest by the Manchukuo authorities, he fled back to his hometown. In the spring of 1945, he returned to Harbin and was arrested.
62 Zhi Yuan, "Bai tenghua" [White vine flower], *Huawen Daban meiri* [Chinese Osaka daily], 1943, reprinted in Liang Shanding, ed., *Zhuxin ji* [Candlewick collection] (Shenyang: Chunfeng wenyi chubanshe, 1989), 349-62.
63 Ibid., 351.
64 Ibid., 356
65 Ibid., 350
66 Ibid., 351.
67 Baudelaire (1821-67) was a French poet. See ibid., 353.
68 Ibid., 355.
69 Ibid., 359.
70 Ibid.
71 Ibid.
72 Ibid., 360.
73 Zhu Ti, "Yuantian de liuxing" [A shooting star in a faraway sky], *Xin chao* [New tide] 1, 7 (1943), reprinted in *Ying* [Cherry] (Xinjing: Guomin tushu zhushi huishe, 1945), 82-98.
74 Ibid., 92.
75 Ibid., 94.
76 Zuo Di wrote the novella in 1943, and it was published two years later. Zuo Di, *Meiyou guang de xing* [A lustreless star], *Chuangzuo liancong* [Creative collection], February 1945, reprinted in Liang Shanding, ed., *Changye yinghuo* [Fireflies of the long night] (Shenyang: Chunfeng wenyi chubanshe, 1986), 446.
77 Ibid., 442.
78 Ibid., 445.
79 Ibid., 442.
80 Ibid., 452.
81 Ibid.
82 Lan Ling, "Guxiang de jia" [Native place home], *Daban Huawen meiri* [Chinese Osaka daily], 10.1, 1943, 34-38.
83 Ibid., 36.
84 Ibid., 37.
85 Ibid., 35.
86 Xu and Huang, *Zhongguo,* 267.
87 Gu Ding, "Ji mie" [Attack, extinguish], *Qilin* [Unicorn], September 1944, 21.
88 Xiao Song, "Yiwenjia gankuai wuzhuang qilai" [Writers and artists militarize quickly], *Qilin* [Unicorn], November 1944, 48.
89 Mark Driscoll describes a 1944 campaign designed by Furumi Tadayuki that required 2 million addicts to report to detox clinics, from which registrants were reputedly shuttled

out the back doors to labour camps. See Mark Driscoll, *Absolute Erotic, Absolute Grotesque* (Durham, NC: Duke University Press, 2010), 231.

90 Shu Shi, "Zui" [Intoxication], *Qingnian wenhua* [Youth culture] 2, 6 (1944): 42-43.

91 Ibid., 42.

92 Ibid.

93 Ibid.

94 Ibid.

95 Ibid.

96 Yang Xu, "Laomazi riji" [Nanny's diary], in *Wo de riji* [My diary] (Xinjing: Kaiming tushu gongsi, 1944), 37.

97 Ibid., 36.

98 Ibid., 40.

99 Ibid., 43.

100 Jin Yin, "Muchang shang de xueyuan" [Blood ties on the pasture], in Jin Yin, ed., *Manzhou zuojia xiaoshuoji* [Collected novels of Manchukuo writers] (Xinjing: Wuxing shulin, 1944), reprinted in Liang Shanding, ed., *Zhuxin ji* [Candlewick collection] (Shenyang: Chunfeng wenyi chubanshe, 1989), 307.

101 Ibid., 321.

102 Ibid., 331.

103 Qiu Ying, "Lou xiang" [Vulgar alley], *Chuangzuo liancong* [Creative crowd] 2 (1944), reprinted in Liang Shanding, ed., *Zhuxin ji* [Candlewick collection] (Shenyang: Chunfeng wenyi chubanshe, 1989), 111.

104 Ibid., 116.

105 Ibid., 119.

106 Ibid., 112.

107 Ibid., 131.

108 Ibid., 127.

109 Ibid., 120.

110 Ibid., 141.

111 Zhang Chunyuan, *Hen zhong hua* [Flowers among the hate] (Fengtian: Guandong shuju chubanshe, 1944), 63.

112 Ibid., 102-3.

113 Ibid., 94.

114 Ibid., 166.

115 Mei Niang, "Wo de qingshao nian shiqi: 1920-1938" [My childhood, 1920-1938], in Zhang Quan, ed., *Xunzhao Mei Niang* [Searching for Mei Niang] (Beijing: Mingjing chubanshe, 1998), 127.

Chapter 6: The Hostess Scare

1 Zheng Tiantian, *Red Lights: The Lives of Sex Workers in Post-Socialist China* (Minneapolis: University of Minnesota Press, 2009), 22.

2 Ibid., 20.

3 The term *lingmaisuo* is translated as opium "retail outlet" to differentiate it as a licensed business from the less official "opium shop" *[yan guan]* and from the more prejudicial English term "opium den."

4 K.C. Chang, *Food in Chinese Culture: Anthropological and Historical Perspectives* (New Haven, CT: Yale University Press, 1977), 137.

5 A writer using the pseudonym "Beiping city hostess" argued that hostess work was the lowest type of profession but a profession nonetheless. See Ping shi yi zhaodai, "Women de jianglai" [Our future], in Yu Zhizhu, ed., *Nü zhaodai quan ji* [Hostess complete collection] (Tianjin: Lanhua guanggao she, 1933), 49.

6 For example, see "Nü zhaodai ai yun: Bu jing yan guan zhi fan guan, yi jiang shou chedi qudi" [Hostesses have bad luck: Not only banned in opium dens but immediately in restaurants, also will eventually be completely banned], *Shengjing shibao* [Shengjing times], 13 January 1934, 4. It should be noted that *yao*, the first of the two characters in *yaoyan*, has meanings beyond "coquettish," including "goblin," "demon," and "evil and fraudulent"; see *Han-Ying cidian* [Chinese-English dictionary] (Beijing: Shangwu yingshuguan, 1999), 802.

7 You You, "Mingri huang hua" [Tomorrow's yellow flower], in Yu Zhizhu, ed., *Nü zhaodai quan ji* [Hostess complete collection] (Tianjin: Lanhua guanggao she, 1933), 5.

8 Blaine Chiasson notes the "fluid situation," in terms of ethnicity, and "the very newness of Harbin." See Blaine R. Chiasson, *Administering the Colonizer: Manchuria's Russians under Chinese Rule, 1918-29* (Vancouver: UBC Press, 2010), 155.

9 Diana Lary and Thomas R. Gottschwang, *Swallows and Settlers: The Great Migration from North China to Manchuria* (Ann Arbor: University of Michigan Press, 2000), 77. Zheng cites the statistic of 194 men per 100 women in 1948 Dalian, then the greatest disparity in China; see Zheng, *Red Lights*, 40.

10 See Norman Smith, *Resisting Manchukuo: Chinese Women Writers and the Japanese Occupation* (Vancouver: UBC Press, 2007), 61-84.

11 See Shen Kechang, "Nü zhaodai riji" [Hostess diary], in Yu Zhizhu, ed., *Nü zhaodai quan ji* [Hostess complete collection] (Tianjin: Lanhua guanggao she, 1933), 20.

12 Prasenjit Duara, *Sovereignty and Authenticity: Manchukuo and the East Asian Modern* (Oxford: Rowman and Littlefield, 2003), 140-41.

13 For details, see Norman Smith, "Disguising Resistance in Manchukuo: Feminism as Anti-Colonialism in the Collected Works of Zhu Ti," *International History Review* 28, 3 (2006): 515-36.

14 The writer Dan Di wrote about her experiences with advanced education in Japan. See Norman Smith, "The Difficulties of Despair: Dan Di and Chinese Cultural Production in Manchukuo," *Journal of Women's History* 18, 1 (2006): 71-100.

15 For an insightful analysis of hostesses in Canton in the 1930s, see Xavier Paulès, "Drogue et transgressions sociales: Les femmes et l'opium à Canton dans les années 1930," *Clio: Histoire, femmes et sociétés* 28 (2008): 223-42. Paulès's thesis is that the hostesses, called "smoke flowers" *[yanhua]*, caused more critical reflection than women who smoked opium given their potential for social disruption, namely the downfall of rich patrons and their own rise. As in Manchukuo, they were also blamed for disrupting family relations and not fulfilling "proper" women's roles; see ibid., 223-24.

16 *Manchoukuo: A Pictorial Record* (Tokyo and Osaka: Asahi Shimbun, 1934), 74.

17 "Sikai yan guan qiangjian yanke: Shaonü zao roulin" [The rape of a guest in a private opium den: A young girl meets with devastation], *Shengjing shibao* [Shengjing times], 18 August 1935, 2.

18 Tani Barlow, "Theorizing Woman: *Funü, Guojia, Jiating*," *Genders* 10 (1991): 132-60.

19 *Han-Ying cidian*, 879.

20 Ibid., 131.

21 Lü Yonghua, *Wei Man shiqi de dongbei yandu* [Opium poison in the Northeast during the bogus Manchukuo era] (Changchun: Jilin renmin chubanshe, 2004), 85.

22 See Hua Jiangrong, "Yan lou suohua: Ge lingmaisuo nü zhaodai sumiao, di'liu" [Trivial talk about opium dens: Sketches of opium retail outlet hostesses, part six], *Shengjing shibao* [Shengjing times], 7 May 1936, 7.

23 "Yan guan nü zhaodai shangfeng baisu: Wushun dangju yinhe bu gan?" [Opium den hostesses corrupt public morals: Wushun authorities – Why can't they ban them?], *Shengjing shibao* [Shengjing times], 3 August 1935, 11.

24 For example, see Hua Jiangrong, "Yan lou suohua: Ge lingmaisuo nü zhaodai sumiao, di'er" [Trivial talk about opium dens: Sketches of opium retail outlet hostesses, part two], *Shengjing shibao* [Shengjing times], 10 April 1936, 7.

25 Vespa Amleto, *Secret Agent of Japan: A Handbook to Japanese Imperialism* (London: Victor Gollancz, 1938), 101.

26 This report notes that only forty-nine hostesses showed up for exams and that trachoma – not venereal diseases or opium addiction – was the most common ailment they suffered. See "Shenyang jingcha ting Kangde san nian weisheng nianjian, qi'er" [Shenyang police office 1936 hygiene yearbook, part two], *Dongfang yixue zazhi* [Far Eastern medical journal] 15, 3 (1937): 199, 202.

27 Hua, "Yan lou suohua: di'er," 7.

28 "Lingmaisuo nü zhaodai: Ji qin, ji zong – shi wei quidi!" [Opium retail outlet hostesses: Several times captured, several times set free – The so-called ban!], *Shengjing shibao* [Shengjing times], 6 March 1935, 7. Ling Hua argued that hostesses worked like magnets and attracted everything; see Ling Hua, "Wei *Nü zhaodai quan ji* zuo xu" [Preface to *Hostess Complete Collection*], in Yu Zhizhu, ed., *Nü zhaodai quan ji* [Hostess complete collection] (Tianjin: Lanhua guanggao she, 1933), 3.

29 Hua, "Yan lou suohu: di'er," 7.

30 For a recent account, see Lü, *Wei Man shiqi*, 95.

31 Zheng, *Red Lights*, 40.

32 Ruo Xue, "Xie zai *Nü zhaodai quanji* zhi qian" [Writing preceding the *Hostess Complete Collection*], in Yu Zhizhu, ed., *Nü zhaodai quan ji* [Hostess complete collection] (Tianjin: Lanhua guanggao she, 1933), 1.

33 Zheng Zhi, "Nü zhaodai de shouce" [A hostess handbook], *Shengjing shibao* [Shengjing times], 21 January 1936, 5.

34 Ibid.

35 Ibid.

36 Hua Jiangrong, "Yan lou suohua: Ge lingmaisuo nü zhaodai sumiao, di'qi" [Trivial talk about opium dens: Sketches of opium retail outlet hostesses, part seven], *Shengjing shibao* [Shengjing times], 14 May 1936, 7.

37 Karl Gerth argues that in the early 1930s "women became models of how not to consume." See Karl Gerth, *China Made: Consumer Culture and the Creation of the Nation* (Cambridge, MA: Harvard University Press, 2003), 286, 300.

38 Some 700 of Harbin's hostesses lived in hotels. See Hua Jiangrong, "Yan lou suohua: Ge lingmaisuo nü zhaodai sumiao, di'san" [Trivial talk about opium dens: Sketches of opium retail outlet hostesses, part three], *Shengjing shibao* [Shengjing times], 17 April 1936, 7.

39 Hua Jiangrong, "Yan lou suohua: Ge lingmaisuo nü zhaodai sumiao, di'si" [Trivial talk about opium dens: Sketches of opium retail outlet hostesses, part four], *Shengjing shibao* [Shengjing times], 23 April 1936, 7.

40 Hua, "Yan lou suohu: di'er" 7.

41 Ibid.

42 Hua Jiangrong, "Yan lou suohua: Ge lingmaisuo nü zhaodai sumiao, di'wu" [Trivial talk about opium dens: Sketches of opium retail outlet hostesses, part five], *Shengjing shibao* [Shengjing times], 29 April 1936, 7.

43 "Lingmaisuo quxiao nü zhaodai" [Opium retail outlets abolish hostesses], *Shengjing shibao* [Shengjing times], 30 December 1933, 4.

44 Jun Jun, "Xuediao huaping de chiyu ba" [Wipe out the shame of vases], *Qilin* [Unicorn], March 1942, 137.

45 Hua, "Yan lou suohua: di'san," 7.

46 Ibid.

47   Hua, "Yan lou suohua: di'si," 7.

48   Hua, "Yan lou suohua: di'san," 7.

49   Hua Jiangrong, "Yan lou suohua: Ge lingmaisuo nü zhaodai sumiao, di'shi" [Trivial talk about opium dens: Sketches of opium retail outlet hostesses, part ten], *Shengjing shibao* [Shengjing times], 4 June 1936, 7.

50   Hua Jiangrong, "Yan lou suohua: Ge lingmaisuo nü zhaodai sumiao, di'jiu" [Trivial talk about opium dens: Sketches of opium retail outlet hostesses, part nine], *Shengjing shibao* [Shengjing times], 28 May 1936, 7.

51   For one account, see Lü, *Wei Man shiqi*, 94.

52   Fu Chen argued that hostesses were wicked and that they "intoxicated" *(mizui)* the men under their spell while making those who witnessed the scene feel sick. See Fu Chen, "You yuan guilai" [Return from touring the garden], in Yu Zhizhu, ed., *Nü zhaodai quan ji* [Hostess complete collection] (Tianjin: Lanhua guanggao she, 1933), 33.

53   Hua, "Yan lou suohu: di'er," 7.

54   Fu, "You yuan guilai," 33.

55   "Nü zhaodai jian ying fu ye, yin chu cha jin" [Hostesses holding jobs as a side business, should be quickly investigated and forbidden], *Shengjing shibao* [Shengjing times], 14 July 1935, 11.

56   Lian Zhi's popularity is suggested by the inclusion in the article of a photograph of her. See Hua, "Yan lou suohua: di'wu," 7.

57   Hua, "Yan lou suohua: di'liu," 7.

58   Hua, "Yan lou suohua: di'qi," 7.

59   For example, see Wei Zhonglan, "Xin Zhongguo nüxing do dongjing" [Sounds of the new Chinese women's movement], *Qingnian wenhua* [Youth culture] 1, 3 (1943): 35.

60   Hua, "Yan lou suohua: di'er," 7.

61   "Yapian xiao maisuo jie genü zhao ji ke" [Small opium retail outlets use singing girls to attract guests], *Shengjing shibao* [Shengjing times], 5 June 1931, 5.

62   "Xu Biyun deng qiman li lian, nü zhaodaimen ye jiang ying zhi, dasa fengjing de liang chun shi" [Xu Biyun, awaiting the time contracted to depart Dalian: Hostesses will soon be disappearing: Big murder scenery, two events], *Shengjing shibao* [Shengjing times], 13 April 1936, 3.

63   "Nü zhaodai ai yun," 4.

64   "Qudi yapian lingmaisuo: Nü zhaodai zhi wengao" [Banned in the opium retail outlets: Proclamation of the hostesses], *Shengjing shibao* [Shengjing times], 27 February 1934, 3.

65   "Nü zhaodai ai yun," 4.

66   "Xu Biyun deng qiman li lian," 3.

67   Ibid.

68   Hua Jiangrong, "Yan lou suohua: Ge lingmaisuo nü zhaodai sumiao, di'shiyi" [Trivial talk about opium dens: Sketches of opium retail outlet hostesses, part eleven], *Shengjing shibao* [Shengjing times], 10 June 1936, 7.

69   "Shenyang jingcha ting Kangde yuan nian weisheng nianjian" [Shenyang police office 1934 hygiene yearbook], *Dongfang yixue zazhi* [Far Eastern medical journal] 13, 6 (1935): 250.

70   Hua, "Yan lou suohua: di'wu," 7.

71   "Lingmaisuo nü zhaodai," 7.

72   Hua, "Yan lou suohua: di'wu," 7.

73   *Manchoukuo: A Pictorial Record,* 280.

74   Hua, "Yan lou suohua: di'san," 7.

75   "Nü zhaodai shi ye hou, ji han jiaobo, shang yi er ci huyu" [After hostesses lose their profession, hunger and cold together compel them to yet propose a second appeal], *Shengjing shibao* [Shengjing times], 7 December 1933, 4.

76 "Nü zhaodai quxiao hou, yan guan za shou daji: Dong Guxuan lingxian chengqing zhong" [After hostesses were banned, opium dens were struck down: Dong Guxuan took a leading role in applying to the authorities for approval], *Shengjing shibao* [Shengjing times], 10 December 1933, 4.

77 "Lingmaisuo qing huifu nü zhaodai you bei bo" [Opium retail outlets' pleas to resume hostesses were refuted], *Shengjing shibao* [Shengjing times], 20 November 1935, 4.

78 "Nü zhaodai kai hui fandui na juan" [Hostesses hold a meeting to oppose paying contributions], *Shengjing shibao* [Shengjing times], 27 December 1935, 12.

79 For further details on Mei Niang, see Norman Smith, "'Only Women Can Change This World into Heaven': Mei Niang, Male Chauvinist Society, and the Japanese Cultural Agenda in North China, 1939-1941," *Modern Asian Studies* 40, 1 (2006): 81-107.

80 Mei Niang, "Zhui" [The chase], in *Di'er dai* [The second generation] (Xinjing: Wencong han xinghui, 1940), 129-44.

81 Ibid., 136.

82 Ibid., 135.

83 Ibid., 136.

84 Ibid.

85 Ibid., 144.

86 This story was written in 1939 and published in 1944. See Ye Li, "San ren" [Three people], in *Hua zhong* [Flower tomb] (Xinjing: Zhushi huishe dadi tushu gongsi, 1944), reprinted in Liang Shanding, ed., *Zhuxin ji* [Candlewick collection] (Shenyang: Chunfeng wenyi chubanshe, 1989), 254-68.

87 Ibid., 261.

88 Ibid., 264.

89 Ibid., 261.

90 Ibid., 263.

91 Wei Cheng, "Kuilan de du shi" [The festering, poisoned tongue], *Qilin* [Unicorn], July 1942, 142-49.

92 Ibid., 143.

93 Ibid., 146.

94 Ibid., 148.

95 Zhizhu, "Xie zai qian ye" [Writing on the front page], in Yu Zhizhu, ed., *Nü zhaodai quan ji* [Hostess complete collection] (Tianjin: Lanhua guanggao she, 1933), 4.

96 You You, "Mingri huang hua" [Tomorrow's yellow flower], in Yu Zhizhu, ed., *Nü zhaodai quan ji* [Hostess complete collection] (Tianjin: Lanhua guanggao she, 1933), 6.

97 Zheng, *Red Lights*, 5.

Chapter 7: Reasoning Addiction, Taking the Cures

Epigraph: "Jie yan geyao" [Quit smoking ballad], *Shengjing shibao* [Shengjing times], 17 November 1938, 4.

1 Alan Baumler, *The Chinese and Opium under the Republic: Worse than Floods and Wild Beasts* (Albany: State University of New York Press, 2007).

2 For example, see "Fengtian jieyansuo fangwen ji" [Notes on an interview at the Fengtian Quit Smoking Centre], *Xin qingnian* [New youth] 8, 5 (1939): 10.

3 Wang Luo, "Manzhouguo zhi yapian zhidu, di'er pian" [The Manchukuo opium system, part two], *Dongfang yixue zazhi* [Far Eastern medical journal] 12, 12 (1934): 483.

4 On the difficulties of achieving a ban, see "Yinzhe fuyin" [Glad tidings for addicts], *Shengjing shibao* [Shengjing times], 24 May 1940, 4. On the need to eradicate, see Wang Shigong, "Manzhouguo yapian wenti, di'yi" [Manchukuo's opium question, part one: Fengtian city medical doctor conference special speech draft], *Shengjing shibao* [Shengjing times], 30 December 1936, 5.

5   Xiang Naixi, "Jie yan yu jie yan yao" [Quit smoking and quit smoking medicine], *Shengjing shibao* [Shengjing times], 22 October 1935, 9. Xiang, a Manchu, was born in Fengtian in 1903 and earned his medical degree at South Manchuria Medical University.

6   Wang, "Manzhouguo yapian wenti, di'yi," 5.

7   Wang Shigong, "Fengtian shi yapian yinzhe tongji de guancha" [Survey of Fengtian city opium addicts' statistics], *Dongfang yixue zazhi* [Far Eastern medical journal] 13, 3 (1935): 96.

8   Bai Chun, "Yan fei tan" [Sigh over opium and morphine], *Shengjing shibao* [Shengjing times], 4 May 1941, 8.

9   Bai Chun, "Zhi jin yan tong yin shu" [Promoting the popular book banning opium], *Shengjing shibao* [Shengjing times], 20 April 1941, 8.

10   Bai Chun, "Jin yan chuyan" [Brief introduction to ban smoking], *Shengjing shibao* [Shengjing times], 4 May 1941, 8.

11   Of the 4,286 patients, 1,674 were around the age of twenty, 1,693 around thirty, and 590 around forty. See "Xin guomin yundong de quchu yapian zuotanhui" [New Citizens' Movement to Get Rid of Opium Forum], *Xin Manzhou* [New Manchuria], August 1941, 28.

12   This representation is also noted in Miriam Lynn Kingsberg, "The Poppy and the Acacia: Opium and Imperialism in Japanese Dairen and the Kwantung Leased Territory, 1905-1945" (PhD diss., History Department, University of California at Berkeley, 2009), 146. For further discussion of the lives of coolies, see ibid., 109-25.

13   "Xin guomin yundong," 30.

14   Wang, "Manzhouguo yapian wenti, di'yi," 5.

15   Ru Gai, "Su zhi jie yan jingyan tan, san" [Discussion of my experience quitting smoking, three], *Shengjing shibao* [Shengjing times], 14 November 1930, 7.

16   Yong Boping, "Yapian yu renti" [Opium and the human body], *Shengjing shibao* [Shengjing times], 25 August 1936, 9.

17   Bai Chun, "Yan fei tan, di'yi" [Opium and morphine sigh, part one], *Shengjing shibao* [Shengjing times], 10 April 1941, 7.

18   T. Nagashima, "Opium Administration in Manchoukuo," *Contemporary Manchuria* 3, 1 (1939): 23.

19   Liu Guojun, "Jin yan yu juewu" [Ban opium and consciousness], *Datong bao* [Great unity herald], 23 October 1941, 4.

20   Su Jianxun, "Yinshi" [Addicts], *Shengjing shibao* [Shengjing times], 17 October 1941, 8.

21   Qiu Shan, "Yapian huo zai Manzhou de jinhou, shang" [Opium calamity in Manchuria from now on, first], *Datong bao* [Great unity herald], 15 February 1939, 15.

22   Feng Shuo noted that the excitement of trying new things was the primary motivating factor for youth starting to smoke opium. See Feng Shuo, "Qingnian yi ruhe fangzhi xi chi yapian" [How youth should prevent smoking opium], *Xin qingnian* [New youth] 5.11 (August 1937): 25.

23   Jin Long, "Yapian yin zhi yanjiu" [Opium addiction research], *Shengjing shibao* [Shengjing times], 11 January 1930, 9. Miriam Kingsberg cites additional studies that document medical reasons for first starting to consume drugs; see Kingsberg, "Poppy and the Acacia," 150.

24   Ni Fuzhi, "Shen lun zhi de jiao xing tan" [Talking about a degenerate's awakening], *Shengjing shibao* [Shengjing times], 17 October 1940, 5.

25   Chikamori Kansuke, "Sekai o fūbe suru ahen oyobi mayakuka to Manshūkoku no dankin hōsaku" [The Trouble of Opium and Morphine that Spread All over the World and the Prohibition Policy of Manchukuo], *Minsei* [People's livelihood], January 1938, 29.

26   "Jie yin zhi huanxin zuotan hui, yi" [Exultant Forum on Resolving Addiction, one], *Shengjing shibao* [Shengjing times], 20 October 1940, 4.

27   Ibid. The women's Russian names are not provided, only the transliterations, Dalasuo and Liubinaijia.

28 Ibid.
29 Ibid.
30 Zhang Guochen, "Yaowuxue shiyezhong de yapian" [Opium in the field of vision of phar-macology], *Jiankang Manzhou* [Healthy Manchuria] 3.4 (1941): 13.
31 "Xin guomin yundong," 30.
32 Qiu, "Yapian huo zai Manzhou," 15.
33 "Xiang guomin zhuwei ji ju hua" [A few words to citizens], *Shengjing shibao* [Shengjing times], 10 April 1941, 7.
34 Wang, "Fengtian shi yapian yinzhe," 96.
35 "Xin guomin yundong," 30.
36 Yong Shanqi, "Jin yan judu zhi juti fangce, xu" [Concrete directives for banning smoking and refusing poison, continued], *Shengjing shibao* [Shengjing times], 19 December 1940, 8. Wang Shigong argued that 17 percent of opium addicts were women; see Wang, "Fengtian shi yapian yinzhe," 96.
37 Xiang noted that 80 to 90 percent of female opium addicts no longer had periods. See Xiang Naixi, "Manxing mayao zhong duzhe xinli de guancha, qi'er" [Survey of the psychol-ogy of chronic morphine drug users, part two], *Dongfang yixue zazhi* [Far Eastern medical journal] 15, 9 (1937): 501.
38 For example, see "Kangsheng yuan Daode hui hezuo" [Co-operation between Healthy Life Institutes and the Morality Society], *Shengjing shibao* [Shengjing times], 15 September 1944, 2.
39 "Xuanming ahpian duanjin guoce" [Announcing the opium prohibition national policy], *Shengjing shibao* [Shengjing times], 27 August 1942, 2.
40 Yu Li, "Funü xiyan zhi hai" [The harm of women's smoking], *Jiankang Manzhou* [Healthy Manchuria] 2.7 (1940): 3-5.
41 Ibid., 4.
42 Ibid., 3.
43 Jin, "Yapian yin zhi yanjiu," 12 January 1930, 9.
44 Ibid., 13 January 1930, 5.
45 Ibid., 14 January 1930, 9.
46 "Xin guomin yundong," 30.
47 "Shoudu jinyan xuanchuan dahui" [Capital city forbid opium publicity meeting], *Shengjing shibao* [Shengjing times], 29 April 1943, 4.
48 For a present-day discussion of terms such as *yan gui*, see Yi Bi, "Jiu min zhong zhong" [A variety of alcohol people], in Li Tongfeng and Zou Changshun, eds., *Jiu zhi yun* [The charm of alcohol] (Shenyang: Liaohai chubanshe, 2007), 105-7.
49 Bao Kun, "Yapian yinzhe shenjing, yi" [The condition of opium addicts' nerves, one], *Shengjing shibao* [Shengjing times], 5 September 1941, 5.
50 For example, see Yong, "Yapian yu renti," 9.
51 Su, "Yinshi," 8.
52 Qu Kezhong, "Jin yan bai zi ci" [Banning smoking one hundred word poem], *Shengjing shibao* [Shengjing times], 7 June 1941, 8.
53 Bao, "Yapian yinzhe shenjing, yi," 5.
54 Quoted in Edward R. Slack Jr., *Opium, State, and Society: China's Narco-Economy and the Guomindang, 1924-1937* (Honolulu: University of Hawai'i Press, 2001), 47.
55 "Xin guomin yundong," 30.
56 Bai, "Yan fei tan," 8. Women turning to sex work because of addiction is discussed in Yang Chaohui and An Linhai, "Wei Man shiqi de Rehe yapian" [Rehe opium during the bogus Manchukuo era], in Sun Bang, ed., *Wei Man wenhua* [Bogus Manchukuo culture], in *Wei Man shiliao congshu* [Collection of historical materials on bogus Manchukuo], 10 vols. (Changchun: Jilin renmin chubanshe, 1993), vol. 6, 428.

57 Jin, "Yapian yin zhi yanjiu," 12 January 1930, 9.
58 "Yan hai tan" [Discussion of the harm of smoke], *Shengjing shibao* [Shengjing times], 16 March 1935, 7.
59 Studies on morphine by researchers such as Nishigishi Shingen are discussed in Kingsberg, "Poppy and the Acacia," 325-26.
60 "Jie yan qike da mayao zhen" [Quit smoking should not involve morphine injections], *Shengjing shibao* [Shengjing times], 24 October 1939, 4.
61 For example, see "Si yu mafei" [Dead from morphine], *Shengjing shibao* [Shengjing times], 13 December 1916, 5; and "Mafei wei lu" [The dead end of morphine], *Shengjing shibao* [Shengjing times], 10 January 1917, 5.
62 Zhao Kuiru, "Dongtian de mafei ke" [Winter morphine wanderer], *Shengjing shibao* [Shengjing times], 25 February 1934, 5.
63 Zhao Min, "Yapian duanjinzhe tiyan ji" [Personal notes on abstaining from opium], *Shengjing shibao* [Shengjing times], 19 December 1940, 8.
64 Itō Ryōichi, "Yinzhe zhiliao zhi genben linian, si" [The basic theory of curing addicts, four], *Shengjing shibao* [Shengjing times], 19 December 1940, 8. For more on Itō's career, see Kingsberg, "Poppy and the Acacia," 330.
65 Jin, "Yapian yin zhi yanjiu," 14 January 1930, 9.
66 Wang, "Manzhouguo yapian wenti, di'yi," 5.
67 Zhang Jiyou, "Yapian" [Opium], *Jiankang Manzhou* [Healthy Manchuria] 1.3 (1939): 12.
68 Ibid.
69 Ibid.
70 Wang, "Manzhouguo zhi yapian zhidu," 482. Xiang also discussed "gewöhnung" [habituation] and "sucht" [addiction/obsession]; see Xiang, "Manxing mayao zhong duzhe," 510.
71 "Jie yin zhi huanxin zuotan hui," 20 October 1940, 4. Mariana Valverde provides a fascinating study of Western understandings of relationships between addiction and the body, soul, and will. See Mariana Valverde, *Diseases of the Will: Alcohol and the Dilemmas of Freedom* (Cambridge, UK: Cambridge University Press, 1998).
72 Zhang, "Yapian," 12.
73 Xiang, "Jie yan yu jie yan yao," 9.
74 Bai, "Jin yan chuyan," 8; Liu Lang, "Jieyan yu jieyan yao" [Quit smoking and quit smoking medicine], *Shengjing shibao* [Shengjing times], 18 August 1935, 9.
75 Takeo Akiyoshi, "Jie yan baihua, xuqian" [Plain talk about quitting smoking, continued], *Shengjing shibao* [Shengjing times], 14 October 1906, 2.
76 Ibid.
77 Ibid.
78 Takeo Akiyoshi, "Jie yan baihua" [Plain talk about quitting smoking], *Shengjing shibao* [Shengjing times], 13 October 1906, 2.
79 Ru Gai, "Su zhi jie yan jingyan tan, si" [Discussion of my experience quitting smoking, four], *Shengjing shibao* [Shengjing times], 20 November 1930, 7.
80 Yong Boping, "Yapian yu renti, xu" [Opium and the human body, continued], *Shengjing shibao* [Shengjing times], 29 August 1936, 9.
81 Further discussion of product names and advertising techniques can be found in Kingsberg, "Poppy and the Acacia," 344-48.
82 For example, see Ebosi [Aibiaosi] ad, *Qilin* [Unicorn], December 1942, 23.
83 Liu, "Jieyan yu jieyan yao," 9.
84 "Treating an addict," *Daily Times*, 26 February 1937.
85 Anqimaoqin ad, *Shengjing shibao* [Shengjing times], 10 September 1925, 8.
86 Nie'ou'moxi'en [Neo-Mohyn] ad, *Shengjing shibao* [Shengjing times], 12 June 1936, 10.
87 Puluojiabing ad, *Shengjing shibao* [Shengjing times], 6 June 1934, 14. The dangers of red pills had long been warned against. For example, see Zhai Wenxuan, "Ji cheng fujian"

[Memorial plan attachment], *Fengtian guomin gongbao* [Fengtian national bulletin], 24 April 1912, 15.

88 Qiao Enrun, "Yapian zhi hai shenyu hongshuimengshou" [The harm of opium is worse than fierce floods and savage beasts], *Shengjing shibao* [Shengjing times], 15 October 1944, 2. Mark Driscoll notes that in a 1944 anti-addiction campaign, 200,000 of the most addicted users were injected with the amphetamine Dongguang ji to maximize their hard labour; see Mark Driscoll, *Absolute Erotic, Absolute Grotesque* (Durham, NC: Duke University Press, 2010), 303.

89 Itō, "Yinzhe zhiliao zhi genben linian, si," 8.

90 Xiang, "Jie yan yu jie yan yao," 9. For the seventy-nine methods, see Xiang Naixi, "Xiandai Hanyi suo yong zhi jieyan fang" [Modern Chinese medicine methods of quitting smoking], *Dongfang yixue zazhi* [Far Eastern medical journal] 15, 8 (1937): 441-64.

91 Wang Shaoxian, "Wo guo jin zheng gaikuang" [Survey of my country's prohibit opium policy], *Shengjing shibao* [Shengjing times], 6 March 1941, 8.

92 "Jie yan xisheng" [Quit smoking sacrifice], *Shengjing shibao* [Shengjing times], 27 November 1930, 5.

93 In January 1933 the Society for Nutrition and Raising Children was established as a limited company. In July 1943 the trade name was changed to Wakamoto Pharmaceutical. For additional information, see the company's website: http://www.wakamoto-pharm.co.jp.

94 Ruosu [Basic Element] ad, *Qilin* [Unicorn], December 1943, back cover. See also "Fangzhi yapian zhong du yu yancao jiejue zhi kutong" [Defend against the pain of opium poison and tobacco withdrawal], *Shengjing shibao* [Shengjing times], 7 January 1936, 10.

95 Ruosu [Basic Element] ad, *Shengjing shibao* [Shengjing times], 26 November 1932, 8.

96 "Bujiu yapian yin suozhi zhuzheng you ke jianqing jieyan de kutong" [Mend and save opium addicts from their sickness and lighten the quit smoking pain], *Shengjing shibao* [Shengjing times], 29 June 1937, 10.

97 Jiao Runming, *Jindai Dongbei shehui zhu wenti yanjiu* [Research on various questions in modern Northeast society] (Beijing: Zhongguo shehui kexue chubanshe, 2004), 225.

98 "Qingzhu chengren Manzhouguo" [Celebrate the recognition of Manchukuo], *Shengjing shibao* [Shengjing times], 16 September 1932, 6.

99 Ruosu [Basic Element] ad, *Shengjing shibao* [Shengjing times], 26 November 1932, 8.

100 "Zengjin jingli hulihua yundong" [A rational movement to promote energy], *Shengjing shibao* [Shengjing times], 26 November 1932, 8.

101 "Ruosu zhi renshou fangfa" [Basic Element's workforce method], *Shengjing shibao* [Shengjing times], 26 November 1932, 8.

102 "Ruosu chengfen you tianran zucheng" [Basic Element ingredients are natural compositions], *Shengjing shibao* [Shengjing times], 26 November 1932, 8.

103 "Rensheng benneng de kuaile bu ru yangyuan daiqi zi yong" [Life's instinctual happiness is not as good as nourishment about to increase], *Shengjing shibao* [Shengjing times], 22 November 1932, 8.

104 See "Wangdao yao gong ke yun weida" [You may say the efficacy of the Kingly Way medicine is mighty], *Shengjing shibao* [Shengjing times], 26 November 1932, 8.

105 Ruosu [Basic Element] ad, *Shengjing shibao* [Shengjing times], 26 November 1932, 8.

106 "Fangzhi yapian zhong du yu yancao," 10.

107 "Yin jiu mei shi shu duan shou ming" [Consuming alcohol and good food can shorten your life], *Shengjing shibao* [Shengjing times], 7 January 1936, 10.

108 "Zhuyi!! Yan du, jiu du, cha du: Yingdang zenyang jiuzhi" [Attention!! You ought to know how to cure tobacco poison, alcohol poison, and tea poison], *Shengjing shibao* [Shengjing times], 5 April 1941, 4.

109 "Yan, jiu, cha yu jiankang de yinxiang" [The influence of tobacco, alcohol, and tea on health], *Shengjing shibao* [Shengjing times], 9 January 1940, 2.

110   "Yin jiu mei shi shu duan shou ming," 10.
111   Ruosu ad, *Qilin* [Unicorn], July 1944, back cover.
112   Ruosu ad, *Shengjing shibao* [Shengjing times], 22 November 1932, 8.
113   Ruosu child's ad, *Qilin* [Unicorn], September 1944, 12.
114   "Huo baobei: Tianmi de wen" [Live baby: Sweet kiss], *Shengjing shibao* [Shengjing times], 28 June 1940, 5.
115   "Xin sheng qu" [New life melody], *Qilin* [Unicorn], July 1944, 22.
116   Ruosu [Basic Element] ad, *Qilin* [Unicorn], February/March 1945, back cover.
117   Ibid., November 1941, 16.
118   "Qudi de juewu" [Consciousness of the ban], *Shengjing shibao* [Shengjing times], 10 April 1941, 7.
119   See Zhang, "Yapian," 12; and Xiang, "Jie yan yu jie yan yao," 9.
120   Jin Long, "Yan ke bao jian" [Smoke wanderer encyclopedia], *Shengjing shibao* [Shengjing times], 18 June 1930, 9.
121   Yong, "Jin yan judu zhi juti fangce," 17 October 1940, 8.
122   In 1939 T. Nagashima reported on the costs, real and projected, of administering Healthy Life Institutes: establishment was 1 million yuan in 1938 and 300,000 yuan in 1939; upkeep was 1,330,000 yuan in 1938, 3,370,000 yuan in 1939, and 4,040,000 yuan in 1940; equipment for the guidance and treatment of addicts was 1 million yuan for each year from 1938 to 1940; upkeep of training facilities was 67,500 yuan for 1938, 337,500 yuan for 1939, and 607,500 yuan for 1940 (including 2,400 yuan for one section head and 1,200 yuan each for three instructors); and anti-opium campaigning and general education were 434,000 yuan for each year from 1938 to 1940. See Nagashima, "Opium Administration," 37.
123   Yong, "Jin yan judu zhi juti fangce, xu," 8.
124   For example, see Dongbei jieyan [Northeast Quit Smoking] Hospital ad, *Shengjing shibao* [Shengjing times], 27 June 1930, 9.
125   For example, see "Jie yan qike da mayao zhen" [Quit smoking should not involve morphine injections], *Shengjing shibao* [Shengjing times] (24 October 1939), 4.
126   Zhenhua yiyuan [China Rise with Force and Spirit Hospital], "Jie yan" [Quit smoking] ad, *Shengjing shibao* [Shengjing times], 11 January 1932, 1.
127   Daqian yiyuan [Boundless Hospital] ad, *Shengjing shibao* [Shengjing times], 6 June 1934, 14.
128   Zhenhua yiyuan [China Rise with Force and Spirit Hospital] ad, *Shengjing shibao* [Shengjing times], 9 July 1939, 2.
129   Boji yiyuan [Rich Aid Hospital] ad, *Shengjing shibao* [Shengjing times], 9 July 1939, 2.
130   Nagashima, "Opium Administration," 34.
131   See Yong, "Jin yan judu zhi juti fangce, xu," 8; and "Duanjin zhengce jiji" [Vigorous prohibition policy], *Shengjing shibao* [Shengjing times], 1 July 1940, 2.
132   Nagashima, "Opium Administration," 34; "Xin guomin yundong," 30.
133   "Xin guomin yundong," 31.
134   "Kangsheng yuan Daode hui hezuo," 2.
135   Kangsheng yuan [Healthy Life Institute] ad, *Datong bao* [Great unity herald], 6 December 1941, 4.
136   For details, see Norman Smith, "Disrupting Narratives: Chinese Women Writers and the Japanese Cultural Agenda in Manchuria, 1936-1945," *Modern China* 30, 3 (2004): 295-325.
137   Xu Bochun, "Tiantang de kangsheng yuan" [The heavenly Healthy Life Institute], *Shengjing shibao* [Shengjing times], 20 April 1941, 8.
138   "Jie yin zhi huanxin zuotan hui," 20 October 1940, 4.
139   Xing, Zhang, and Chen recounted their stories together. See "Jie yin zhi huanxin zuotan hui, si," 24 October 1940, 4.

140 Xiang Naixi also discusses this, in "Fengtian jieyansuo fangwen ji," 11.
141 "Jie yin zhi huanxin zuotan hui," 24 October 1940, 6.
142 Ibid.
143 "Jie yin zhi huanxin zuotan hui, er," 22 October 1940, 4.
144 Xiang, "Manxing mayao zhong duzhe," 498-511.
145 Ibid., 499-500.
146 Ibid., 504.
147 "Ji shi kangsheng yuan da gexin" [Jilin city Healthy Life Institute innovation], *Shengjing shibao* [Shengjing times], 24 May 1940, 4.
148 "Fengtian jieyansuo fangwen ji," 12.
149 "Chedi yapian duanjin" [Thoroughly prohibit opium], *Shengjing shibao* [Shengjing times], 1 March 1940, 2. In Fengtian's Quit Smoking Centre, in 1939, patients had to produce 200 matchboxes every day after lunch; see "Fengtian jieyansuo fangwen ji," 12.
150 Chen Li, "Kangsheng yuan de xinfu ji" [Notes on the laborious blessings of Healthy Life Institutes], *Shengjing shibao* [Shengjing times], 21 November 1941, 4.
151 Food costs paid by Chinese patients in Fengtian in 1939 averaged 6 *jiao*. See "Fengtian jieyansuo fangwen ji," 11.
152 Bai Yu, "Kuhai huitou ji" [Repentant notes on the sea of bitterness], *Shengjing shibao* [Shengjing times], 5 September 1941, 5.
153 For the open letter, see Ying, "Quan fuqin jinyan shu" [Persuade father to quit smoking letter], *Shengjing shibao* [Shengjing times], 17 October 1941, 8. For the father's response, see Liu Jingliang, "Kangsheng zhong de wo" [Me in the Healthy Life Institute], *Shengjing shibao* [Shengjing times], 17 October 1941, 8.
154 Xiang Naixi, director of the Fengtian Quit Smoking Centre, argued that the average patient first had to report to the police before entering rehabilitation. Quoted in "Fengtian jieyansuo fangwen ji," 11.
155 Ma Ji, "Tiantang de kangsheng yuan" [The heavenly Healthy Life Institute], *Shengjing shibao* [Shengjing times], 20 March 1941, 8.
156 "Lao yinshi bu ting quangao, xiao yingxiong jinggao dangguan" [Old addict does not listen to advice, little hero warns officials], *Qilin* [Unicorn], June 1941, 85.
157 *Manchoukuo Yearbook: 1941* (Hsinking: Manchoukuo Yearbook Company, 1942), 725.
158 Ibid., 722. For details of the 1939 plans, see T. Nagashima, "Opium Administration in Manchoukuo," *Contemporary Manchuria* 3, 1 (1939): 33-36.
159 Literally, "To hang up a sheep's head and sell dogmeat." See Wang Xianwei, "Jin yan zhengce de qipian xing" [The fraudulent nature of the smoking prohibition], in Sun Bang, ed., *Jingji lüeduo* [Plundering the economy], in *Wei Man shiliao congshu* [Collection of historical materials on bogus Manchukuo], 10 vols. (Changchun: Jilin renmin chubanshe, 1993), vol. 4, 712.
160 Ibid., 709.
161 See Driscoll, *Absolute Erotic*, 231; and Wang, "Jin yan zhengce de qipian xing," 713.
162 Wang, "Jin yan zhengce de qipian xing," 711.
163 Mou Jianping, "Wei Man de dupin zhengce" [The narcotic policies of bogus Manchukuo], in Sun Bang, ed., *Jingji lüeduo* [Plundering the economy], in *Wei Man shiliao congshu* [Collection of historical materials on bogus Manchukuo], 10 vols. (Changchun: Jilin renmin chubanshe, 1993), vol. 4, 723.
164 For example, see Han Yu, "Zong du zhengce xia de Benxi" (Benxi village under the narcotics policies), in Sun Bang, ed., *Wei Man wenhua* [Bogus Manchukuo culture], in *Wei Man shiliao congshu* [Collection of historical materials on bogus Manchukuo], 10 vols. (Changchun: Jilin renmin chubanshe, 1993), vol. 6, 449.
165 For more information on Xiang's career researching Kashin-Beck disease and radition, see http://baike.baidu.com/.

166   See the company's official website: http://www.wakamoto-pharm.co.jp/.
167   http://www.wakamoto-pharm.co.jp/.
168   Ibid.
169   Rana Mitter, "Evil Empire? Competing Constructions of Japanese Imperialism in Manchuria, 1928-1937," in Li Narangoa and Robert Cribb, eds., *Imperial Japan and National Identities in Asia, 1895-1945* (London: RoutledgeCurzon, 2003), 156.
170   Ibid., 155.

Chapter 8: The Opium Monopoly's "Interesting Discussion"

1   No mention is made of French involvement in the Second Opium War, likely owing to Manchukuo's relationship with German-occupied France.
2   "Jinlin de Zhao laoyezi" [Neighbour Master Zhao], in Kakegawa Akikuni, ed., *Qu tan conglin, di'yi ji* [Interesting discussion thicket, volume number 1] (Fengtian: Xing Ya yinshua zhushi huishe, 1942), 2.
3   For discussion of what area constituted the Manchu homelands, see Shao Dan, *Remote Homeland, Recovered Borderland: Manchus, Manchoukuo, and Manchuria, 1907-1985* (Honolulu: University of Hawai'i Press, 2011), 25-30.
4   "Jinlin de Zhao laoyezi," 5.
5   Ibid., 6.
6   Ibid., 7.
7   "Ahpian zhanzheng yu Yinguo de dong Ya qinlüe" [Opium War and England's East Asia aggression], in Kakegawa Akikuni, ed., *Qu tan conglin, di'yi ji* [Interesting discussion thicket, volume number 1] (Fengtian: Xing Ya yinshua zhushi huishe, 1942), 35.
8   "Jinlin de Zhao laoyezi," 7.
9   "Ahpian zhanzheng yu Yinguo," 42.
10   "Jinlin de Zhao laoyezi," 7.
11   "Ahpian zhanzheng yu Yinguo," 34.
12   Ibid., 37. The 20,283 chests contained approximately 1.2 million kilograms of opium.
13   Ibid., 41.
14   The title of the page with this historical account and illustration is "Zhengyi Riben de fenqi" [The righteous Japanese rise with force and spirit], in ibid., 44.
15   Ibid., 45.
16   Ibid., 44.
17   Examples include cinema produced under the Ministry of Information in England and cartoons produced by Warner Brothers in the United States.
18   "Ahpian fa bugao" [Opium Law Proclamation], in Kakegawa Akikuni, ed., *Qu tan conglin, di'yi ji* [Interesting discussion thicket, volume number 1] (Fengtian: Xing Ya yinshua zhushi huishe, 1942), 22.
19   "Jinlin de Zhao laoyezi," 7.
20   "Guowuyuan bugao" [State Proclamation], in Kakegawa Akikuni, ed., *Qu tan conglin, di'yi ji* [Interesting discussion thicket, volume number 1] (Fengtian: Xing Ya yinshua zhushi huishe, 1942), 72.
21   "Jinlin de Zhao laoyezi," 6.
22   Ibid., 7.
23   "Xiguan wu" [Custom error], in Kakegawa Akikuni, ed., *Qu tan conglin, di'yi ji* [Interesting discussion thicket, volume number 1] (Fengtian: Xing Ya yinshua zhushi huishe, 1942), 46.
24   Ibid., 47.
25   "Gu bei tan" [Sigh for an age-old stele], in Kakegawa Akikuni, ed., *Qu tan conglin, di'yi ji* [Interesting discussion thicket, volume number 1] (Fengtian: Xing Ya yinshua zhushi huishe, 1942), 92.

26 Ibid., 94.
27 Ibid.
28 Ibid., 95.
29 "Mayao yinzhe de wang'en" [The ingratitude of anaesthetic addicts], in Kakegawa Akikuni, ed., *Qu tan conglin, di'yi ji* [Interesting discussion thicket, volume number 1] (Fengtian: Xing Ya yinshua zhushi huishe, 1942), 51.
30 Ibid.
31 "Tang Xinji de shi gong" [Tang Xinji's true confession], in Kakegawa Akikuni, ed., *Qu tan conglin, di'yi ji* [Interesting discussion thicket, volume number 1] (Fengtian: Xing Ya yinshua zhushi huishe, 1942), 14.
32 Ibid., 17.
33 Ibid., 15.
34 Ibid., 19.
35 Ibid., 21.
36 "Chun guang zailai" [Spring scenery returns], in Kakegawa Akikuni, ed., *Qu tan conglin, di'yi ji* [Interesting discussion thicket, volume number 1] (Fengtian: Xing Ya yinshua zhushi huishe, 1942), 30.
37 Ibid., 32.
38 "Zhang Dexin xiansheng" [Mr. Zhang Dexin], in Kakegawa Akikuni, ed., *Qu tan conglin, di'yi ji* [Interesting discussion thicket, volume number 1] (Fengtian: Xing Ya yinshua zhushi huishe, 1942), 97.
39 Ibid., 98.
40 Ibid.
41 Ibid., 99.
42 Ibid., 98.
43 Ibid., 99.
44 The opening of Morality Society branches, the numbers of acres, and their worth for Harbin (700 yuan) and for Xinjing's headquarters (600 yuan) are cited in "Zhang Dexin xiansheng," 100.
45 "Tang Xinji de shi gong," 21.
46 Ibid.
47 "Chun guang zailai," 32.
48 "Qin'ai de Liu Zheng xian di" [Dear first brother Liu Zheng], in Kakegawa Akikuni, ed., *Qu tan conglin, di'yi ji* [Interesting discussion thicket, volume number 1] (Fengtian: Xing Ya yinshua zhushi huishe, 1942), 102.
49 Ibid., 105.
50 Ibid., 107.
51 Ibid., 107-8.
52 Ibid., 111.
53 Ibid., 112.
54 Ibid.
55 "Qingtian zai lai di shang" [Sunny days come again to the land], in Kakegawa Akikuni, ed., *Qu tan conglin, di'yi ji* [Interesting discussion thicket, volume number 1] (Fengtian: Xing Ya yinshua zhushi huishe, 1942), 118.
56 Ibid., 119.
57 Ibid.
58 Ibid., 120.
59 Ibid., 122.
60 Ibid., 124.
61 *Manchoukuo Yearbook: 1941* (Hsinking: Manchoukuo Yearbook Company, 1942), 725.

62   "Xiaozhang xiansheng" [Mr. Principal], in Kakegawa Akikuni, ed., *Qu tan conglin, di'yi ji* [Interesting discussion thicket, volume number 1] (Fengtian: Xing Ya yinshua zhushi huishe, 1942), 57-58.

63   Ibid., 59.

64   Ibid., 62.

65   "Yu shaonian de qi ji" [Young Yu's surprise plan], in Kakegawa Akikuni, ed., *Qu tan conglin, di'yi ji* [Interesting discussion thicket, volume number 1] (Fengtian: Xing Ya yinshua zhushi huishe, 1942), 90.

Conclusion

1   Bob Wakabayashi notes that the Guomindang executed 149 imperial Japanese subjects on drug-related charges. See Bob Tadashi Wakabayashi, "'Imperial Japanese' Drug Trafficking in China: Historiographic Perspectives," 277, http://chinajapan.org/articles/13.1/13.1wakabayashi3-19.pdf.

2   For example, see Lu Shouxin, "Ha'erbin de yapian yandu" [Harbin's poisonous opium smoke], in Sun Bang, ed., *Wei Man wenhua* [Bogus Manchukuo culture], in *Wei Man shiliao congshu* [Collection of historical materials on bogus Manchukuo], 10 vols. (Changchun: Jilin renmin chubanshe, 1993), vol. 6, 446.

3   For details on the post-occupation industry, see *Ha'erbin shi zhi: Fushi pinshang ye zhi* [Harbin city records: Nonstaple food commodity trade records], http://218.10.232.41:8080/.

4   For an incisive discussion of the impact of domestic Japanese left-wing politics on understandings of imperial Japan's opium operations, see Wakabayashi, "'Imperial Japanese,'" 8-15. For discussion of "Japan's empire of the living dead," see Mark Driscoll, *Absolute Erotic, Absolute Grotesque* (Durham, NC: Duke University Press, 2010), 310.

5   Cheryl Krasnick Warsh, "'John Barleycorn Must Die': An Introduction to the Social History of Alcohol," in Cheryl Krasnick Warsh, ed., *Drink in Canada: Historical Essays* (Montreal and Kingston: McGill-Queen's University Press, 1993), 11-12.

6   Feng Qi, "Jiu ren shuo jiu hua: Dongbei jiu wenhua he xiaofei xiguan yanjiu" [Drinkers talk drink talk: Research on Northeast alcohol culture and consumption habits], http://www.cnbm.net.cn/.

7   For example, see Yang Jun, "Dongbeiren yu dongbei jiu wenhua" [Northeasterners and Northeast alcohol culture], http://tieba.baidu.com/.

8   The other two are to eat "bread as big as a lid" *(da mianbao xiang guogai)* and to "eat big pancakes outside" *(dabingzi chi zai wai)*. See Chi Xiucai, *Laoxiang hua Dongbei* [Fellow townsfolk talk: The Northeast] (Changchun: Jilin renmin chubanshe, 2007), 215.

9   Chung Kyoon Lee, "Alcoholism in Korea," in John E. Helzer and Glorisa J. Canino, eds., *Alcoholism in North America, Europe, and Asia* (Oxford: Oxford University Press, 1992), 247.

10   Amy Borovy, *The Too-Good Wife: Alcohol, Codependency, and the Politics of Nurturance in Postwar Japan* (Berkeley: University of California Press, 2005), 47.

11   Ibid., 50.

12   W.J. Rorabaugh, *The Alcoholic Republic: An American Tradition* (New York: Oxford University Press, 1979), 246.

13   For an illuminating introduction to alcohol history in Canada, see Warsh, "'John Barleycorn Must Die,'" 10.

14   Tsung-Yi Lin and David T.C. Lin, "Alcoholism among the Chinese: Further Observations of a Low-Risk Population," *Culture, Medicine and Psychiatry* 6, 2 (1982): 112.

15   Catherine Carstairs, *Jailed for Possession: Illegal Drug Use, Regulation, and Power in Canada, 1920-1961* (Toronto: University of Toronto Press, 2006), 161.

16   Quoted original text is in English. Gong Li, *Yin jiu shihua* [History of alcohol drinking] (Beijing: Zhongguo da bailiao quanshu chubanshe, 2009), 77.

17 http://www.abc.net.au/.

18 Li Zhengping, *Zhongguo jiu wenhua* [Chinese alcohol culture] (Beijing: Shishi chubanshe, 2006), 123.

19 The other two most popular beer festivals are in Dalian and Qingdao. The Harbin municipal government has boasted that at the 2010 festival nearly 500,000 people consumed 800,000 litres of beer. See http://www.harbin.gov.cn/.

20 Karl Gerth also argues that China is the fastest-growing market for the finest Scotch whiskeys – which are sometimes consumed with ice and green tea, just as fine wines are often consumed with carbonated beverages. See Karl Gerth, *As China Goes, So Goes the World: How Chinese Consumers Are Transforming Everything* (New York: Hill and Wang, 2010), 47, 130.

21 In 1876 Wujiapi wine won its first gold medal in Singapore. See Pieter Eijkhoff, "Wine in China: Its History and Contemporary Developments" (2000), 136, http://www.eykhoff.nl/Wine%20in%20China.pdf.

22 The 7 January 2011 edition of *China Economic Review* cites an annual sales volume of 520 million nine-litre cases. See http://www.chinaeconomicreview.com/node/24511.

23 Li Lili has even argued that men and alcohol are comparable to fish in water. See Li Lili, "Wen jiu shi nanren" [Smell wine, know men], in Li Tongfeng and Zou Changshun, eds., *Jiu zhi yun* [The charm of alcohol] (Shenyang: Liaohai chubanshe, 2007), 89.

Bibliography

Non-English language sources

A You. "Putaojiu" [Grape wine]. *Shengjing shibao* [Shengjing times], 18 October 1936, 14.

Ah Ling. "Yinzhe de xin" [An addict's letter]. *Shengjing shibao* [Shengjing times], 3 October 1941, 5.

"Ahpian fa bugao" [Opium Law Proclamation]. In Kakegawa Akikuni, ed., *Qu tan conglin, di'yi ji* [Interesting discussion thicket, volume number 1], 22. Fengtian: Xing Ya yinshua zhushi huishe, 1942.

"Ahpian zhanzheng yu Yinguo de dong Ya qinlüe" [Opium war and England's East Asia aggression]. In Kakegawa Akikuni, ed., *Qu tan conglin, di'yi ji* [Interesting discussion thicket, volume number 1], 33-35. Fengtian: Xing Ya yinshua zhushi huishe, 1942.

An Longzhen. *Modai de huanghou Wanrong* [The last empress Wanrong]. Beijing: Huaxia chubanshe, 1994.

Anqimaoqin ad. *Shengjing shibao* [Shengjing times], 10 September 1925, 8.

Ao Shuang'an. "Mei jin jiu gan yan" [Moving words about American Prohibition]. *Shengjing shibao* [Shengjing times], 10 March 1922, 1.

Asahi [Chinese: Riguang; English: Sunlight] ad. *Shengjing shibao* [Shengjing times], 19 June 1912, 8.

Asahi [Chinese: Taiyang; English: Sun] ad. *Shengjing shibao* [Shengjing times], 1 June 1915, 4.

Asahi [Chinese: Taiyang; English: Sun], Fu shen [Good Fortune Spirit], and Sapporo [Zha huang] ad. *Shengjing shibao* [Shengjing times], 6 June 1920, 8.

Asahi [Chinese: Xu; English: Brilliance of the Rising Sun] ad. *Shengjing shibao* [Shengjing times], 11 June 1909, 1.

Asahi [Chinese: Xu; English: Brilliance of the Rising Sun] and Sapporo [Zha huang] ad. *Shengjing shibao* [Shengjing times], 15 February 1907, 1.

Asahi [Chinese: Xu; English: Brilliance of the Rising Sun] and Sapporo [Zha huang] ad. *Shengjing shibao* [Shengjing times], 23 April 1908, 6.

Bai Chun. "Jin yan chuyan" [Brief introduction to ban smoking]. *Shengjing shibao* [Shengjing times], 4 May 1941, 8.

—. "Yan fei tan" [Sigh over opium and morphine]. *Shengjing shibao* [Shengjing times], 4 May 1941, 8.

—. "Yan fei tan, di'yi" [Opium and morphine sigh, part one]. *Shengjing shibao* [Shengjing times], 10 April 1941, 7.

—. "Zhi jin yan tong yin shu" [Promoting the popular book banning opium]. *Shengjing shibao* [Shengjing times], 20 April 1941, 8.

Bai He. "Lun yan jiu zhi hai (xia)" [Discussing the harm of alcohol and opium (second)]. *Xin Manzhou* [New Manchuria], June 1939, 38-40.

Bai Lang. "Panni de erzi" [Rebellious son]. In Liang Shanding, ed., *Changye yinghuo* [Fireflies of the long night], 37-50. Shenyang: Chunfeng wenyi chubanshe, 1986.

Bai Yu. "Kuhai huitou ji" [Repentant notes on the sea of bitterness]. *Shengjing shibao* [Shengjing times], 5 September 1941, 5.

"Bairi jian jin jiu duanxing: Bin sheng aiguo jingshen zuoxing" [One hundred days' practice of prohibiting alcohol: Patriotic spirits are up in Bin province]. *Shengjing shibao* [Shengjing times], 17 February 1938, 9.

Bao jing [Precious Mirror] ad. *Shengjing shibao* [Shengjing times], 13 November 1937, 11.

Bao Kun. "Yapian yinzhe shenjing, yi" [The condition of opium addicts' nerves, one]. *Shengjing shibao* [Shengjing times], 5 September 1941, 5.

Boji yiyuan [Rich Aid Hospital] ad. *Shengjing shibao* [Shengjing times], 9 July 1939, 2.

"Bujiu yapian yin suozhi zhuzheng you ke jianqing jieyan de kutong" [Mend and save opium addicts from their sickness and lighten the quit smoking pain]. *Shengjing shibao* [Shengjing times], 29 June 1937, 10.

"Chedi yapian duanjin" [Thoroughly prohibit opium]. *Shengjing shibao* [Shengjing times], 1 March 1940, 2.

Chen Li. "Kangsheng yuan de xinfu ji" [Notes on the laborious blessings of Healthy Life Institutes]. *Shengjing shibao* [Shengjing times], 21 November 1941, 4.

"Chengxiang shu na si yanguan" [Chengxiang office takes firm hold of private opium dens]. *Shengjing shibao* [Shengjing times], 4 September 1936, 12.

Chi Xiucai. *Laoxiang hua Dongbei* [Fellow townsfolk talk: The Northeast]. Changchun: Jilin renmin chubanshe, 2007.

Chi yu [Red Ball] ad. *Datong bao* [Great unity herald], 3 March 1939, 7.

–. *Datong bao* [Great unity herald], 26 March 1939, 4.

–. *Shengjing shibao* [Shengjing times], 16 November 1917, 8.

–. *Shengjing shibao* [Shengjing times], 27 August 1919, 8.

–. *Shengjing shibao* [Shengjing times], 10 September 1921, 3.

Chikamori Kansuke. "Sekai o fūbe suru ahen oyobi mayakuka to Manshūkoku no dankin hōsaku" [The trouble of opium and morphine that spread all over the world and the prohibition policy of Manchukuo]. *Minsei* [People's livelihood], January 1938, 22-38.

Chu Guoqing. "Nüren yu jiu" [Women and alcohol]. In Li Tongfeng and Zou Changshun, eds., *Jiu zhi yun* [The charm of alcohol], 11-16. Shenyang: Liaohai chubanshe, 2007.

"Chun guang zailai" [Spring scenery returns]. In Kakegawa Akikuni, ed., *Qu tan conglin, di'yi ji* [Interesting discussion thicket, volume number 1], 23-32. Fengtian: Xing Ya yinshua zhushi huishe, 1942.

"'Ci Liu Ling': Zui jiu shou fu chi yi nu jiu huazuo diaosigui" ['Female Liu Ling': Intoxicated and reprimanded by husband, suddenly angry and becomes a hung dead ghost]. *Shengjing shibao* [Shengjing times], 27 February 1942, 4.

Cui Yu. "*Taosu* yu taofu" [*Taosu* and spring festival couplets]. *Qilin* [Unicorn], January 1942, 7.

Da yang [Big Sun] ad. *Shengjing shibao* [Shengjing times], 18 May 1925, 8.

Da Yong. "Shuang zhi yan" [A pair of swallows]. *Qilin* [Unicorn], December 1941, 26.

Daqian yiyuan [Boundless Hospital] ad. *Shengjing shibao* [Shengjing times], 6 June 1934, 14.

"Datong gongsuo quan jie yan jiu" [Datong government office persuades to quit smoking and drinking]. *Shengjing shibao* [Shengjing times], 5 August 1931, 5.

Dongbei jieyan [Northeast Quit Smoking] Hospital ad. *Shengjing shibao* [Shengjing times], 27 June 1930, 9.

Dongbei lunxian shisi nian shi zong bian shi and Riben zhimin di wenhua yanjiu hui, eds. *Wei Manzhouguo de zhenxiang* [The real truth of the puppet Manchukuo]. Beijing: Shehui kexue wenxian chubanshe, 2010.

"Duanjin zhengce jiji" [Vigorous prohibition policy]. *Shengjing shibao* [Shengjing times], 1 July 1940, 2.

Ebosi [Aibiaosi] ad. *Qilin* [Unicorn], December 1942, 23.

Fan Ying. "Beidi lian'ge" [Northern love story]. *Qilin* [Unicorn], October 1941, 82-87.

Fang Fei. "Jin jiu jin du" [Ban alcohol, ban gambling]. *Shengjing shibao* [Shengjing times], 10 February 1936, 5.

"Fangzhi yapian zhong du yu yancao jiejue zhi kutong" [Defend against the pain of opium poison and tobacco withdrawal]. *Shengjing shibao* [Shengjing times], 7 January 1936, 10.

"Fasheng xing Ya zhi zhuangli" [Strong prosperous Asia]. *Jiankang Manzhou* [Healthy Manchuria] 2, 2 (1940): back outside cover.

Feng Qi. "Jiu ren shuo jiu hua: Dongbei jiu wenhua he xiaofei xiguan yanjiu" [Drinkers talk drink talk: Research on Northeast alcohol culture and consumption habits]. http://www. cnbm.net.cn/.

Feng Sen. "Yin jiu mantan, yi" [Informal discussion of drinking alcohol, one]. *Shengjing shibao* [Shengjing times], 7 July 1937, 9.

–. "Yin jiu mantan, er" [Informal discussion of drinking alcohol, two. *Shengjing shibao* [Shengjing times], 8 July 1937, 9.

–. "Yin jiu mantan, san" [Informal discussion of drinking alcohol, three]. *Shengjing shibao* [Shengjing times], 9 July 1937, 9.

Feng Shuo. "Qingnian yi ruhe fangzhi xi chi yapian" [How youth should prevent smoking opium]. *Xin qingnian* [New youth] 5.11 (August 1937): 24-31.

"Fengtian jieyansuo fangwen ji" [Notes on an interview at the Fengtian Quit Smoking Centre]. *Xin qingnian* [New youth] 8, 5 (1939): 10-13.

Fu Chen. "You yuan guilai" [Return from touring the garden]. In Yu Zhizhu, ed., *Nü zhaodai quan ji* [Hostess complete collection], 33-36. Tianjin: Lanhua guanggao she, 1933.

"Fu qiaohui kaishi jin jiu yundong" [Women's society starts a prohibit alcohol movement]. *Shengjing shibao* [Shengjing times], 3 September 1938, 5.

Fuji Kyūta. Yangming jiu [Life Support Wine] ad. *Qilin* [Unicorn], April 1942, 4.

"Funü yin jiu yingxiang ertong jiankang" [Women who drink alcohol influence children's health]. *Shengjing shibao* [Shengjing times], 29 January 1942, 2.

Gong Li. *Yin jiu shihua* [History of alcohol drinking]. Beijing: Zhongguo da bailiao quanshu chubanshe, 2009.

"Gu bei tan" [Sigh for an age-old stele]. In Kakegawa Akikuni, ed., *Qu tan conglin, di'yi ji* [Interesting discussion thicket, volume number 1], 92-96. Fengtian: Xing Ya yinshua zhushi huishe, 1942.

Gu Ding. "Ji mie" [Attack, extinguish]. *Qilin* [Unicorn], September 1944, 21.

Gui pai haomeng putaojiu [Essence of Turtle] ad. *Jiankang Manzhou* [Healthy Manchuria] 1, 4 (1939): back outside cover.

Guo Panxi. *Zhongguo yin jiu xisu* [Chinese drinking alcohol customs]. Taibei: Wenhua chubanshe, 1989.

"Guowuyuan bugao" [State Proclamation]. In Kakegawa Akikuni, ed., *Qu tan conglin, di'yi ji* [Interesting discussion thicket, volume number 1], 72. Fengtian: Xing Ya yinshua zhushi huishe, 1942.

Ha'erbin shi zhi: Fushi pinshang ye zhi [Harbin city records: Nonstaple food commodity trade records]. http://218.10.232.41:8080/.

Han Hu. "Yan jiu suo hua" [Trivial words about smoke and alcohol]. *Qilin* [Unicorn], April 1943, 118-21.

Han-Ying cidian [Chinese-English dictionary]. Beijing: Shangwu yinshuguan, 1999.

Han Yu. "Zong du zhengce xia de Benxi" [Benxi village under the narcotics policies]. In Sun Bang, ed., *Wei Man wenhua* [Bogus Manchukuo culture], in *Wei Man shiliao congshu* [Collection of historical materials on bogus Manchukuo], 10 vols., vol. 6, 449. Changchun: Jilin renmin chubanshe, 1993.

"Hao jiu de ren wei shenme bu ai chi tian de?" [Why don't people who are fond of alcohol like to eat sweet things?]. *Shengjing shibao* [Shengjing times], 17 January 1937, 5.

Hei [Black] ad. *Shengjing shibao* [Shengjing times], 17 July 1921, 3.

Hei'ermisi [Hermes] ad. *Shengjing shibao* [Shengjing times], 18 May 1918, 8.

—. *Shengjing shibao* [Shengjing times], 25 June 1919, 6.

Higashimoto Hide. Yangming jiu [Life Support Wine] ad. *Qilin* [Unicorn], December 1942, 4.

Hong Nian. "Tan yin jiu" [Discussion of drinking alcohol]. *Shengjing shibao* [Shengjing times], 26 July 1938, 4.

Hong xing [Red Star] ad. *Shengjing shibao* [Shengjing times], 18 July 1937, 8.

Hua Jiangrong. "Yan lou suohua: Ge lingmaisuo nü zhaodai sumiao, di'er" [Trivial talk about opium dens: Sketches of opium retail outlet hostesses, part two]. *Shengjing shibao* [Shengjing times], 10 April 1936, 7.

—. "Yan lou suohua: Ge lingmaisuo nü zhaodai sumiao, di'san" [Trivial talk about opium dens: Sketches of opium retail outlet hostesses, part three]. *Shengjing shibao* [Shengjing times], 17 April 1936, 7.

—. "Yan lou suohua: Ge lingmaisuo nü zhaodai sumiao, di'si" [Trivial talk about opium dens: Sketches of opium retail outlet hostesses, part four]. *Shengjing shibao* [Shengjing times], 23 April 1936, 7.

—. "Yan lou suohua: Ge lingmaisuo nü zhaodai sumiao, di'wu" [Trivial talk about opium dens: Sketches of opium retail outlet hostesses, part five]. *Shengjing shibao* [Shengjing times], 29 April 1936, 7.

—. "Yan lou suohua: Ge lingmaisuo nü zhaodai sumiao, di'liu" [Trivial talk about opium dens: Sketches of opium retail outlet hostesses, part six]. *Shengjing shibao* [Shengjing times], 7 May 1936, 7.

—. "Yan lou suohua: Ge lingmaisuo nü zhaodai sumiao, di'qi" [Trivial talk about opium dens: Sketches of opium retail outlet hostesses, part seven]. *Shengjing shibao* [Shengjing times], 14 May 1936, 7.

—. "Yan lou suohua: Ge lingmaisuo nü zhaodai sumiao, di'jiu" [Trivial talk about opium dens: Sketches of opium retail outlet hostesses, part nine]. *Shengjing shibao* [Shengjing times], 28 May 1936, 7.

—. "Yan lou suohua: Ge lingmaisuo nü zhaodai sumiao, di'shi" [Trivial talk about opium dens: Sketches of opium retail outlet hostesses, part ten]. *Shengjing shibao* [Shengjing times], 4 June 1936, 7.

—. "Yan lou suohua: Ge lingmaisuo nü zhaodai sumiao, di'shiyi" [Trivial talk about opium dens: Sketches of opium retail outlet hostesses, part eleven]. *Shengjing shibao* [Shengjing times], 10 June 1936, 7.

Huai Yin. "Junfa yu yapian" [Warlords and opium]. *Shengjing shibao* [Shengjing times], 19 November 1924, 1.

Hugu huashe yaojiu [Tiger Bone, Flower Snake Medicinal Wine] ad. *Shengjing shibao* [Shengjing times], 6 October 1937, 6

"Huo baobei: Tianmi de wen" [Live baby: Sweet kiss]. *Shengjing shibao* [Shengjing times], 28 June 1940, 5.

Imamura Masu. Yangming jiu [Life Support Wine] ad. *Qilin* [Unicorn], October 1942, 4.

Itō Ryōichi. "Guanyu xi hailuoying (heroin) shi yixing yu yan zhong de youxiao chengfen liang" [Regarding measurements of active ingredients in heroin when smoking]. *Dongfang yixue zazhi* [Far Eastern medical journal] 14, 10 (1935): 376-96.

—. "Yinzhe zhiliao zhi genben linian, si" [The basic theory of curing addicts, four]. *Shengjing shibao* [Shengjing times], 19 December 1940, 8.

"Ji shi kangsheng yuan da gexin" [Jilin city Healthy Life Institute innovation]. *Shengjing shibao* [Shengjing times], 24 May 1940, 4.

Jia Xiao. "Mantan yan jiu" [Informal discussion of opium and alcohol]. *Qilin* [Unicorn], July 1942, 72.

Jiang Hai. *Jiu de gushi* [The story of alcohol]. Jinan: Shandong renmin yinshuachang, 2006.

Jiao Runming. *Jindai Dongbei shehui zhu wenti yanjiu* [Research on various questions in modern Northeast society]. Beijing: Zhongguo shehui kexue chubanshe, 2004.

Jie Xueshi. "Ri Wei shiqi de wenhua tongzhi zhengce" [State policies of cultural domination during the Japanese occupation]. In Feng Weiqun, Wang Jianzhong, Li Chunyan, and Li Shuquan, eds., *Dongbei lunxian shiqi wenxue guoji xueshu yantaohui lunwenji* [Collection of papers from the International Symposium on Literature of the Enemy-Occupied Northeast], 182-98. Shenyang: Shenyang chubanshe, 1992.

"Jie yan ge" [Get off opium song]. Words by Li Juanqing, music by Liang Leyin. On *Li Xianglan Collection*. Taipei: Zhonghua Records, 1999.

"Jie yan geyao" [Quit smoking ballad]. *Shengjing shibao* [Shengjing times], 17 November 1938, 4.

"Jie yan qike da mayao zhen" [Quit smoking should not involve morphine injections]. *Shengjing shibao* [Shengjing times], 24 October 1939, 4.

"Jie yan xisheng" [Quit smoking sacrifice]. *Shengjing shibao* [Shengjing times], 27 November 1930, 5.

"Jie yin zhi huanxin zuotan hui, yi" [Exultant Forum on Resolving Addiction, one]. *Shengjing shibao* [Shengjing times], 20 October 1940, 4.

"Jie yin zhi huanxin zuotan hui, er" [Exultant Forum on Resolving Addiction, two]. *Shengjing shibao* [Shengjing times], 22 October 1940, 4.

"Jie yin zhi huanxin zuotan hui, san" [Exultant Forum on Resolving Addiction, three]. *Shengjing shibao* [Shengjing times], 23 October 1940, 4.

"Jie yin zhi huanxin zuotan hui, si" [Exultant Forum on Resolving Addiction, four]. *Shengjing shibao* [Shengjing times], 24 October 1940, 4.

Jin Long. "Yan ke bao jian" [Smoke wanderer encyclopedia]. *Shengjing shibao* [Shengjing times], 18 June 1930, 9.

–. "Yapian yin zhi yanjiu" [Opium addiction research]. *Shengjing shibao* [Shengjing times], 11 January 1930, 9.

–. "Yapian yin zhi yanjiu" [Opium addiction research]. *Shengjing shibao* [Shengjing times], 12 January 1930, 9.

–. "Yapian yin zhi yanjiu" [Opium addiction research]. *Shengjing shibao* [Shengjing times], 13 January 1930, 5.

–. "Yapian yin zhi yanjiu" [Opium addiction research]. *Shengjing shibao* [Shengjing times], 14 January 1930, 9.

Jin Yin. "Muchang shang de xueyuan" [Blood ties on the pasture]. In Jin Yin, ed., *Manzhou zuojia xiaoshuoji* [Collected novels of Manchurian writers] (Xinjing: Wuxing shulin, 1944). Reprinted in Liang Shanding, ed., *Zhuxin ji* [Candlewick collection], 306-32. Shenyang: Chunfeng wenyi chubanshe, 1989.

Jing Chun. "Jie yan ge" [Quit smoking song]. *Shengjing shibao* [Shengjing times], 10 April 1941, 7.

"Jingli de yuanquan" [Source of energy]. *Datong bao* [Great unity herald], 3 November 1941, 4.

"Jinlin de Zhao laoyezi" [Neighbour Master Zhao]. In Kakegawa Akikuni, ed., *Qu tan conglin, di'yi ji* [Interesting discussion thicket, volume number 1], 1-8. Fengtian: Xing Ya yinshua zhushi huishe, 1942.

"Jiu, yanjuan, cha neng qi xueyagao yu jingli: Shenghuo zhi guanxi" [Alcohol, rolled tobacco, and tea can raise high blood pressure and energy: The relationship with life]. *Shengjing shibao* [Shengjing times], 31 January 1935, 5.

"Jiu, yanpao, tangtou: Suitong shuilu tigao jiage, ershi ba qian suo zhe buxu zhangti" [Alcohol, tobacco, and sugar: Following taxes, prices rise: Those before the 28th are not allowed to raise prices]. *Shengjing shibao* [Shengjing times], 28 December 1940, 7.

"Jiu hou wude, ou bi renming" [After drinking, no morality, beats and drives out person]. *Shengjing shibao* [Shengjing times], 7 October 1936, 12.

"Jiu hou wude hu qiangqiang hu: Bai Linfu chu tuxing shi nian" [After drinking, no morality rob by force: Bai Lingfu sentenced to prison for ten years]. *Shengjing shibao* [Shengjing times], 12 November 1937, 2.

"Jiu jin kai hou, Mei jing qiguan" [After Prohibition ended, the American environment has strange vision]. *Shengjing shibao* [Shengjing times], 18 April 1933, 3.

"Jiu ke wuli nao" [Drunkard is a nuisance]. *Shengjing shibao* [Shengjing times], 4 October 1938, 5.

"Jiu lun" [Discussion of alcohol]. *Shengjing shibao* [Shengjing times], 9 April 1931, 3.

"Jiu luo, liang zhang, shui zhong" [Alcohol down, grains rise, taxes heavy]. *Shengjing shibao* [Shengjing times], 20 October 1934, 9.

"Jiu shou wai jiu yingxiang: Jiu jia yi pi zai pi" [Alcohol influenced by nonlocal alcohol: Alcohol prices lower again and again]. *Shengjing shibao* [Shengjing times], 20 July 1941, 6.

"Jiu shui fa gongbu" [Alcohol tax law proclamation]. *Shengjing shibao* [Shengjing times], 29 July 1935, 2.

"Jiu wei xing Ya zhi di" [Alcohol is the enemy of a prospering Asia]. *Shengjing shibao* [Shengjing times], 2 September 1941, 7.

"Jiu yu fang die zhi guanxi" [Relationship between alcohol and guarding against espionage]. *Jian'guo jiaoyu* [Building the country's education] 9, 11 (1943): 47.

"Jiu yu shensi" [Alcohol and development of the state of mind]. *Shengjing shibao* [Shengjing times], 26 February 1941, 3.

"Jiu yu yousheng zhi guanxi" [The relationship between alcohol and eugenics]. *Shengjing shibao* [Shengjing times], 29 April 1943, 4.

"Jiu zhi bie ming kao" [Different names for alcohol test]. *Shang gong yuekan* [Commerce and industry monthly] 7 (1942): 66.

"Jiu zui shenye gui jia: Zhuchu fa qi you nü" [In the deep of the night, a drunk returns home and chases out his original wife and young daughter]. *Shengjing shibao* [Shengjing times], 31 May 1937, 3.

Jun Jun. "Xuediao huaping de chiyu ba" [Wipe out the shame of vases]. *Qilin* [Unicorn], March 1942, 136-37.

Jun Qing. "Tan pijiu, shang" [Talking beer, first]. *Shengjing shibao* [Shengjing times], 21 August 1937, 4.

Kakegawa Akikuni, ed. *Qu tan conglin, di'yi ji* [Interesting discussion thicket, volume number 1]. Fengtian: Xing Ya yinshua zhushi huishe, 1942.

Kangsheng yuan [Healthy Life Institute] ad. *Datong bao* [Great unity herald], 6 December 1941, 4.

"Kangsheng yuan Daode hui hezuo" [Co-operation between Healthy Life Institutes and the Morality Society]. *Shengjing shibao* [Shengjing times], 15 September 1944, 2.

Kawabe Taichi. "Kunao zhi weichang shuairuo" [The distress of gastrointestinal weakness]. Yangming jiu [Life Support Wine] ad. *Shengjing shibao* [Shengjing times], 4 October 1935, 3.

Ke Chang. "Zhou Zuoren Xiansheng yulu" [Quotations of Mr. Zhou Zuoren]. *Qilin* [Unicorn], March 1943, 84-85.

Ke Ju. *Xiang huai* [Homesickness]. Xinjing: Zongdai shusuo, 1941.

Kin Mitsunari. Yangming jiu [Life Support Wine] ad. *Qilin* [Unicorn], September 1941, 4.

Kirin [Unicorn] ad. *Shengjing shibao* [Shengjing times], 11 May 1911, supplement.

–. *Shengjing shibao* [Shengjing times], 10 July 1933, supplement.
–. *Shengjing shibao* [Shengjing times], 20 June 1934, 3.
–. *Shengjing shibao* [Shengjing times], 6 May 1937, 6.
Kunito Sadao. "Manzhou weisheng xue dayao, qi'san" [Main points of Manchurian hygiene studies, part three]. *Dongfang yixue zazhi* [Far Eastern medical journal] 16, 4 (1938): 155-72.
Lan Ling. "Guxiang de jia" [Native place home]. *Daban Huawen meiri* [Chinese Osaka daily], 10.1, 1943, 34-38.
"Lao yinshi bu ting quangao, xiao yingxiong jinggao dangguan" [Old addict does not listen to advice, little hero warns officials]. *Qilin* [Unicorn], June 1941, 85.
Leng Fo. "Jin yan wenti" [Opium prohibition question]. *Shengjing shibao* [Shengjing times], 24 March 1929, 7.
–. "Shang sheng de jiu" [The harmful nature of alcohol]. *Shengjing shibao* [Shengjing times], 20 January 1931, 4.
–. "Shang sheng de jiu" [The harmful nature of alcohol]. *Shengjing shibao* [Shengjing times], 30 January 1931, 4.
Leng Mei. "Putaojiu" [Grape wine]. *Shengjing shibao* [Shengjing times], 1 January 1933, 2.
Li Lili. "Wen jiu shi nanren" [Smell wine, know men]. In Li Tongfeng and Zou Changshun, eds., *Jiu zhi yun* [The charm of alcohol], 89-90. Shenyang: Liaohai chubanshe, 2007.
Li Qiao. *Xue ren tu* [Bloody sword scheme]. *Wensuan* [Literary collective] 2 (1940). Reprinted in Zhang Yumao, ed., *Dongbei xiandai wenxue daxi, 1919-1949: Xiju juan* [Compendium of modern northeastern literature, 1919-49: Volume of plays], 14 vols., vol. 13, 237-80. Shenyang: Shenyang chubanshe, 1996.
Li Shixun. "Jin yan xingzheng zhi zhongdian" [Serious points regarding the official policy of banning smoking]. *Shengjing shibao* [Shengjing times], 4 May 1941, 8.
Li Tongfeng and Zou Changshun, eds. *Jiu zhi yun* [The charm of alcohol]. Shenyang: Liaohai chubanshe, 2007.
Li Xianglan. *Zai Zhongguo de rizi: Wo de ban sheng* [Days in China: My half-life]. Hong Kong: Baixing wenhua shirong youxian gongshi, 1988.
Li Zhengping. *Zhongguo jiu wenhua* [Chinese alcohol culture]. Beijing: Shishi chubanshe, 2006.
Li Zhiting, ed. *Zhongguo bianjiang tongshi congshu: Dongbei bianshi* [A complete history of China's borders: Northeast borderland]. Zhengzhou: Zhengzhou guji chubanshe, 2003.
Lian. "Tan jiu (shang)" [Discussion of alcohol (first)]. *Shengjing shibao* [Shengjing times], 24 September 1938, 4.
–. "Tan jiu (xia)" [Discussion of alcohol (second)]. *Shengjing shibao* [Shengjing times], 25 September 1938, 5.
Lin Lu. "Yin jiu you yi tan" [Discussion of the benefits of drinking alcohol]. *Shengjing shibao* [Shengjing times], 28 July 1936, 5.
Ling Hua. "Wei *Nü zhaodai quan ji* zuo xu" [Preface to *Hostess Complete Collection*]. In Yu Zhizhu, ed., *Nü zhaodai quan ji* [Hostess complete collection], 3-4. Tianjin: Lanhua guanggao she, 1933.
"Lingmaisuo nü zhaodai: Ji qin, ji zong – shi wei quidi!" [Opium retail outlet hostesses: Several times captured, several times set free – the so-called ban!]. *Shengjing shibao* [Shengjing times], 6 March 1935, 7.
"Lingmaisuo qing huifu nü zhaodai you bei bo" [Opium retail outlets' pleas to resume hostesses were refuted]. *Shengjing shibao* [Shengjing times], 20 November 1935, 4.
"Lingmaisuo quxiao nü zhaodai" [Opium retail outlets abolish hostesses]. *Shengjing shibao* [Shengjing times], 30 December 1933, 4.

Liu Guojun. "Jin yan yu juewu" [Ban opium and consciousness]. *Datong bao* [Great unity herald], 23 October 1941, 4.

Liu Jinghui. *Minzu, xingbie yu jieceng* [Nation, gender, and social stratum]. Beijing: Shehui kexue wenxian chubanshe, 2004.

Liu Jingliang. "Kangsheng zhong de wo" [Me in the Healthy Life Institute]. *Shengjing shibao* [Shengjing times], 17 October 1941, 8.

Liu Lang. "Jieyan yu jieyan yao" [Quit smoking and quit smoking medicine]. *Shengjing shibao* [Shengjing times], 18 August 1935, 9.

Lu Shouxin. "Ha'erbin de yapian yandu" [Harbin's poisonous opium smoke]. In Sun Bang, ed., *Wei Man wenhua* [Bogus Manchukuo culture], in *Wei Man shiliao congshu* [Collection of historical materials on bogus Manchukuo], 10 vols., vol. 6, 445-46. Changchun: Jilin renmin chubanshe, 1993.

Lü Yonghua. *Wei Man shiqi de dongbei yandu* [Opium poison in the northeast during the bogus Manchukuo era]. Changchun: Jilin renmin chubanshe, 2004.

Ma Ji. "Tiantang de kangsheng yuan" [The heavenly Healthy Life Institute]. *Shengjing shibao* [Shengjing times], 20 March 1941, 8.

"Mafei hai ren" [Morphine harms people]. *Shengjing shibao* [Shengjing times], 23 August 1916, 5.

"Mafei wei lu" [The dead end of morphine]. *Shengjing shibao* [Shengjing times], 10 January 1917, 5.

"Mafei zhi hai" [The harm of morphine]. *Shengjing shibao* [Shengjing times], 30 December 1933, 4.

"Maijiu shiye zhi hua qi: Nanbei Manzhou zhi daibiao Fengtian ji Ha shi" [Planning stage of the beer business: The representative cities of south and north Manchuria, Fengtian and Harbin]. *Shengjing shibao* [Shengjing times], 8 December 1936, 12.

Manshu [Manchuria] ad. *Shengjing shibao* [Shengjing times], 26 June 1920, 8.

"Mayao yinzhe de wang'en" [The ingratitude of anaesthetic addicts]. In Kakegawa Akikuni, ed., *Qu tan conglin, di'yi ji* [Interesting discussion thicket, volume number 1], 49-54. Fengtian: Xing Ya yinshua zhushi huishe, 1942.

Mei Niang. "Bang" [Clam]. In *Yu* [Fish]. Beijing: Xinmin yinshuguan, 1943. Reprinted in Liang Shanding, ed., *Changye yinghuo* [Fireflies of the long night], 158-216. Shenyang: Chunfeng wenyi chubanshe, 1986.

—. "Wo de qingshao nian shiqi: 1920-1938" [My childhood: 1920-1938]. In Zhang Quan, ed., *Xunzhao Mei Niang* [Searching for Mei Niang], 97-128. Beijing: Mingjing chubanshe, 1998.

—. "Zhui" [The chase]. In *Di'er dai* [The second generation], 129-44. Xinjing: Wencong han xinghui, 1940.

—. "Zuihou de qiuzhenzhe" [The last patient]. In *Di'er dai* [The second generation], 87-92. Xinjing: Wencong han xinghui, 1940.

Mei Shan. "Jiu you hai?" [Alcohol has harm?]. *Shengjing shibao* [Shengjing times], 17 March 1933, 5.

"Meiguo jiujin chong kai hou" [After American Prohibition began]. *Shengjing shibao* [Shengjing times], 22 February 1933, 3.

Miura Keiko. Yangming jiu [Life Support Wine] ad. *Qilin* [Unicorn], January 1943, 8.

Mou Jianping. "Wei Man de dupin zhengce" [The narcotic policies of bogus Manchukuo). In Sun Bang, ed., *Jingji lüeduo* [Plundering the economy], in *Wei Man shiliao congshu* [Collection of historical materials on bogus Manchukuo], 10 vols., vol. 4, 721-24. Changchun: Jilin renmin chubanshe, 1993.

Nakamura Kōjirō. "Kessenka no sake to tabako" [Sake and tobacco under the condition of total war]. *Manshū kōron* [Manchuria debate], March 1945, 58-61.

Ni Fuzhi. "Shen lun zhi de jiao xing tan" [Talking about a degenerate's awakening]. *Shengjing shibao* [Shengjing times], 17 October 1940, 5.

"Niangjiu gongye zhi jingsui" [The quintessence of the fermented alcohol business]. *Shengjing shibao* [Shengjing times], 18 June 1936, 13.

Nie'ou'moxi'en [Neo-Mohyn] ad. *Shengjing shibao* [Shengjing times], 12 June 1936, 10.

"Nü shifan chuangban yan jiu zizhi hui zhi xian sheng" [Women's teacher training institute heralds the establishment of a smoke and alcohol self-cure association]. *Shengjing shibao* [Shengjing times], 13 April 1916, 4.

"Nü yinzhi: Xing xing ba!" [Female addicts: Wake up!]. *Shengjing shibao* [Shengjing times], 5 September 1941, 5.

"Nü zhaodai ai yun: Bu jing yan guan zhi fan guan, yi jiang shou chedi qudi" [Hostesses have bad luck: Not only banned in opium dens but immediately in restaurants, also will eventually be completely banned]. *Shengjing shibao* [Shengjing times], 13 January 1934, 4.

"Nü zhaodai jian ying fu ye, yin chu cha jin" [Hostesses holding jobs as a side business, should be quickly investigated and forbidden]. *Shengjing shibao* [Shengjing times], 14 July 1935, 11.

"Nü zhaodai kai hui fandui na juan" [Hostesses hold a meeting to oppose paying contributions]. *Shengjing shibao* [Shengjing times], 27 December 1935, 12.

"Nü zhaodai quxiao hou, yan guan za shou daji: Dong Guxuan lingxian chengqing zhong" [After hostesses were banned, opium dens were struck down: Dong Guxuan took a leading role in applying to the authorities for approval]. *Shengjing shibao* [Shengjing times], 10 December 1933, 4.

"Nü zhaodai shi ye hou, ji han jiaobo, shang yi er ci huyu" [After hostesses lose their profession, hunger and cold together compel them to yet propose a second appeal]. *Shengjing shibao* [Shengjing times], 7 December 1933, 4.

"Nüren de nashou shiqing" [Women's expertise matters]. *Qilin* [Unicorn], August 1941, 59.

Ōuchi Takao. "Shi jiu ji qi ta" [Poetry, alcohol, and the others]. *Xin Manzhou* [New Manchuria], January 1943, 68.

Ouzika gaoliang jiu er'shi wu hao de jiu [Gaoliang Vodka Alcohol, Brand No. 25] ad. *Shengjing shibao* [Shengjing times], 12 February 1935, 3.

"Paichu yapian mayao liudu" [Eliminate the pernicious influence of opium and morphine]. *Shengjing shibao* [Shengjing times], 27 October 1940, 4.

"Pang!" [Fat!]. *Shengjing shibao* [Shengjing times], 22 April 1938, 3.

Paulès, Xavier. "Drogue et transgressions sociales: Les femmes et l'opium à Canton dans les années 1930" [Drugs and social transgressions: Women and opium in 1930s Canton]. *Clio: Histoire, femmes et sociétés* [Clio: History, women, and societies] 28 (2008): 223-42.

Pei Ru. "Weisheng: Wo zhi jin jiu dongji" [Hygiene: My motivation for quitting drinking]. *Shengjing shibao* [Shengjing times], 4 February 1923, 5.

–. "Weisheng: Wo zhi jin jiu dongji" [Hygiene: My motivation for quitting drinking]. *Shengjing shibao* [Shengjing times], 6 February 1923, 5.

–. "Weisheng: Wo zhi jin jiu dongji" [Hygiene: My motivation for quitting drinking]. *Shengjing shibao* [Shengjing times], 8 February 1923, 5.

"Pijiu peiji fangfa gaishan: Yi minzhong xuyong wei zhudian" [Beer ration method improvements: The main point is the needs of the common people]. *Shengjing shibao* [Shengjing times], 1 July 1941, 5.

Ping shi yi zhaodai. "Women de jianglai" [Our future]. In Yu Zhizhu, ed., *Nü zhaodai quan ji* [Hostess complete collection], 48-51. Tianjin: Lanhua guanggao she, 1933.

"Pohuai jiankang de si da dusu: Bianbidu, jiehedu, jiudu, yandu" [The four big poisons that destroy health: Constipation, tuberculosis, alcohol, and smoking]. *Jiankang Manzhou* [Healthy Manchuria] 2, 5 (1940): 36.

Puluojiabing ad. *Shengjing shibao* [Shengjing times], 6 June 1934, 14.

"Putaojiu yu putaojiu zhi shuo" [Grape wine and talk of grape wine]. *Shengjing shibao* [Shengjing times], 30 April 1939, supplement.

Qi Jinchang. "Jie yan jiu lun" [Discussion of quitting smoking and drinking]. *Shengjing shibao* [Shengjing times], 31 January 1942, 2.

Qiao Enrun. "Yapian zhi hai shenyu hongshuimengshou" [The harm of opium is worse than fierce floods and savage beasts]. *Shengjing shibao* [Shengjing times], 15 October 1944, 2.

"Qifo'a'nadunai: Jiu se zhi cheng" [Tijuana: Alcohol-coloured city]. *Shengjing shibao* [Shengjing times], 15 May 1937, 6.

"Qin'ai de Liu Zheng xian di" [Dear first brother Liu Zheng]. In Kakegawa Akikuni, ed., *Qu tan conglin, di'yi ji* [Interesting discussion thicket, volume number 1], 101-16. Fengtian: Xing Ya yinshua zhushi huishe, 1942.

"Qingtian zai lai di shang" [Sunny days come again to the land]. In Kakegawa Akikuni, ed., *Qu tan conglin, di'yi ji* [Interesting discussion thicket, volume number 1], 117-25. Fengtian: Xing Ya yinshua zhushi huishe, 1942.

"Qingzhu chengren Manzhouguo" [Celebrate the recognition of Manchukuo]. *Shengjing shibao* [Shengjing times], 16 September 1932, 6.

Qiu Shan. "Yapian huo zai Manzhou de jinhou, shang" [Opium calamity in Manchuria from now on, first]. *Datong bao* [Great unity herald], 15 February 1939, 15.

Qiu Ying. *He liu de diceng* [The bottom of the river]. Dalian: Shiye yanghang chubanbu faxing, 1941. Reprinted under name of Wang Qiuying, in Kong Fanjin, ed., *Zhongguo xiandai wenxue buyi shuxi* [Addendum of modern Chinese literature series], 8 vols., vol. 5, 720-849. Jinan: Mingtian chubanshe, 1990.

–. "Lou xiang" [Vulgar alley]. *Chuangzuo liancong* [Creative crowd] 2 (1944). Reprinted in Liang Shanding, ed., *Zhuxin ji* [Candlewick collection], 111-42. Shenyang: Chunfeng wenyi chubanshe, 1989.

Qu Bingshan. "Yapian zhuanmai yu duhai" [The Opium Monopoly and poison]. In Sun Bang, ed., *Jingji lüeduo* [Plundering the economy], in *Wei Man shiliao congshu* [Collection of historical materials on bogus Manchukuo], 10 vols., vol. 4, 687-92. Changchun: Jilin renmin chubanshe, 1993.

Qu Kezhong. "Jin yan bai zi ci" [Banning smoking one hundred word poem]. *Shengjing shibao* [Shengjing times], 7 June 1941, 8.

"Qudi de juewu" [Understanding the ban]. *Shengjing shibao* [Shengjing times], 10 April 1941, 7.

"Qudi yapian lingmaisuo: Nü zhaodai zhi wengao" [Banned in the opium retail outlets: Proclamation of the hostesses]. *Shengjing shibao* [Shengjing times], 27 February 1934, 3.

Ren Ji. "Jin jiu zhi yi" [The benefit of banning alcohol]. *Shengjing shibao* [Shengjing times], 11 April 1934, 11.

"Rensheng benneng de kuaile bu ru yangyuan daiqi zi yong" [Life's instinctual happiness is not as good as nourishment about to increase]. *Shengjing shibao* [Shengjing times], 22 November 1932, 8.

"Ri jin jiu tongmeng paiyuan lai Man" [The Japanese Prohibit Alcohol Alliance members come to Manchukuo]. *Shengjing shibao* [Shengjing times], 8 September 1933, 4.

"Riben pijiu jie: Shengchan jizeng" [Japanese beer world: Production increases]. *Shengjing shibao* [Shengjing times], 13 August 1933, 7.

Ru Gai. "Su zhi jie yan jingyan tan, san" [Discussion of my experience quitting smoking, three]. *Shengjing shibao* [Shengjing times], 14 November 1930, 7.

–. "Su zhi jie yan jingyan tan, si" [Discussion of my experience quitting smoking, four]. *Shengjing shibao* [Shengjing times], 20 November 1930, 7.

−. "Yu zhi jie yan jingyan" [After quitting smoking experience]. *Shengjing shibao* [Shengjing times], 30 November 1930, 7.

Ruo Xue. "Xie zai *Nü zhaodai quan ji* zhi qian" [Writing preceding the *Hostess Complete Collection*]. In Yu Zhizhu, ed., *Nü zhaodai quan ji* [Hostess complete collection], 1. Tianjin: Lanhua guanggao she, 1933.

Ruosu [Basic Element] ad. *Qilin* [Unicorn], November 1941, 16.

−. *Qilin* [Unicorn], December 1943, back cover.

−. *Qilin* [Unicorn], July 1944, back cover.

−. *Qilin* [Unicorn], February/March 1945, back cover.

−. *Shengjing shibao* [Shengjing times], 2 November 1932, 8.

−. *Shengjing shibao* [Shengjing times], 26 November 1932, 8.

−. *Shengjing shibao* [Shengjing times], 28 June 1940, 5.

"Ruosu chengfen you tianran zucheng" [Basic Element ingredients are natural compositions]. *Shengjing shibao* [Shengjing times], 26 November 1932, 8.

"Ruosu zhi renshou fangfa" [Basic Element's workforce method]. *Shengjing shibao* [Shengjing times], 26 November 1932, 8.

Sakura [Cherry] ad. *Shengjing shibao* [Shengjing times], 2 September 1915, 4.

−. *Shengjing shibao* [Shengjing times], 16 June 1936, supplement.

San Lang. "Zhuxin" [Candlewick]. In San Lang and Qiao Yin, *Bashe* [Trek]. Harbin: Wuri huakan yinshuashe, 1933. Reprinted in Liang Shanding, ed., *Zhuxin ji* [Candlewick collection], 1-20. Shenyang: Chunfeng wenyi chubanshe, 1989.

Sapporo and Asahi ad. *Manchuria*, 1 November 1937, 759.

Shangguan Ying. "Zhang Chunyuan he *Hua zhong hen*" [Zhang Chunyan and *Flowers among the Hate*]. In *Dongbei lunxian qu wenxue shihua* [Talking about the literary history of the Northeast enemy-occupied area], 149-51. Changchun: Changchun shi zhengxie wenshi ziliao weiyuanhui, 2006.

Shao Guanzhi. "Yan, jiu yu renti" [Tobacco, alcohol, and the human body]. *Jiankang Manzhou* [Healthy Manchuria] 3.5 (1941): 14-15.

Shen Kechang. "Nü zhaodai riji" [Hostess diary]. In Yu Zhizhu, ed., *Nü zhaodai quan ji* [Hostess complete collection], 16-20. Tianjin: Lanhua guanggao she, 1933.

Shen rong hugu yanshou jiu [Ginseng, Antler, Tiger Bone Prolong Life Wine] ad. *Shengjing shibao* [Shengjing times], 21 July 1938, 3.

Shenxiao hugu yaojiu [Magic Tiger Bone Medicinal Wine] ad. *Shengjing shibao* [Shengjing times], 19 October 1911, 6.

"Shenyang jingcha ting Kangde san nian weisheng nianjian, qi'er" [Shenyang police office 1936 hygiene yearbook, part two]. *Dongfang yixue zazhi* [Far Eastern medical journal] 15, 3 (1937): 178-226.

"Shenyang jingcha ting Kangde yuan nian weisheng nianjian" [Shenyang police office 1934 hygiene yearbook]. *Dongfang yixue zazhi* [Far Eastern medical journal] 13, 6 (1935): 215-62.

Shenyang shi Lao long kou jiuchang bianzuan bangongshi, ed. *Shenyang shi Lao long kou jiuchangzhi* [Shenyang city's Lao long kou (Old Dragon Mouth) wine factory records]. Shenyang: Shenyang chubanshe, 1993.

Shi Zhizi. "Ou'gan ou'ji bingyu tan" [A discussion of occassional feelings, occassional memories]. *Xin qingnian* [New youth] October (1937). Reprinted in Qian Liqun, ed., *Zhongguo lunxianqu wenxue daxi: Pinglun juan* [Compendium of the literature of China's enemy-occupied territories: Volume of commentary], 390-94. Nanling, Guangxi: Guangxi jiaoyu chubanshe, 2000.

"Shoudu jinyan xuanchuan dahui" [Capital city forbid opium publicity meeting]. *Shengjing shibao* [Shengjing times], 29 April 1943, 4.

Shu Shi. "Zui" [Intoxication]. *Qingnian wenhua* [Youth culture] 2, 6 (1944): 42-43.

"Shuzhang zhao ji lingmaisuo huiyi" [Director calls for meeting with retail stores]. *Shengjing shibao* [Shengjing times], 4 September 1936, 12.

"Si yu mafei" [Dead from morphine]. *Shengjing shibao* [Shengjing times], 13 December 1916, 5.

"Sikai yan guan qiangjian yanke: Shaonü zao roulin" [The rape of a guest in a private opium den: A young girl meets with devastation]. *Shengjing shibao* [Shengjing times], 18 August 1935, 2.

Su Jianxun. "Yinshi" [Addicts]. *Shengjing shibao* [Shengjing times], 17 October 1941, 8.

Takeo Akiyoshi. "Jie yan baihua" [Plain talk about quitting smoking]. *Shengjing shibao* [Shengjing times], 13 October 1906, 2.

–. "Jie yan baihua, xuqian" [Plain talk about quitting smoking, continued]. *Shengjing shibao* [Shengjing times], 14 October 1906, 2.

"Tang Xinji de shi gong" [Tang Xinji's true confession]. In Kakegawa Akikuni, ed., *Qu tan conglin, di'yi ji* [Interesting discussion thicket, volume number 1], 9-21. Fengtian: Xing Ya yinshua zhushi huishe, 1942.

Tsai Yu. "Cong yin jiu dao ziran: Yi Tao shi wei hexin tantao" [From drinking to nature: A study on the poetry of Tao Yuan-Ming]. *Taida zhongwen xuebao* [National Taiwan University Chinese journal] (22 June 2005): 223-68.

Wang Chengli. *Zhongguo Dongbei lunxian shisi nian shi gangyao* [Compendium of the fourteen-year history of the Northeast of China's enemy occupation]. Beijing: Zhongguo da bai liao chuan shu chubanshe, 1991.

Wang Dashan. "Jin yan ganyan" [Ban smoking heartfelt words]. *Shengjing shibao* [Shengjing times], 5 December 1940, 8.

Wang Luo. "Manzhouguo zhi yapian zhidu, di'er pian" [The Manchukuo opium system, part two]. *Dongfang yixue zazhi* [Far Eastern medical journal] 12, 12 (1934): 482-92.

Wang Shaoxian. "Wo guo jin zheng gaikuang" [Survey of my country's prohibit opium policy]. *Shengjing shibao* [Shengjing times], 6 March 1941, 8.

Wang Shigong, "Fengtian shi yapian yinzhe tongji de guancha" [Survey of Fengtian city opium addicts' statistics]. *Dongfang yixue zazhi* [Far Eastern medical journal] 13, 3 (1935): 85-98.

–. "Manzhouguo yapian wenti, di'yi: Fengtian shi yishi jiangxihui tebie jianyan yanchi" [The Manchukuo opium question, part one: Fengtian city medical doctor conference special speech draft]. *Shengjing shibao* [Shengjing times], 30 December 1936, 5.

Wang Xianwei. "Jin yan zhengce de qipian xing" [The fraudulent nature of the smoking prohibition]. In Sun Bang, ed., *Jingji lüeduo* [Plundering the economy], in *Wei Man shiliao congshu* [Collection of historical materials on bogus Manchukuo], 10 vols., vol. 4, 709-13. Changchun: Jilin renmin chubanshe, 1993.

"Wangdao yao gong ke yun weida" [You may say the efficacy of the Kingly Way medicine is mighty]. *Shengjing shibao* [Shengjing times], 26 November 1932, 8.

Wanling fenghan hugu jiu [Cold Souls Tiger Bone Wine] ad. *Shengjing shibao* [Shengjing times], 8 December 1922, 8.

"Wei baoquan jiu lei, shi shi xuke ji" [To protect various kinds of alcohol, implementation of permit system]. *Shengjing shibao* [Shengjing times], 28 December 1940, 7.

Wei Cheng. "Kuilan de du shi" [The festering, poisoned tongue]. *Qilin* [Unicorn], July 1942, 142-49.

Wei Zhonglan. "Xin Zhongguo nüxing de dongjing" [Sounds of the new Chinese women's movement]. *Qingnian wenhua* [Youth culture] 1, 3 (1943): 33-35.

Wen Long, ed. *Zhongguo jiu dian* [Chinese alcohol code]. Changchun: Jilin chuban jituan youxian guiren gongsi, 2010.

Wu Lang. "Women de wenxue de shiti yu fangxiang" [The substance and direction of our literature], *Daban Huawen meiri* [Chinese Osaka daily], 15 January 1941. Reprinted in

Qian Liqun, ed., *Zhongguo lunxianqu wenxue daxi: Pinglun juan* [Compendium of the literature of China's enemy-occupied territories: Volume of commentary], 395-401. Nanling, Guangxi: Guangxi jiaoyu chubanshe, 2000.

Wu Ying. "Gui" [Deceit]. In *Liang ji* [Two extremes], 93-105. Xinjing: Wenyi conghan hanxinghui, 1939.

—. "Jiu li chunhou" [Alcohol's strength is rich]. *Qilin* [Unicorn], September 1942, 26.

"Wuye gong yin jiuzui dongwu" [Drinking until midnight, start a fight]. *Shengjing shibao* [Shengjing times], 10 January 1935, 4.

Xian you [Virtuous Friend] and Ju quan [Chrysanthemum Spring] ad. *Shengjing shibao* [Shengjing times], 20 June 1934, 8.

—. *Shengjing shibao* [Shengjing times], 24 July 1934, 3.

"Xiang guomin zhuwei ji ju hua" [A few words to citizens]. *Shengjing shibao* [Shengjing times], 10 April 1941, 7.

Xiang Naixi. "Jie yan yu jie yan yao" [Quit smoking and quit smoking medicine]. *Shengjing shibao* [Shengjing times], 22 October 1935, 9.

—. "Manxing mayao zhong duzhe xinli de guancha, qi'er" [Survey of the psychology of chronic morphine drug users, part two]. *Dongfang yixue zazhi* [Far Eastern medical journal] 15, 9 (1937): 498-511.

—. "Xiandai Hanyi suo yong zhi jieyan fang" [Modern Chinese medicine methods of quitting smoking]. *Dongfang yixue zazhi* [Far Eastern medical journal] 15, 8 (1937): 441-64.

Xiao Ling. "Tan jiu yu tang" [Discussion of alcohol and sugar]. *Qilin* [Unicorn], January 1942, 151.

Xiao Song. "Yiwenjia gankuai wuzhuang qilai" [Writers and artists militarize quickly]. *Qilin* [Unicorn], November 1944, 48.

"Xiaozhang xiansheng" [Mr. principal]. In Kakegawa Akikuni, ed., *Qu tan conglin, di'yi ji* [Interesting discussion thicket, volume number 1], 55-72. Fengtian: Xing Ya yinshua zhushi huishe, 1942.

"Xiguan wu" [Custom error]. In Kakegawa Akikuni, ed., *Qu tan conglin, di'yi ji* [Interesting discussion thicket, volume number 1], 46-48. Fengtian: Xing Ya yinshua zhushi huishe, 1942.

"Xin guomin yundong de quchu yapian zuotanhui" [New citizens' movement to get rid of opium forum]. *Xin Manzhou* [New Manchuria], August 1941, 26-31.

"Xin sheng qu" [New life melody]. *Qilin* [Unicorn], July 1944, 22.

"Xin shui fa shi yi, di'jiu" [New tax laws explanation, part nine]. *Shengjing shibao* [Shengjing times], 10 September 1941, 1.

"Xu Biyun deng qiman li lian, nü zhaodaimen ye jiang ying zhi, dasa fengjing de liang chun shi" [Xu Biyun, awaiting the time contracted to depart Dalian: Hostesses will soon be disappearing: Big murder scenery, two events]. *Shengjing shibao* [Shengjing times], 13 April 1936, 3.

Xu Bochun. "Tiantang de kangsheng yuan" [The heavenly Healthy Life Institute]. *Shengjing shibao* [Shengjing times], 20 April 1941, 8.

Xu Naixiang and Huang Wanhua. *Zhongguo kangzhan shiqi lunxianqu wenxue shi* [History of the literature of the enemy-occupied territories during China's war of resistance]. Fuzhou: Fujian jiaoyu chubanshe, 1995.

Xuan Bingshan. *Minjian yinshi xisu* [Popular food and drink customs]. Beijing: Zhongguo shehui chubanshe, 2006.

"Xuanming ahpian duanjin guoce" [Announcing the opium prohibition national policy]. *Shengjing shibao* [Shengjing times], 27 August 1942, 2.

Yamada Goichi. *Manshūkoku No Ahensenbai* [Opium monopoly in Manchuria]. Tokyo: Kyuko Shoen, 2002.

"Yan, jiu, cha, xiangliao gei ni de haochu?" [Smoke, alcohol, tea, and perfume give you a benefit?]. *Shengjing shibao* [Shengjing times], 12 October 1940, 4.

"Yan, jiu, cha yu jiankang de yinxiang" [The influence of tobacco, alcohol, and tea on health]. *Shengjing shibao* [Shengjing times], 9 January 1940, 2.

"Yan guan nü zhaodai shangfeng baisu: Wushun dangju yinhe bu gan?" [Opium den hostesses corrupt public morals: Wushun authorities – why can't they ban them?] *Shengjing shibao* [Shengjing times], 3 August 1935, 11.

"Yan hai tan" [Discussion of the harm of smoke]. *Shengjing shibao* [Shengjing times], 16 March 1935, 7.

"Yan jiu qunian shengchan liang" [Last year's production of tobacco and alcohol]. *Shengjing shibao* [Shengjing times], 31 March 1937, 7.

"Yan xun zhifu" [Opium patrol uniforms]. *Shengjing shibao* [Shengjing times], 21 August 1927, 5.

Yang Chaohui and An Linhai. "Wei Man shiqi de Rehe yapian" [Rehe opium during the bogus Manchukuo era]. In Sun Bang, ed., *Wei Man wenhua* [Bogus Manchukuo culture], in *Wei Man shiliao congshu* [Collection of historical materials on bogus Manchukuo], 10 vols., vol. 6. Changchun: Jilin renmin chubanshe, 1993.

Yang Jun. "Dongbeiren yu dongbei jiu wenhua" [Northeasterners and Northeast alcohol culture]. http://tieba.baidu.com/.

Yang Xu. "Gongkai de zuizhuang" [Open indictment]. In *Wo de riji* [My diary], 89-113. Xinjing: Kaiming tushu gongsi, 1944.

–. "Laomazi riji" [Nanny's diary]. In *Wo de riji* [My diary], 34-48. Xinjing: Kaiming tushu gongsi, 1944.

–. "Zui" [Intoxication]. In *Luoying ji* [Collection of fallen petals], 124-25. Xinjing: Kaiming tushu gongsi, 1943.

Yangming jiu [Life Support Wine] ad. *Qilin* [Unicorn], August 1943, 4.

–. *Shengjing shibao* [Shengjing times], 4 October 1935, 3.

–. *Shengjing shibao* [Shengjing times], 19 December 1935, 13.

–. *Shengjing shibao* [Shengjing times], 20 June 1937, 12.

Yao Jibin. *Jiankang zhi dao* [The Path of Health]. Shenyang: Yao Shi yiyuan, 1948.

–. "Weisheng: Jiu de duhai (xia)" [Hygiene: The poisonous harm of alcohol (second)]. *Shengjing shibao* [Shengjing times], 15 March 1935, 9.

"Yapian xiao maisuo jie genü zhao ji ke" [Small opium retail outlets use singing girls to attract guests]. *Shengjing shibao* [Shengjing times], 5 June 1931, 5.

Ye Fengsheng. Yangming jiu [Life Support Wine] ad. *Shengjing shibao* [Shengjing times], 19 February 1941, 5.

Ye Li. "San ren" [Three people]. In *Hua zhong* [Flower tomb]. Xinjing: Zhushi huishe dadi tushu gongsi, 1944. Reprinted in Liang Shanding, ed., *Zhuxin ji* [Candlewick collection], 254-68. Shenyang: Chunfeng wenyi chubanshe, 1989.

Ye Xing. "Jiu yu nüren" [Wine and women]. *Shengjing shibao* [Shengjing times], 30 November 1941, 7.

"'Yi bei jiu jie qian chou,' danshi zheyang shihou, qing nin bu yao yin jiu" ['One cup of alcohol can relieve a thousand worries,' but in these times please do not drink alcohol]. *Shengjing shibao* [Shengjing times], 18 July 1937, 5.

Yi Bi. "Jiu min zhong zhong" [A variety of alcohol people]. In Li Tongfeng and Zou Changshun, eds., *Jiu zhi yun* [The charm of alcohol], 105-7. Shenyang: Liaohai chubanshe, 2007.

Yi Chi. "Guanyu wo de chuangzuo" [Concerning my creative work]. In *Hua yue ji* [The flower moon collection]. Xinjing: Yishu yanjiu hui, 1938. Reprinted in Zhang Yumao, ed., *Dongbei xiandai wenxue daxi, 1919-49: Sanwen juan* [Compendium of modern northeastern literature, 1919-49: Volume of prose], 14 vols., vol. 10, 729-32. Shenyang: Shenyang chubanshe, 1996.

Yi Mei. "Jiu yu ji" [Alcohol and prostitutes]. *Shengjing shibao* [Shengjing times], 11 May 1933, 9.

Yi Xi. "Jiu de ziwei" [The taste of alcohol]. *Shengjing shibao* [Shengjing times], 20 February 1933, 3.

Yi Yuan, ed. *Jiu mo: Jiu fengqing xiaopinji* [Alcohol mystics: Collection of essays on amorous feelings for alcohol]. Taibei: Yeqiang chuban, 1994.

Yin. "Tan yin jiu" [Discussion of drinking alcohol]. *Shengjing shibao* [Shengjing times], 29 May 1938, 4.

"Yin jiu mei shi shu duan shou ming" [Consuming alcohol and good food can shorten your life]. *Shengjing shibao* [Shengjing times], 7 January 1936, 10.

Yin Zhengping. "'Zui'e zhi hua' zai Dongbei – Riben zai Dongbei shixing de yan du zhengci" [The "pattern of crime" in the Northeast: Japan's implementation in the Northeast of an opium poison policy]. 2008. http://www.minge.gov.cn/.

Ying. "Quan fuqin jinyan shu" [Persuade father to quit smoking letter]. *Shengjing shibao* [Shengjing times], 17 October 1941, 8.

"Yinzhe denglu jiang jiezhi" [Addict registry about to be cut off]. *Shengjing shibao* [Shengjing times], 11 June 1938, 9.

"Yinzhe fuyin" [Glad tidings for addicts]. *Shengjing shibao* [Shengjing times], 24 May 1940, 4.

Yong Boping. "Yapian yu renti" [Opium and the human body]. *Shengjing shibao* [Shengjing times], 25 August 1936, 9.

–. "Yapian yu renti, xu" [Opium and the human body, continued]. *Shengjing shibao* [Shengjing times], 29 August 1936, 9.

Yong Shanqi. "Jin yan judu zhi juti fangce, si" [Concrete directives for banning smoking and refusing poison, four]. *Shengjing shibao* [Shengjing times], 17 October 1940, 5.

–. "Jin yan judu zhi juti fangce, qi" [Concrete directives for banning smoking and refusing poison, seven]. *Shengjing shibao* [Shengjing times], 5 December 1940, 8.

–. "Jin yan judu zhi juti fangce, xu" [Concrete directives for banning smoking and refusing poison, continued]. *Shengjing shibao* [Shengjing times], 19 December 1940, 8.

You You. "Mingri huang hua" [Tomorrow's yellow flower]. In Yu Zhizhu, ed., *Nü zhaodai quan ji* [Hostess complete collection], 5-14. Tianjin: Lanhua guanggao she, 1933.

You'ni'en [Union] ad. *Shengjing shibao* [Shengjing times], 17 July 1921, 3.

–. *Shengjing shibao* [Shengjing times], 16 May 1926, 8.

Yu Lei. "Ziliao" [Data]. *Dongbei wenxue yanjiu shiliao* [Historical research materials of northeastern literature] 6 (1987): 171-81.

Yu Li. "Funü xiyan zhi hai" [The harm of women's smoking]. *Jiankang Manzhou* [Healthy Manchuria] 2.7 (1940): 3-5.

"Yu shaonian de qi ji" [Young Yu's surprise plan]. In Kakegawa Akikuni, ed., *Qu tan conglin, di'yi ji* [Interesting discussion thicket, volume number 1], 73-91. Fengtian: Xing Ya yinshua zhushi huishe, 1942.

Yu Xuebin. *Dongbei zhaohuang* [Old signboards of the Northeast]. Shanghai: Shanghai shudian chubanshe, 2002.

"Yu zhi yan jiu jie jiekuan guan" [My point of view on borrowing money for opium and alcohol]. *Shengjing shibao* [Shengjing times], 16 September 1919, 1.

Yu Zhizhu, ed. *Nü zhaodai quan ji* [Hostess complete collection]. Tianjin: Lanhua guang-gao she, 1933.

Yue Ai. "Jin yan lun" [Discussion of opium prohibition]. *Shengjing shibao* [Shengjing times], 3 October 1941, 5.

"Zengjin jingli hulihua yundong" [A rational movement to promote energy]. *Shengjing shibao* [Shengjing times], 26 November 1932, 8.

Zhai Wenxuan. "Ji cheng fujian" [Memorial plan attachment]. *Fengtian guomin gongbao* [Fengtian national bulletin], 24 April 1929, 15-16.

Zhang Chunyuan. *Hen zhong hua* [Flowers among the hate]. Fengtian: Guandong shuju chubanshe, 1944.

"Zhang Dexin xiansheng" [Mr. Zhang Dexin]. In Kakegawa Akikuni, ed., *Qu tan conglin, di'yi ji* [Interesting discussion thicket, volume number 1], 97-100. Fengtian: Xing Ya yinshua zhushi huishe, 1942.

Zhang Feng. "Yin jiu xianhua" [Chatting about drinking alcohol]. *Shengjing shibao* [Shengjing times], 6 December 1935, 8.

Zhang Guochen. "Yaowuxue shiye zhong de yapian" [Opium in the view of pharmacology]. *Jiankang Manzhou* [Healthy Manchukuo] 3.4 (1941): 6-13.

Zhang Huinuan. *Beifang shaoshu minzu de jiu wenhua* [Northern national minority alcohol culture]. Huhhot: Nei Menggu daxue chubanshe, 2008.

Zhang Jiyou. "Yapian" [Opium]. *Jiankang Manzhou* [Healthy Manchuria] 1.3 (1939): 12-14.

Zhang Nianhui. "Jie yan si ji ge" [Four seasons of quitting smoking song]. *Shengjing shibao* [Shengjing times], 20 April 1941, 8.

Zhao Kuiru. "Dongtian de mafei ke" [Winter morphine wanderer]. *Shengjing shibao* [Shengjing times], 25 February 1934, 5.

Zhao Min. "Yapian duanjinzhe tiyan ji" [Personal notes on abstaining from opium]. *Shengjing shibao* [Shengjing times], 19 December 1940, 8.

Zheng Zhi. "Nü zhaodai de shouce" [A hostess handbook]. *Shengjing shibao* [Shengjing times], 21 January 1936, 5.

"Zhengli yinzhe suqing si yan guan: Wei jin yan zhengci de yaowu, Yu Sheng, weisheng chuzhang fabiao tanhua" [Straighten out addicts, eliminate private opium dens: Important items for the government policies of prohibiting opium, Yu Sheng, section chief of the hygiene department, publishes a statement]. *Shengjing shibao* [Shengjing times], 2 September 1941, 11.

Zhenhua yiyuan [China Rise with Force and Spirit Hospital]. "Jie yan" [Quit smoking] ad. *Shengjing shibao* [Shengjing times], 11 January 1932, 1.

Zhenhua yiyuan [China Rise with Force and Spirit Hospital] ad. *Shengjing shibao* [Shengjing times], 9 July 1939, 2.

Zhi Jing. "Tan yin jiu" [Discussion of drinking alcohol]. *Shengjing shibao* [Shengjing times], 30 July 1937, 4.

Zhi Xing. "Jiu yu tianzhen" [Alcohol and innocence]. *Shengjing shibao* [Shengjing times], 23 May 1937, 9.

Zhi Yuan. "Bai tenghua" [White vine flower]. *Huawen Daban meiri* [Chinese Osaka daily], 1943. Reprinted in Liang Shanding, ed., *Zhuxin ji* [Candlewick collection], 349-62. Shenyang: Chunfeng wenyi chubanshe, 1989.

Zhizhu. "Xie zai qian ye" [Writing on the front page]. In Yu Zhizhu, ed., *Nü zhaodai quan ji* [Hostess complete collection], 4. Tianjin: Lanhua guanggao she, 1933.

Zhong Xin. "Tan yin jiu" [Discussion of drinking alcohol]. *Shengjing shibao* [Shengjing times], 25 August 1935, 5.

Zhou Zuoren. "Mazui li zan" [Praise for anaesthesia]. In Yi Yuan, ed., *Jiumo: Jiu fengqing xiaopinji* [Alcohol mystics: Collection of essays on amorous feelings for alcohol], 22-25. Taibei: Yeqiang chuban, 1994.

–. "Tan jiu" [Talk alcohol]. In Yi Yuan, ed., *Jiumo: Jiu fengqing xiaopinji* [Alcohol mystics: Collection of essays on amorous feelings for alcohol], 18-21. Taibei: Yeqiang chuban, 1994.

Zhu Jiqing. "Canjia Meiguo gonggong weisheng xuehui di'liushi ci nianhui gan yan" [Moving words on participating in the American Public Health Association's 60th annual meeting]. *Dongfang yixue zazhi* [Far Eastern medical journal] 11, 1 (1933): 18-31.

Zhu Ruimei. *Yin jiu qudian* [Interesting quotations on drinking alcohol]. Taipei: Shixueshe chuban gufen youxian gongsi, 2004.

Zhu Ti. "Yuantian de liuxing" [A shooting star in a faraway sky]. *Xin chao* [New tide] 1, 7 (1943). Reprinted in *Ying* [Cherry], 82-98. Xinjing: Guomin tushu zhushi huishe, 1945.

"Zhuyi!! Yan du, jiu du, cha du: Yingdang zenyang jiuzhi" [Attention!! You ought to know how to cure tobacco poison, alcohol poison, and tea poison]. *Shengjing shibao* [Shengjing times], 5 April 1941, 4.

"Zi su ri: Jiu zheng ainao lixing jieyue, yan jin yan jiu du" [Self-respect time: Solemnly encouraging economizing: A serious ban on smoking, alcohol, and gambling]. *Shengjing shibao* [Shengjing times], 10 January 1940, 4.

Zuo Di. "Meiyou guang de xing" [A lustreless star], *Chuangzuo liancong* [Creative collection], February 1945, reprinted in Liang Shanding, ed., *Changye yinghuo* [Fireflies of the long night] (Shenyang: Chunfeng wenyi chubanshe, 1986), 436-56. Shenyang: Chunfeng wenyi chubanshe, 1986.

English-language sources

Amleto, Vespa. *Secret Agent of Japan: A Handbook to Japanese Imperialism*. London: Victor Gollancz, 1938.

Armstrong, David E. *Alcohol and Altered States in Ancestor Veneration Rituals of Zhou Dynasty China and Iron Age Palestine*. Lewiston, NY: Edwin Mellen, 1998.

Assemblies of God, Foreign Missions Department. *Gospel Rays in Manchoukuo*. Springfield, MO: Assemblies of God, 1937.

Bakich, Olga. "Did You Speak Harbin Sino-Russian." *Itinerario* 35.3 (March 2012): 23-36.

Barlow, Tani. "Theorizing Woman: *Funü, Guojia, Jiating*." *Genders* 10 (1991): 132-60.

Barnhart, Michael A. *Japan Prepares for Total War: The Search for Economic Security, 1919-41*. Ithaca, NY: Cornell University Press, 1987.

Baumler, Alan. *The Chinese and Opium under the Republic: Worse than Floods and Wild Beasts*. Albany: State University of New York Press, 2007.

Bello, David Anthony. *Opium and the Limits of Empire: Drug Prohibition in the Chinese Interior, 1729-1850*. Cambridge, MA: Harvard University Press, 2005.

Benedict, Carol. *Golden-Silk Smoke: A History of Tobacco in China, 1550-2010*. Berkeley: University of California Press, 2011.

Bix, Herbert. "Japanese Imperialism and the Manchurian Economy, 1900-31." *China Quarterly* 51 (1972): 425-43.

Borovy, Amy. *The Too-Good Wife: Alcohol, Codependency, and the Politics of Nurturance in Postwar Japan*. Berkeley: University of California Press, 2005.

"The Brewing Industry in Manchoukuo." *Contemporary Manchuria* 3.4 (1939): 63-78.

Brook, Timothy, and Bob Tadashi Wakabayashi. "Introduction: Opium's History in China." In Timothy Brook and Bob Tadashi Wakabayashi, eds., *Opium Regimes: China, Britain, and Japan, 1839-1952*, 1-29. Berkeley: University of California Press, 2000.

–. *Opium Regimes: China, Britain, and Japan, 1839-1952*. Berkeley: University of California Press, 2000.

Bufo Yamamuro. "Notes on Drinking in Japan." In Mac Marshall, ed., *Beliefs, Behaviors, and Alcoholic Beverages: A Cross-Cultural Survey*, 270-77. Ann Arbor: University of Michigan Press, 1979.

Bunting, Chris. *Drinking Japan: A Guide to Japan's Best Drinks and Drinking Establishments*. North Clarendon, VT: Tuttle Publishing, 2011.

Carstairs, Catherine. *Jailed for Possession: Illegal Drug Use, Regulation, and Power in Canada, 1920-1961*. Toronto: University of Toronto Press, 2006.

Carter, James H. *Creating a Chinese Harbin: Nationalism in an International City, 1916-1932*. Ithaca, NY: Cornell University Press, 2002.

Chang Chiung-fang. "Two Thousand Years of Tippling." Trans. Chris Findler. *Taiwan Panorama*, 7 June 2002. http://www.sino.gov.tw/.

Chang Hsin-pao. *Commissioner Lin and the Opium War*. Cambridge, MA: Harvard University Press, 1964.

Chang, K.C. *Food in Chinese Culture: Anthropological and Historical Perspectives*. New Haven, CT: Yale University Press, 1977.

Chiasson, Blaine R. *Administering the Colonizer: Manchuria's Russians under Chinese Rule, 1918-29*. Vancouver: UBC Press, 2010.

Chung, Tan. *China and the Brave New World*. Durham, NC: Carolina Academic Press, 1978.

Cochran, Sherman. *Chinese Medicine Men: Consumer Culture in China and Southeast Asia*. Cambridge, MA: Harvard University Press, 2006.

Cooper, Arthur. *Li Po and Tu Fu: Poems, Selected and Translated*. Harmondsworth, UK: Penguin, 1973.

Courtwright, David T. *Forces of Habit: Drugs and the Making of the Modern World*. Cambridge, MA: Harvard University Press, 2001.

Culver, Annika A. "Two Japanese Avant-Garde Writers' Views of Gender Relations and Colonial Oppression in Manchuria, 1921-31." *US-Japan Women's Journal* 37 (2009): 3-28.

Dikötter, Frank. *Things Modern: Material Culture and Everyday Life in China*. London: Hurst, 2007.

Dikötter, Frank, Lars Laamann, and Zhou Xun. *Narcotic Culture: A History of Drugs in China*. Chicago, IL: University of Chicago Press, 2004.

Driscoll, Mark. *Absolute Erotic, Absolute Grotesque*. Durham, NC: Duke University Press, 2010.

Duara, Prasenjit. *Sovereignty and Authenticity: Manchukuo and the East Asian Modern*. New York: Rowman and Littlefield, 2003.

Eijkhoff, Pieter. "Wine in China: Its History and Contemporary Developments." 2000. http://www.eykhoff.nl/Wine%20in%20China.pdf.

Fairchild, L.N. *Nelson Fairchild*. Boston, MA: Merrymount, 1907.

Francks, Penelope. "Inconspicuous Consumption: Sake, Beer, and the Birth of the Consumer in Japan." *Journal of Asian Studies* 68, 1 (2009): 135-64.

Gamsa, Mark. "Harbin in Comparative Perspective." *Urban History* 37, 1 (2010): 136-49.

Gayn, Mark. *Journey from the East*. New York: Alfred A. Knopf, 1944.

Gerth, Karl. *As China Goes, So Goes the World: How Chinese Consumers Are Transforming Everything*. New York: Hill and Wang, 2010.

–. *China Made: Consumer Culture and the Creation of the Nation*. Cambridge, MA: Harvard University Press, 2003.

Helzer, John E., and Glorisa J. Canino, eds. *Alcoholism in North America, Europe, and Asia*. Oxford: Oxford University Press, 1992.

Jennings, John M. *The Opium Empire: Japanese Imperialism and Drug Trafficking in Asia, 1895-1945*. London: Praeger, 1997.

Jones, F.C. *Manchuria since 1931*. London: Royal Institute of International Affairs, 1949.

Kang Chao. *The Economic Development of Manchuria: The Rise of a Frontier Economy*. Ann Arbor: Center for Chinese Studies, University of Michigan, 1983.

Kingsberg, Miriam Lynn. "The Poppy and the Acacia: Opium and Imperialism in Japanese Dairen and the Kwantung Leased Territory, 1905-1945." PhD diss., History Department, University of California at Berkeley, 2009.

Kinney, Ann Rasmussen. *Japanese Investment in Manchurian Manufacturing, Mining, Transportation and Communications, 1931-1945.* New York: Garland, 1982.

Lary, Diana, and Thomas R. Gottschwang. *Swallows and Settlers: The Great Migration from North China to Manchuria.* Ann Arbor: University of Michigan Press, 2000.

Lee, Chung Kyoon. "Alcoholism in Korea." In John E. Helzer and Glorisa J. Canino, eds., *Alcoholism in North America, Europe, and Asia,* 247-63. Oxford: Oxford University Press, 1992.

Lin Tsung-Yi and David T.C. Lin. "Alcoholism among the Chinese: Further Observations of a Low-Risk Population." *Culture, Medicine and Psychiatry* 6, 2 (1982): 109-16.

Lo Cheng-Pang. "The Fight against Opium." *Pan Pacific* 3, 4 (1939): 71-72.

Madancy, Joyce A. *The Troublesome Legacy of Commissioner Lin: The Opium Trade and Opium Suppression in Fujian Province, 1820s to 1920s.* Cambridge, MA: Harvard University Asia Centre, 2003.

Manchoukuo: A Pictorial Record. Tokyo and Osaka: Asahi Shimbun, 1934.

Manchoukuo Yearbook: 1941. Hsinking: Manchoukuo Yearbook Company, 1942.

Manchuria: Land of Opportunities. New York: South Manchuria Railway Company, 1922.

McCormack, Gavin. *Chang Tso-lin in Northeast China, 1911-1928.* Stanford, CA: Stanford University Press, 1977.

Meyer, Kathryn. "Garden of Grand Vision: Economic Life in a Flophouse Complex, Harbin, China, 1940." *Crime, Law and Social Change* 36 (2001): 327-52.

–. "Japan and the World Narcotics Traffic." In Jordan Goodman, Paul E. Lovejoy, and Andrew Sherratt, eds., *Consuming Habits: Drugs in History and Anthropology,* 185-203. London: Routledge, 1995.

–. *Webs of Smoke: Smugglers, Warlords, Spies and the History of the International Drug Trade.* Lanham, MD: Rowman and Littlefield, 1998.

Mitter, Rana. "Evil Empire? Competing Constructions of Japanese Imperialism in Manchuria, 1928-1937." In Li Narangoa and Robert Cribb, eds., *Imperial Japan and National Identities in Asia, 1895-1945,* 146-68. London: RoutledgeCurzon, 2003.

–. *The Manchurian Myth: Nationalism, Resistance, and Collaboration in Modern China.* Berkeley: University of California Press, 2000.

Motohiro Kobayashi. "Drug Operations by Resident Japanese in Tianjin." Trans. Bob Tadashi Wakabayashi. In Timothy Brook and Bob Tadashi Wakabayashi, eds., *Opium Regimes: China, Britain, and Japan, 1839-1952,* 152-66. Berkeley: University of California Press, 2000.

Myers, Ramon H. "Creating a Modern Enclave Economy: The Economic Integration of Japan, Manchuria, and North China, 1932-45." In Peter Duus, Ramon H. Myers, and Mark R. Peattie, eds., *The Japanese Wartime Empire, 1931-45,* 136-70. Princeton, NJ: Princeton University Press, 1996.

Nagashima, T. "Opium Administration in Manchoukuo." *Contemporary Manchuria* 3, 1 (1939): 18-44.

Naotaka Shinfuku. "Japanese Culture and Drinking." In Stanton Peele and Marcus Grant, eds., *Alcohol and Pleasure: A Health Perspective,* 113-21. Philadelphia, PA: Taylor and Francis, 1999.

Newman, R.K. "Opium Smoking in Late Imperial China: A Reconsideration." *Modern Asian Studies* 29, 4 (1995): 765-94.

Pernikoff, Alexandre. *Bushido: The Anatomy of Terror.* New York: Liveright, 1943.

Polachek, James. *The Inner Opium War.* Cambridge, MA: Harvard East Asian Monographs, 1992.

Rorabaugh, W.J. *The Alcoholic Republic: An American Tradition.* New York: Oxford University Press, 1979.

Shao Dan. *Remote Homeland, Recovered Borderland: Manchus, Manchoukuo, and Manchuria, 1907-1985.* Honolulu: University of Hawai'i Press, 2011.

Shinichi Yamaguchi. "Contemporary Literature in Manchuria." In Manchuria Daily News, ed., *Concordia and Culture in Manchoukuo,* 27. Xinjing: Manchuria Daily News, 1938.

Simoons, Frederick J. *Food in China.* Boca Raton, FL: CRC Press, 1991.

Singer, K. "Drinking Patterns and Alcoholism in the Chinese." In Mac Marshall, ed., *Beliefs, Behaviors, and Alcoholic Beverages: A Cross-Cultural Survey,* 313-26. Ann Arbor: University of Michigan Press, 1979.

Slack, Edward R., Jr. *Opium, State, and Society: China's Narco-Economy and the Guomindang, 1924-1937.* Honolulu: University of Hawai'i Press, 2001.

Smith, Norman. "The Difficulties of Despair: Dan Di and Chinese Cultural Production in Manchukuo." *Journal of Women's History* 18, 1 (2006): 71-100.

–. "Disguising Resistance in Manchukuo: Feminism as Anti-Colonialism in the Collected Works of Zhu Ti." *International History Review* 28, 3 (2006): 515-36.

–. "Disrupting Narratives: Chinese Women Writers and the Japanese Cultural Agenda in Manchuria, 1936-1945." *Modern China* 30, 3 (2004): 295-325.

–. "'Only Women Can Change This World into Heaven': Mei Niang, Male Chauvinist Society, and the Japanese Cultural Agenda in North China, 1939-1941." *Modern Asian Studies* 40, 1 (2006): 81-107.

–. *Resisting Manchukuo: Chinese Women Writers and the Japanese Occupation.* Vancouver: UBC Press, 2007.

Snow, Edgar. "Japan Builds a New Colony." *Saturday Evening Post,* 24 February 1934, 12-13, 80-81, 84-87.

Spence, Jonathan. "Opium." In *Chinese Roundabout: Essays in History and Culture,* 228-56. New York: W.W. Norton, 1992.

Stephenson, Shelley. "'Her Traces Are Found Everywhere': Shanghai, Li Xianglan, and the 'Greater East Asia Film Sphere.'" In Yingjin Zhang, ed., *Cinema and Urban Culture in Shanghai, 1922-1943,* 222-45. Stanford, CA: Stanford University Press, 1999.

Suleski, Ronald. *Civil Government in Warlord China: Tradition, Modernization and Manchuria.* New York: Bern, 2002.

Sun Kungtu and Ralph W. Huenemann. *The Economic Development of Manchuria in the First Half of the Twentieth Century.* Cambridge, MA: Harvard University Press, 1969.

Tamanoi, Mariko Asano, ed. *Crossed Histories: Manchuria in the Age of Empire.* Honolulu: University of Hawai'i Press, 2005.

Underwood, John Jr. *Japanese Armour in Manchuria, 1931-1945.* West Chester, OH: Nafziger, 2001.

Valverde, Mariana. *Diseases of the Will: Alcohol and the Dilemmas of Freedom.* Cambridge, UK: Cambridge University Press, 1998.

Wakabayashi, Bob Tadashi. "'Imperial Japanese' Drug Trafficking in China: Historiographic Perspectives." http://chinajapan.org/articles/13.1/13.1wakabayashi3-19.pdf.

Wang Chang-Hua, William T. Liu, Ming-Yuan Zhang, Elena S.H. Yu, Zheng-Yi Xia, Marilyn Fernandez, Ching-Tung Lung, Chang-Lin Xu, and Guang-Ya Qu. "Alcohol Use, Abuse, and Dependency in Shanghai." In John E. Helzer and Glorisa J. Canino, eds., *Alcoholism in North America, Europe, and Asia,* 264-88. Oxford: Oxford University Press, 1992.

Warsh, Cheryl Krasnick. "'John Barleycorn Must Die': An Introduction to the Social History of Alcohol." In Cheryl Krasnick Warsh, ed., *Drink in Canada: Historical Essays,* 3-26. Montreal and Kingston: McGill-Queen's University Press, 1993.

Wolff, David. *To the Harbin Station: The Liberal Alternative in Russian Manchuria, 1898-1914.* Stanford, CA: Stanford University Press, 1999.

Wong, J.Y. *Deadly Dreams: Opium, Imperialism and the Arrow War*. Cambridge, UK: Cambridge University Press, 1998.

Wright, Tim. "The Manchurian Economy and the 1930s World Depression." *Modern Asian Studies* 41, 5 (2007): 1073-112.

Xu Gan Rong and Bao Tong Fa. *Grandiose Survey of Chinese Alcoholic Drinks and Beverages*. http://www.sytu.edu.cn/.

Xu Xiaomin. "Ganbei through the Ages." *Shanghai Star,* 29 May 2003. http://app1.chinadaily.com.cn/.

Yamamuro Shin'ichi. *Manchuria under Japanese Dominion*. Trans. Joshua Fogel. Philadelphia: University of Pennsylvania Press, 2006.

Yeoh Eng-Kung and Hai-Gwo Hwu. "Alcoholism in Taiwan Chinese Communities." In John E. Helzer and Glorisa J. Canino, eds., *Alcoholism in North America, Europe, and Asia*, 214-46. Oxford: Oxford University Press, 1992.

Young, Louise. *Japan's Total Empire: Manchuria and the Culture of Wartime Imperialism*. Berkeley: University of California Press, 1998.

Zheng Tiantian. *Red Lights: The Lives of Sex Workers in Post-Socialist China*. Minneapolis: University of Minnesota Press, 2009.

Zheng Yangwen. *The Social Life of Opium*. Cambridge, UK: Cambridge University Press, 2005.

Zhou, Hellen, and Shannon Roy. "New Wine, Old Stories." *Beijing This Month,* 1 August 2004. http://www.btmbeijing.com/.

Zhou Yongming. *Anti-Drug Crusades in Twentieth Century China: Nationalism, History, and State Building*. Oxford: Rowman and Littlefield, 1999.

Zhu Jianfei. *Chinese Spatial Strategies: Imperial Beijing, 1420-1911*. London: RoutledgeCurzon, 2004.

Index

Note: "(f)" following a number indicates a figure

Contemporary Chinese Studies

Printed and bound in Canada by Friesens

Set in Futura and Warnock by Artegraphica Design Co. Ltd.

Copy editor: Robert Lewis

Proofreader: Frank Chow

Indexer: Noeline Bridge